Practical Introduction to Laser Dermatology

Vishal Madan
Editor

Practical Introduction to Laser Dermatology

Springer

Editor
Vishal Madan
Consultant Dermatologist, Laser and Mohs Surgeon
Salford Royal NHS Foundation Trust, Stott Lane
Salford
UK

ISBN 978-3-030-46450-9 ISBN 978-3-030-46451-6 (eBook)
https://doi.org/10.1007/978-3-030-46451-6

This Springer imprint is published by the registered company Springer Nature Switzerland AG
The registered company address is: Gewerbestrasse 11, 6330 Cham, Switzerland

Contents

1 **Fundamentals of Lasers and Light Devices in Dermatology** 1
Elizabeth Raymond Brown

2 **Lasers for Vascular Indications** 53
Giulia Rinaldi, Samira Batul Syed, and Vishal Madan

3 **Pigment Specific Lasers and Light Devices** 91
Sanjeev Aurangabadkar

4 **Epilation Lasers** 119
Samantha Hills and Daron Seukeran

5 **Ablative Lasers** 143
Vishal Madan

6 **Fractional Laser Technology** 163
Sarah Felton and Vishal Madan

7 **Radiofrequency Devices Including Fractional Radiofrequency** 173
Ileana Afroditi Kleidona, Ali M. Ghanem, and Nicholas J. Lowe

8 **Light Emitting Diodes and Low Level Laser Light Therapy** 201
Caiwei Zheng, Ali Rajabi-Estarabadi, Melanie M. Hirsch, and Keyvan Nouri

9 **Intense Pulsed Light in Dermatology** 219
Sam Hills and Miguel Montero

10 **Cosmeceuticals** 231
Rhonda Meys

11 **Self-Assessment Questionnaire** 249
Vishal Madan

Index 257

Fundamentals of Lasers and Light Devices in Dermatology

1

Elizabeth Raymond Brown

Historical Development of the Laser

The theory describing the properties of light emitted by the process of *stimulated emission* was proposed by Albert Einstein in 1917 [1] but Einstein did not use the term *laser* in his publication.

According to Hecht [2] the development of the laser was 'neither simple nor easy' yet we take lasers and laser applications very much for granted because they are so widely used in the field of medicine, dentistry, veterinary, entertainment, commerce, industry and research.

The first practical laser was demonstrated in 1960 by Theodore H. Maiman at the Hughes Research Laboratory in America [3], using a cylinder of synthetic ruby just 1 cm in diameter and 2 cm long in an arrangement that Maiman referred to as an *optical maser*. The foundation for this incredible achievement was made possible by the fundamental physics studies of Max Planck who in 1900 described light as a form of *energy* and presented the concept of *quanta*, for which he received the Nobel Prize in physics in 1918 [4]. Planck's work inspired Albert Einstein to investigate the interaction of light with matter and in 1905 he too concluded that light delivers energy in discrete *quantum particles* which are now referred to as *photons* [5].

E. Raymond Brown (✉)
Laser Education Limited, Gainsborough, UK
e-mail: admin@laser-ed.co.uk

Table 1.1 summarises the historical landmarks in the development of laser devices.

The 1980s onwards saw a rapid development in lasers capable of delivering new wavelength wavelengths, stable beam and output characteristics and devices that were more compact and efficient. The growth in laser types mirrored the search for new applications and tailoring to specific interventions, e.g. wavelengths for improving absorption by a given target or depth of penetration.

Properties of Light

Light is described as a wave-particle duality, meaning it displays characteristics of *waves* and *particles* (Fig. 1.1). Beams of light being reflected, diffracted or experiencing interference are evidence of light travelling as a wave. Light acting as a particle is evidenced by the *photoelectric* effect that causes a precise and specific removal of materials such as ablation of corneal tissue by excimer lasers. Either concept may be used depending upon the sense of scale, e.g. wavelength versus photon energy and both descriptions are relevant to laser and light interventions and laser safety. For example, light as a *wave* is used to describe spectral output, i.e., *the wavelength* of the output beam, while light as a *particle* explains specific interactions with matter and tissues, i.e. tissue *ablation*.

V. Madan (ed.), *Practical Introduction to Laser Dermatology*,
https://doi.org/10.1007/978-3-030-46451-6_1

Table 1.1 Historical landmarks in laser development

Year	Contributor	Contribution
1917	Albert Einstein [5]	Proposed the conditions required for 'stimulated emission' of light.
1957	Gordon Gould [6]	Proposed the conditions required for stimulated emission at visible wavelengths. Acknowledged to be the first person to use the term 'LASER'. Gould did not immediately patent his concepts and the ideas of Schawlow and Townes were patented first.
1958	Arthur Schawlow and Charles Townes [7]	Demonstrated a maser (microwave amplification by stimulated emission of radiation) using ammonia gas and microwave radiation. Their papers published in 1954 and 1958, led to patents on the theoretical requirements for designing 'optical masers'. While technically they invented the first laser it was referred to as an 'optical maser'.
1960	Theodore Maiman [3]	Demonstrated the visible first laser using a rod of synthetic ruby with reflective coatings on each end surrounded by a helical flashlamp. The publication Physical Review rejected Maiman's original article (June 1960), but the scientific community later recognised it as a discovery that changed the world.
1960	Ali Javan [8]	In 1959 Javan proposed the first gas laser and in 1960 demonstrated a helium-neon (HeNe) gas laser operating continuously rather than in pulses. The HeNe laser initially emitted in the near IR with the 632.8 nm (red) output discovered in 1962, making it one of the most popular early lasers in research and medicine.
1963	Zhores Alferov [9] Herbert Kroemer [10]	In 1963 Alferov and Kromer independently proposed the principles for semiconductor heterostructures to be used to emit light. It took until the 1970s to produce stable, room temperature operated devices and semiconductor lasers are now the commonly used laser types.
1964	William Bridges [11]	Bridges was the first to report ten different laser transitions, including blue and green light, from an argon gas laser.
1964	Kumar Patel [12]	Patel demonstrated the first carbon dioxide (CO_2) laser showing it to be capable of very high continuous-wave and pulsed power output at very high conversion efficiencies.
1964	James Geusic et al. [13]	Demonstrated the first neodymium yttrium aluminium garnet (Nd:YAG) laser. Initially developed in 1961 neodymium-based lasers required the inclusion of yttrium aluminium garnet (YAG) to emit stable and reliable outputs.
1968	Peter Sorokin et al. [14]	Demonstrated the first laser using an organic dye as the active medium.
1970	Nikolai Basov et al. [15]	Basov is generally credited with the initial development of a gas laser using a xenon dimer. However, research groups including IBM developed the technology using noble gases for a family of devices known as *excimer* lasers. Initially designed for photoetching materials, applications extended to human tissue in particular corrective eye surgery.
1983	Rox Anderson and James Parish [16]	Published a paper describing thermal confinement of heat to target tissue thus allowing precise and selective destruction through a process termed selective Photothermolysis. Their publication significantly advanced the understanding of laser and light-tissue interactions.

Light as an Electromagnetic Wave

For safe and effective practice, it is essential that clinicians understand the different types of lasers, the differences between laser and intense light sources (ILS), also known as intense pulsed light (IPL (TM)) devices and the properties of laser and light beams. The starting point is to understand *electromagnetic radiation (EMR)* and the *electromagnetic (EM) spectrum*.

Electromagnetic radiation (EMR) is the continuous range of energies that extends from X-radiation to radio waves. Although these forms of energy are different from one another, they all travel through space as waves thus exhibiting *wavelike* properties. A key feature of EM waves is that they propagate and move without a propagation medium and hence can travel the vast distances of outer space. The electromagnetic spectrum is the term used to describe the range of EMR (Fig. 1.2).

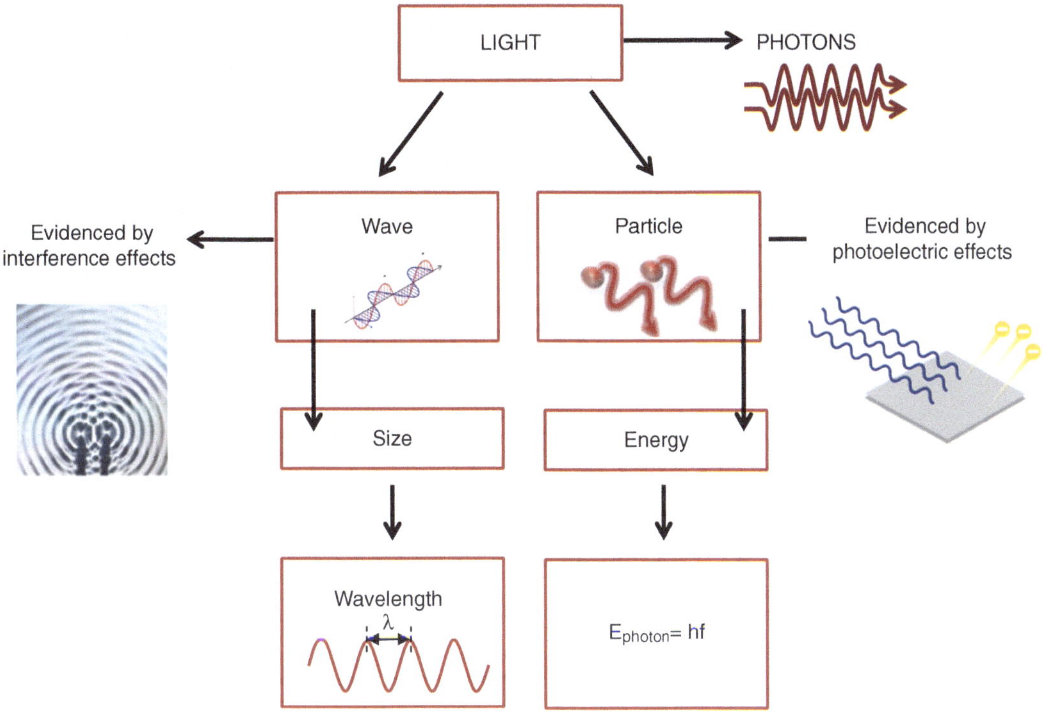

Fig. 1.1 Illustration of the concept of the wave-particle duality of light

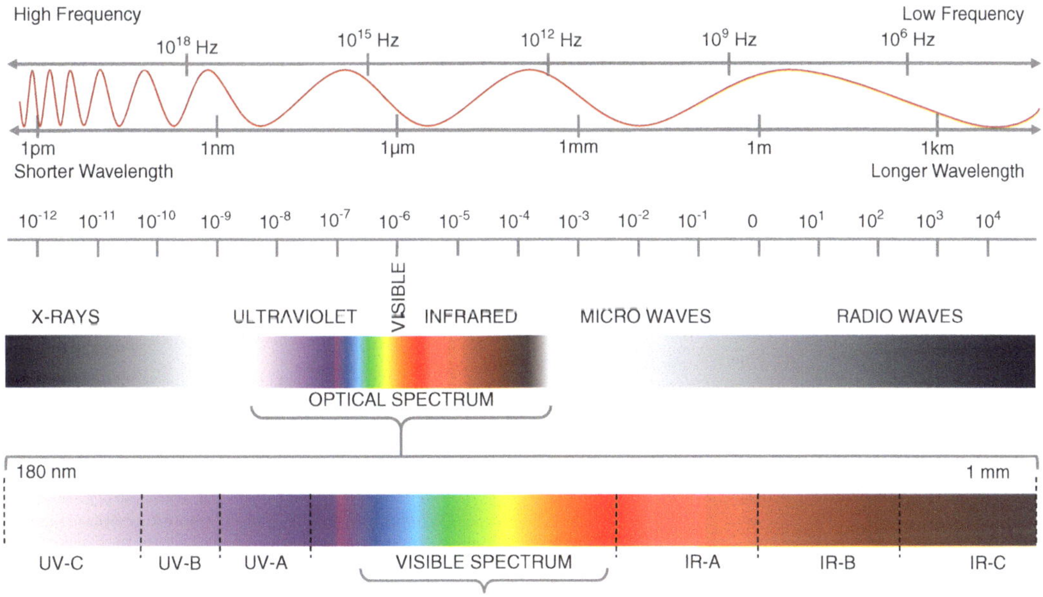

Fig. 1.2 Illustration of the concept of the electromagnetic (EM) spectrum

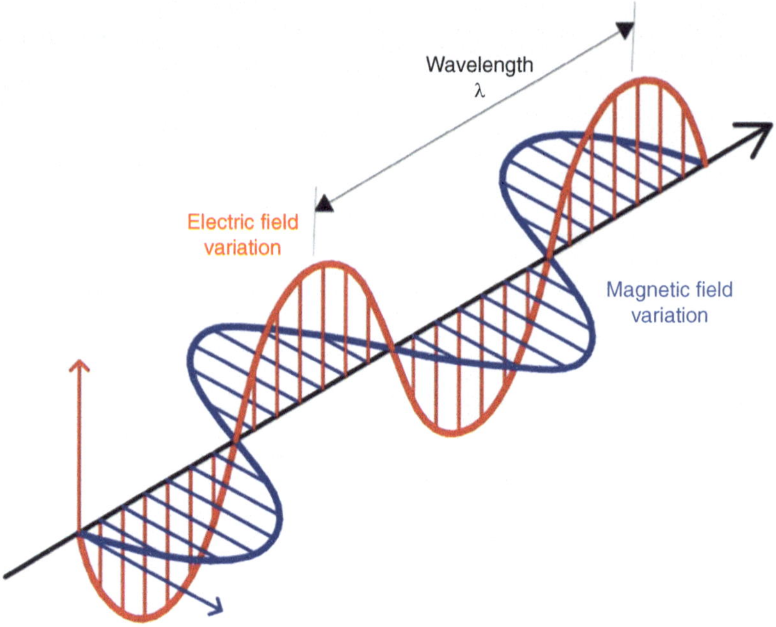

Fig. 1.3 Illustration of the concept of light as an electromagnetic (EM) wave

Many of the properties that electromagnetic radiation demonstrates including reflection, refraction and diffraction are explained by considering a propagating wave compromised of *electric* and *magnetic* fields which are at right angles, both to each other and to the direction of propagation as illustrated (Fig. 1.3).

In layman's terms, EMR can be described in several ways. For example:

- by name e.g., microwave energy
- by wavelength e.g., 755 nanometres (nm) quoted in fractions of a metre (m)
- by frequency e.g., radio waves quoted in Hertz (Hz)
- by photon energy, e.g. amount of energy carried by individual photons (E_{photon}).

The EM spectrum includes a specific wavelength range referred to as the *optical spectrum* that includes *ultraviolet* (UV), *visible* (light) and *infrared* (IR) radiation. The wave nature of EMR allows this range to be categorised into distinctive bands Table 1.2.

Laser and light practitioners should note that ultraviolet and infrared radiation does not invoke the visual response in human eyes and therefore is described as invisible but lasers emitting UV or IR radiation still pose a potential hazard to eyes and skin. Equally the sensitivity of the human eye is not

Table 1.2 Divisions of the *Optical Region* of the EM spectrum [17]

Region of optical spectrum	Division	Wavelength (nm/mm)
Ultraviolet (UV) radiation—'beyond' violet	UV—C	180–280 nm
	UV—B	280–315 nm
	UV—A	315–400 nm
Visible radiation (VIS)—'light'	A sensation of violet coloured light through to red coloured light	400–780 nm*
Infrared (IR) radiation—'Below red'	IR—A (near IR)	780–1400 nm
	IR—B (mid IR)	1400–3000 nm
	IR—C (far IR)	3000 nm –1 mm

*The spectral regions defined by CIE are shorthand notations useful in describing biological effects and may not agree with spectral breakpoints for laser safety calculations. The visible range (light) is quoted as 400–700 nm for laser safety purposes

uniform over the visible spectrum, being a smooth function of wavelength and differing between individuals. For example, the human eye detects approximately 1% of light at 690 nm (red) but only 0.01% at 750 nm (near infrared), effectively making wavelengths longer than 750 nm 'invisible' unless the light source is extremely bright [18].

Light as a Particle

Light has been described as an electromagnetic wave propagating through space yet the development of the laser would not have been possible without the realisation of the *particle properties* postulated by Planck as cited by Nauenberg [19]. Planck observed that matter could only absorb or emit energy in discrete amounts or quanta that cannot be further sub-divided.

The energy of an individual photon is related to the frequency of the corresponding light wave by the relationship:

$$E = hf \text{ or } E = hc / \lambda \qquad (1.1)$$

where

E energy of the photon in Joules (J)

h the Planck's constant (6.626×10^{-34}) in Joule second

f photon frequency (Hz)

λ wavelength

c speed of light (3.00×10^{8} ms^{-1})

This relationship shows that photon energy increases with increasing frequency which is vital in the context of light-tissue interactions. For example, comparing *photothermal* effects induced by longer wavelength, lower frequency radiation, e.g. infrared, with *photochemical* interactions induced by shorter wavelength, higher frequency radiation, e.g. ultraviolet/blue light.

Planck's observations that electromagnetic radiation is quantised proved that light has both wave-like and particle-like properties and subsequently paved the way for the discovery of the *photon* by Albert Einstein. His understanding that atoms and molecules gain energy by *absorption* and lose energy by emitting photons led to his 1917 publication in which Einstein added the concept of *stimulated emission* to the known effects of spontaneous emission and spontaneous absorption [1]. The phenomenon of transferring discrete amounts of photon energy to skin and tissues subsequently led to the medical laser and light interventions available today.

Characteristics of Electromagnetic Radiation

Wavelength

The simplest way to think of optical radiation is as a beam that travels as a wave. Hence the term *wavelength,* which for laser and light therapies is usually quoted in *micrometers* (µm) or *nanometers* (nm).

Wavelength is an important concept to understand because it:

- identifies a particular region of the EM spectrum, e.g., 635 nm (visible radiation)
- determines the 'colour' of the beam, e.g., 532 nm = green light
- determines the light-tissue interactions, e.g., transmission or absorption by tissues
- dictates the lens colour or lens material used in protective eyewear
- relates to the amount of energy carried by the waves.

Figure 1.4 illustrates *wavelength* defined as the horizontal distance of two consecutive troughs or crests on the wave, written as λ (lambda) and expressed in metres (m).

Frequency

Electromagnetic radiation is described as an *oscillating* wave travelling through space. Therefore an alternative way to describe light is by the *frequency* (f or ν) of oscillation of the electromagnetic field. The frequency of a wave refers to the number of wave peaks (full wavelengths) that pass a given point in space every second, expressed in cycles per second (s^{-1}) or *hertz* (Hz).

Wavelength and frequency are inversely proportional, that is the shorter the wavelength the higher the frequency as more wave peaks can

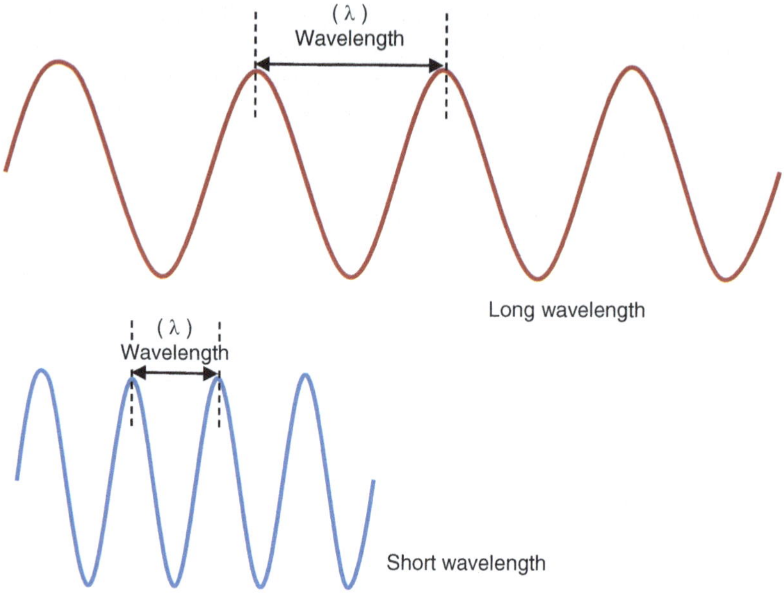

Fig. 1.4 Definition of wavelength showing the concept of long and short wavelengths

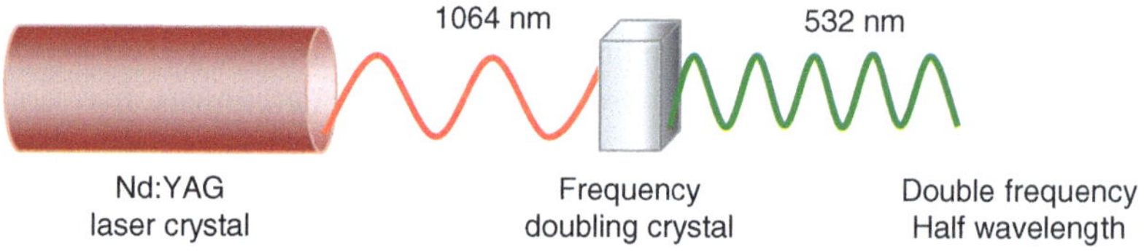

Fig. 1.5 Illustration of the concept of frequency doubling. The fundamental Nd:YAG wavelength is halved to 532 nm

pass a given point in a second and vice versa. This relationship is given by:

$$c = \lambda f \quad (1.2)$$

where

λ wavelength (m)

f photon frequency (Hz)

c speed of light ($3.00 \times 10^8\ ms^{-1}$)

This relationship shows that all electromagnetic radiation, regardless of wavelength or frequency travels at the speed of light.

Note: it is important not to confuse frequency of radiation with the frequency of a pulse emitted from a laser referred to as **pulse repetition frequency (PRF)** or *pulse rate*, i.e., the number of pulses emitted in one second, also expressed in Hz.

Frequency Doubling The relationship between wavelength and frequency explains the concept of *frequency doubling (FD)* (or *second-harmonic generation* (SHG)) often written as FD or F∗2. Doubling the frequency halves the wavelength and the ability to produce a different or additional wavelength from one laser device is an advantageous feature for many clinical applications, but not all types of laser can be frequency doubled.

Frequency doubling is a non-linear optical process in which two photons with the same frequency interact with a non-linear material and are combined to emit a photon with twice the energy of the initial photons (equivalently twice the frequency and half the wavelength). The frequency change is achieved by optics or crystals such as *Potassium Titanyl Phosphate ($KTiOPO_4$, KTP)* or *Lithium Triborate (LiB_3O_5, LBO)* placed within the laser cavity (Fig. 1.5). The red and green bands on the handpiece of a frequency doubled laser is intended to indicate to the practitioner the available outputs.

The Nd:YAG laser is very often designed as a system to emit the fundamental wavelength at 1064 nm (infrared radiation) *alone or in addition* to its frequency doubled output at 532 nm (green) as both are beneficial therapeutic wavelengths, e.g. 1064 nm for deeper vascular lesions and 532 nm for shallow vascular lesions. A KTP crystal is commonly used to achieve the frequency doubling and this is the reason such systems are commonly referred to as *KTP lasers* whereas in fact they are FD Nd:YAG lasers, the Nd:YAG being the *gain medium* of the laser (see section "Gain Medium (Active Medium)").

The laser design and intended application dictates whether both wavelengths (1064 nm *and* 532 nm) or just one of those wavelengths is available as the output beam. Frequency doubling typically reduces the output power of the halved wavelength.

An alternative method to change or shift the output wavelength is via dye impregnated polymers set within a handpiece by a series of wavelength conversions using the laser output(s) to *pump* the polymer and emit at a shifted wavelength (Fig. 1.6). Some laser systems for tattoo removal offer such handpieces to extend the range of tattoo colours that can be treated using one laser device. However, the output power produced by dye handpieces can be significantly lower than the fundamental beam output due to multiple wavelength conversions which introduces losses. Consequently, the spot size from such handpieces is often smaller to compensate for lower output power.

Amplitude

Amplitude is defined as half the height of a wave from the top of one peak to the bottom of the next (Fig. 1.7). Amplitude measures the magnitude or *power* of the wave. The higher the wave, the greater the amplitude (power). The significance of power will be appreciated when discussing the relationship between power and energy and the effect of *pulse duration* on light-tissue interactions (see section "Light Tissue Interactions").

Velocity

Velocity is the rate of speed at which the wave travels. All wavelengths travel at the same speed within a vacuum. The speed of light, c is constant at approximately 300,000 km per second (186,300 miles per second) in a vacuum.

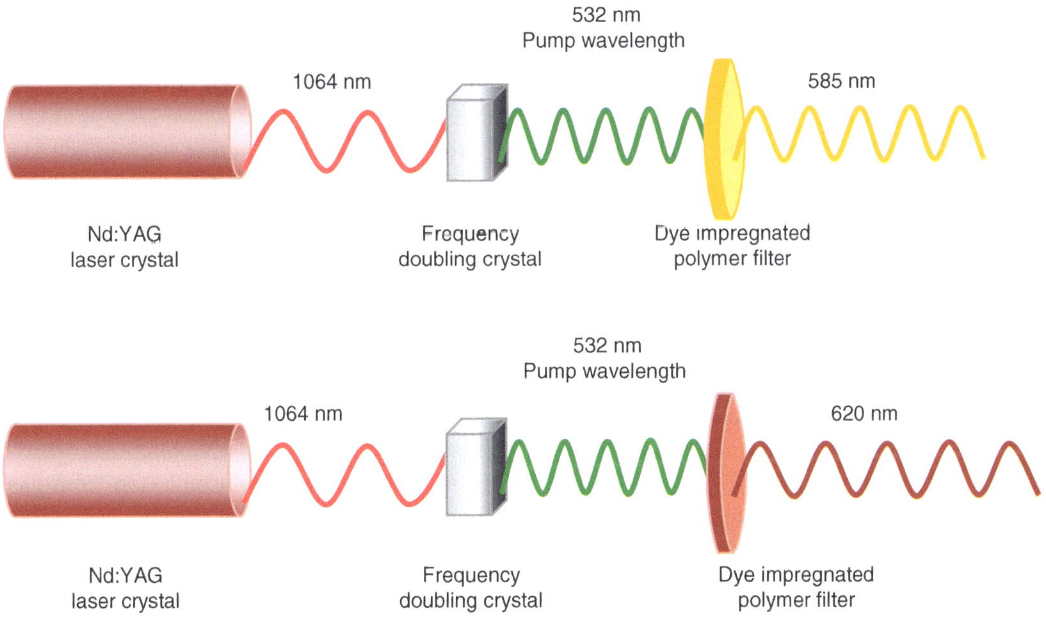

Fig. 1.6 Dye impregnated polymers to shift output wavelength

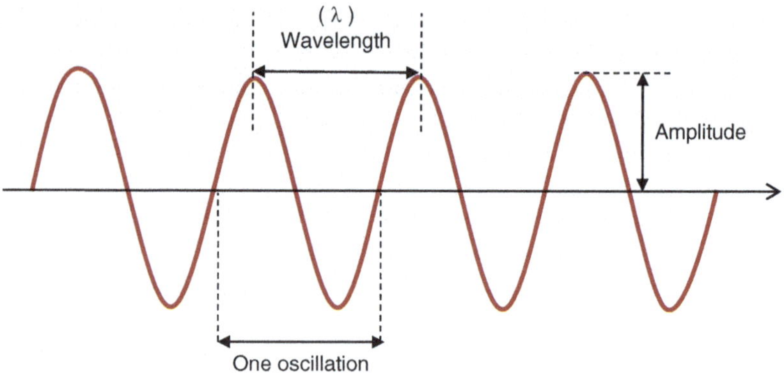

Fig. 1.7 Illustration of a stylised waveform indicating amplitude, wavelength and oscillation

Producing Light and Laser Beams

The purpose of this section is to explain the acronym *LASER* by describing the stages involved in ***L**ight **A**mplification by the **S**timulated **E**mission of **R**adiation.* To understand this process, we need to first describe the operation of other light sources.

Spontaneous Emission of Light

There are several ways to generate photons but all of them require a means of energising electrons that orbit the nucleus of an atom. The electrons (negative charge) circle a nucleus containing protons and neutrons (positive charge) in fixed orbits known as *energy states or levels* (Fig. 1.8).

In physics, the *Bohr model* [20] depicts an atom as a small, positively charged *nucleus* containing protons and neutrons, surrounded by electrons that travel in circular orbits around it in a three-dimensional *cloud*. The orbitals, known as *energy states* or *energy levels* around the nucleus can each hold a specific number of electrons, equal to the number of positive protons in the nucleus, i.e. the atomic number of an atom.

The first energy state can hold a maximum of two electrons in one orbital, the second state can hold a maximum of eight electrons distributed over four orbitals, and the third energy state can contain a maximum of 18 electrons distributed over nine different orbitals. This arrangement is the atom's lowest energy or *ground state*. Different atoms have a different number of energy states, but each is arranged with the lowest energy level closest to the nucleus. It is important to note that the electrons cannot exist *between* energy states. An analogy would be described by rows of seating in a theatre or cinema, a person can sit *in* a particular row but they cannot sit *between* the rows.

It is possible to *pump* or *excite* electrons from a lower energy state to a higher *unfilled* energy state by absorption of a quantum of energy corresponding to the energy difference between the states. Using the previous analogy of theatre seating, the rows or states must fill from the front (lower positions) to the back (higher positions). Excitation from a lower to higher energy state can be via an electric current, a flash of light or another form of energy.

From the instant an electron is promoted to a higher energy state it is intrinsically unstable and can only remain in the higher energy state for a particular *lifetime* before *spontaneously* falling to a lower energy state or its ground state, emitting a photon of light as it falls. The *metastable state* or *upper-state lifetime* depends on the orbital structure of the atom, typically ranging from picoseconds (10^{-12} seconds) to milliseconds (10^{-3} seconds). *Spontaneous emission* is the process of light emission from gas discharge lamps such as neon signs and xenon flash lamps.

An emitted photon has a frequency and wavelength equal to the energy difference between the states to which it was excited and then spontane-

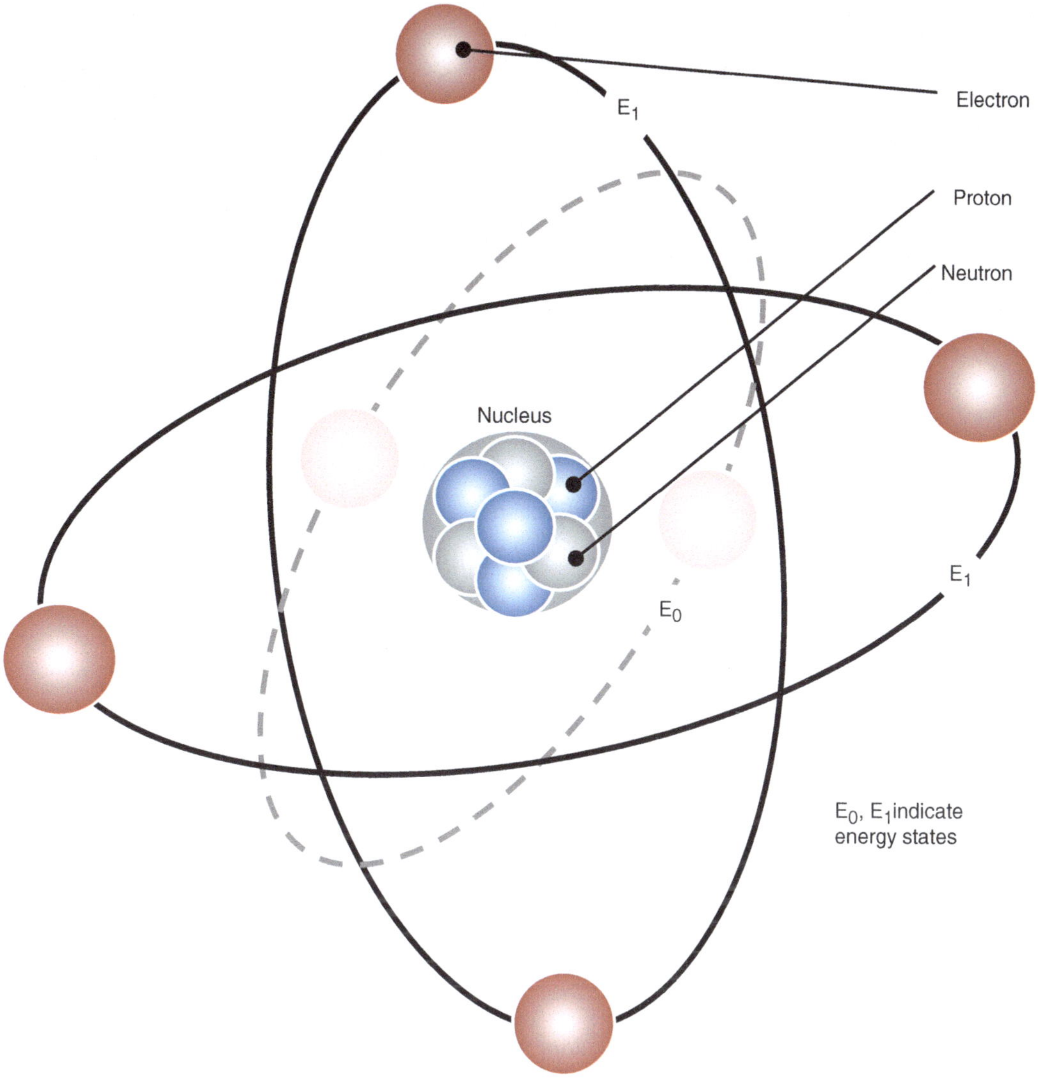

Fig. 1.8 Illustration of orbiting electrons around the nucleus of an atom

ously fell. This continual process of electrons rising and spontaneously falling back to a lower energy state produces a stream or pulse of photons that human eyes perceive as light (assuming it is visible radiation) (Fig. 1.9).

The emission spectra (wavelength(s)) of the emitted radiation depends on the type of source producing it, for example, yellow light from a sodium street lamp, red light from a neon gas lamp. The light is emitted randomly regarding direction and time and hence is described as *incoherent*.

Stimulated Emission of Light

Albert Einstein understood the process of *spontaneous emission* whereby an excited atom (one in a higher energy state) returns to a lower energy state and emits a photon. While studying this process and the interaction of light with matter, Einstein hypothesised a second mechanism to trigger light emission. A process he described as *stimulated emission*. He believed that if an atom in an *excited state* (one having electrons in higher energy state) were to collide with a stray photon

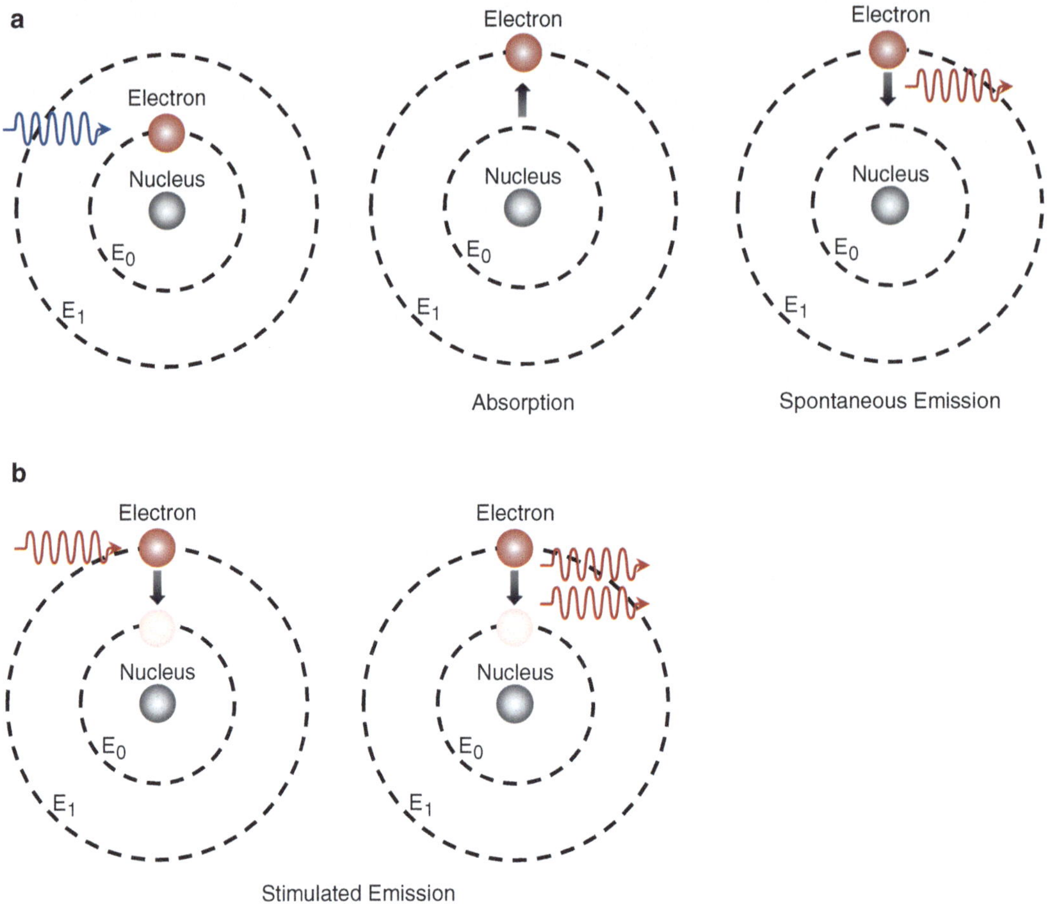

Fig. 1.9 (**a**) Schematic of the process of spontaneous emission of light. (**b**) Schematic of the process of stimulated emission of light

of *identical energy* from another atom, the atom in the excited state could be *stimulated* or triggered to prematurely *decay* (fall to its ground state) and release its photon.

Absorption raises the energy of an electron and in his paper of 1917 [5], Einstein describes the process of *stimulated emission* as the reverse of absorption Stimulated emission lowers electron energy by releasing a photon. More crucially the photon emitted during stimulated emission is *identical* to the photon that *stimulated* its release. It travels in the same direction, has an identical wavelength and oscillates at the same frequency. Thus a single photon interacting with an *excited atom* can produce *two* identical photons and trigger a cascade effect as identical photons move a material containing excited atoms releasing ever more identical photons.

Hence Einstein [5] predicted that light emitted by *stimulated emission* would exhibit the behaviour of waves travelling in the same direction, with identical frequency and with identical phase as the photon that stimulated its release.

However, generating light by *stimulated emission* is a complicated and challenging process because of the natural tendency of electrons to fall *spontaneously* back to a lower energy level. Creating a large number or *population* of atoms in the excited state, known as a metastable state and keeping them there long enough for stimulated emission to occur can overcome this problem. Once the population of electrons in the metastable state exceeds those in a stable state, a

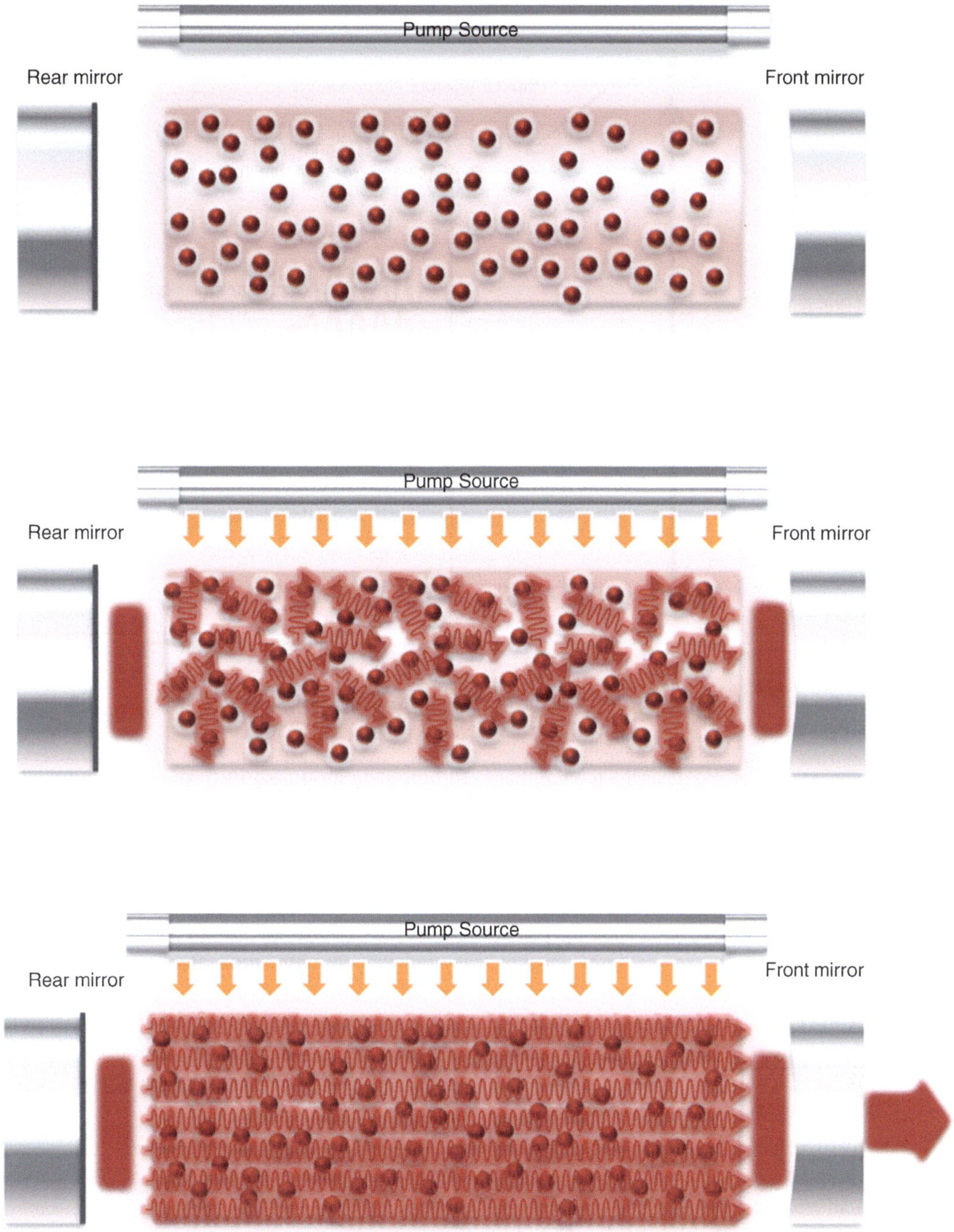

Fig. 1.10 Schematic of the process of lasing

population inversion has occurred and the spontaneously emitted photons, in turn, *stimulate* photon emission, creating a coherent beam of identical photons (Fig. 1.10).

To produce a more *efficient stimulated emission* process by a given laser material (known as the *gain medium)*, multiple *energy level transfers* are used to create the *population inversion. Three*

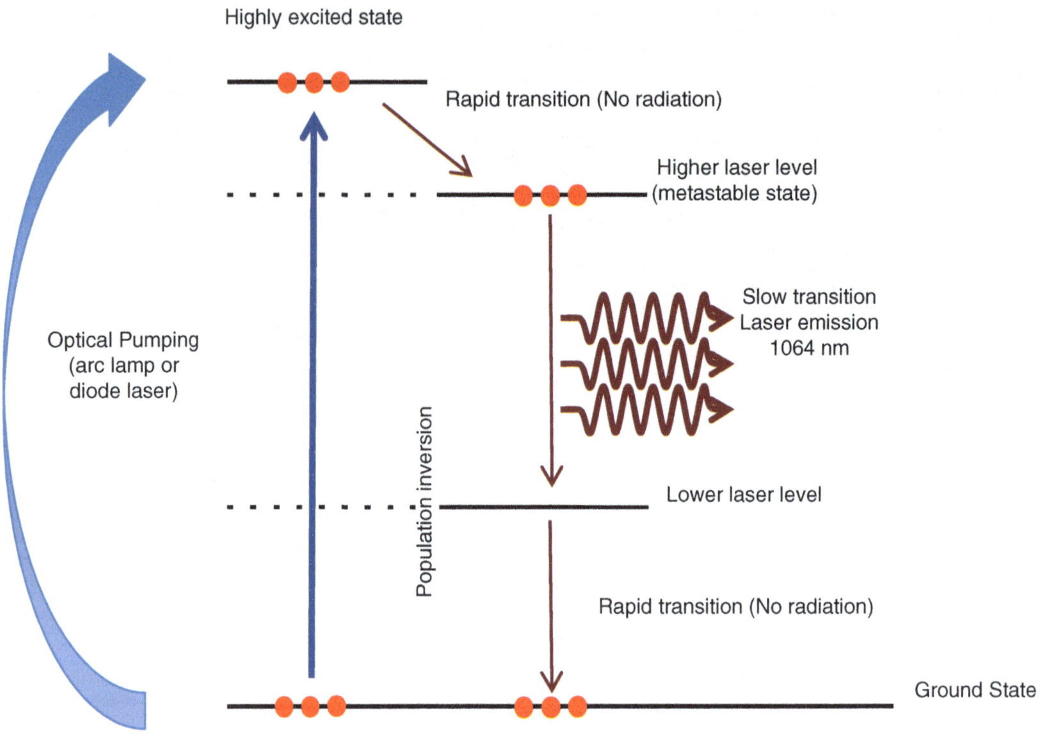

Fig. 1.11 Illustration of a four-level laser system with a solid-state Nd:YAG crystal gain medium

or *four levels* are typical and describe the number of energy level transfers involved in creating the required emission of light. Nd:YAG is a prime example of a *four-level solid state gain medium* (Fig. 1.11).

One advantage of a four-level system over a three-level one is that the *lower laser level* is above the ground state meaning atoms can more easily be excited back to the *metastable state* to maintain the *population inversion* and continue the lasing process.

Although Einstein predicted the properties of the light that could be produced by stimulated emission it took decades before the necessary physical components were assembled in such a way to demonstrate such a beam of light. This took place on 16 May 1960 when Theodore Maiman mounted a 1 cm diameter by 2 cm long synthetic ruby crystal with polished silver-coated ends within a cylindrical photographic flashlamp, all held within a hollow metal cylinder. Applying a voltage to the flashlamp created a flash of white light to excite the ruby crystal, forcing it to emit a short flash of red light. The red light had a wavelength 694.3 nm. Maiman called his apparatus an *optical maser* [3] and not a LASER.

The properties of that flash of red light opened the way to a multitude of applications including medicine, communication and applied research and just 2 years later Maiman's prototype 'laser' was in commercial production by Hughes Aircraft Corporation as the Model 200 ruby laser system, producing 1.5 J pulses at 694.3 nm [21].

Laser Components

This section introduces the components and basics of laser construction. For a comprehensive review of theoretical physics and laser engineering the reader is referred to Photonics and Laser Engineering: Principles, Devices, and Applications [22].

To produce a stable and reliable laser beam requires precision optical, mechanical and elec-

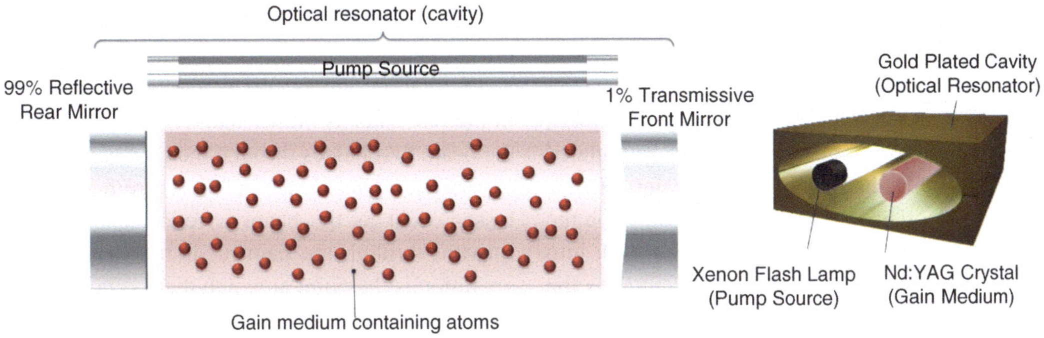

Fig. 1.12 Schematic of a flash lamp excited, solid-state gain medium contained within an optical resonator (cavity)

trical components. Additional some form of internal water or air-cooling is necessary to maintain thermal stability of components due operation.

Nearly all lasers include three essential elements (Fig. 1.12).

Gain Medium (Active Medium)

The *gain medium*, also known as *active medium* is the collection of atoms or materials that can be excited to gain and amplify optical energy.

A *gain medium* may be a:

- solid e.g. Nd:YAG crystal, also known as solid-state
- gas e.g. CO_2
- liquid e.g. organic dye
- semiconductor materials, e.g. diodes and ceramics.

The *gain medium* determines the characteristics of the emitted output. The essential physical properties of a gain medium should include:

- Transitions available in the desired wavelength region, ideally with maximum gain in this region
- High transparency in the emitted wavelength region to reduce loss through absorption by the active medium
- Compatibility with the pump source and appropriate absorption of the pump wavelength(s)
- The ability for high doping with laser-active ions, e.g., crystal or glass doped with rare earth ($Nd^{3+,}$ Er^{3}, Ho^{3+}) or metal ions (Ti^{3+}, Cr^{3+})
- A suitable metastable state lifetime
- Multi-level energy transfer behaviour
- Adequate physical and chemical stability, hardness (solid state media) and robustness

Gas lasers usually contain a gas mixture; for example, a CO_2 laser contains carbon dioxide and helium and nitrogen. Depending on the type of laser, small amounts of other gases such as oxygen (O_2), carbon monoxide (CO), hydrogen (H_2) or xenon (Xe) may be required to improve the efficiency of the excitation process and level of amplification.

Excitation Mechanism or Pump Source

The gain medium (e.g. gas, crystal) requires an external source of energy for it produce the population of excited atoms needed for lasing. The gain medium is energised through a process called *pumping* which must be continuous to sustain lasing. The term *optical pumping* applies if the gain medium is a solid or liquid and the excitation source is typically a flash lamp or another laser (e.g. diode laser) usually operating at shorter wavelengths than the output wavelength(s). *Electrical pumping* describes the excitation of a gas gain medium using an electrical current.

Optical Resonator (Cavity) and Feedback Mechanism

The reader is reminded of the acronym LASER, being **L**ight **A**mplification by the **S**timulated **E**mission of **R**adiation. In pure physics terms a laser is an *optical oscillator* whose output, in the form of electromagnetic waves, is fed back into an *optical resonator* or cavity that *amplifies* the waves. A feedback system allows this process to continue to the point where no further amplification is possible, hence the gain medium is described as *saturated*.

The simplest form of *optical resonator* consists of a pair of mirrors, accurately aligned to allow only photons along the axis of the active medium to reflect back and forth and create the necessary *optical gain*. The combination of optical gain with positive feedback is achieved by a placing the pumped gain medium inside this mirror arrangement. A 99% reflective rear mirror in combined with a 1% transmissive front mirror allows a portion of the coherent radiation to leave the laser in the form of an output beam with may be a continuous or pulsed beam.

Oscillation only occurs when the optical *gain* in the resonator is higher than any *losses*. When the beam first passes through the gain medium, it experiences gain. Once reflected from mirrors, losses occur as the beam is reflected back and forward through the gain medium. Steady-state operation is the point at which there is no change in the beam after one round-trip, i.e. total gain and total losses are balanced. The feedback mechanism keeps the population inversion at this threshold level to maintain this balance.

Cavity design is fundamental to producing stable and efficient outputs, as several loss mechanisms reduce the optical gain, for example, scattering or absorption in the gain medium or cavity mirrors. Cavity design also determines laser compactness, beam mode, quality and radius, pulse duration of a Q switched laser and pulse repetition rate in a mode-locked laser [23].

A stylised optical resonator illustrating gain medium, Q switch, mirror and shutter arrangements is shown (Fig. 1.13).

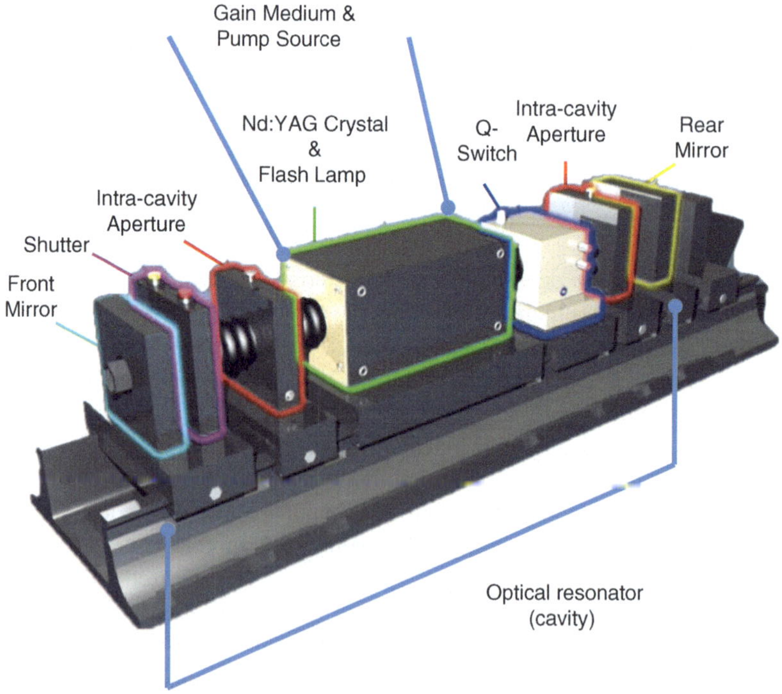

Fig. 1.13 Stylised optical resonator (cavity)

Laser Modes and Beam Quality

Laser oscillation takes place in the optical resonator (cavity) and relative to the emitted wavelength (i.e. nm) the cavity length is significantly larger. As the electromagnetic waves repeatedly travel through the gain medium they interact and interfere with each other. One consequence of this is that oscillations can co-occur on two distinct *modes*, namely *longitudinal* and *transverse electromagnetic modes* (TEM).

Longitudinal modes correspond to different *resonances* along the length of the laser cavity at different frequencies or wavelengths within the gain bandwidth of the active medium. These modes explain why the beam from a laser rarely consists of one pure single wavelength (see Monochromaticity).

The view of a cross section of a *transverse electromagnetic mode* would show different light distributions or patterns across the width of the beam, which affects beam quality.

For the majority of medical applications, controlling the *transverse electromagnetic modes* (TEM) to maintain beam quality is more important than controlling the *longitudinal modes* (so that oscillation is only at one single frequency) [24].

The terminology used to describe these transverse electromagnetic modes comes from the early work of laser development [24]. Modes are classified according to the number of *nulls* that appear within the beam cross-section in two directions. A lower order or *fundamental mode*, where beam intensity peaks at the centre is known as TEM_{00}, e.g., it shows a Gaussian intensity. For many laser applications, this is the preferred output mode as it delivers uniform distribution in a beam that can be focused into a concentrated spot. *Multimode* outputs may which deliver more power, but it usually in a beam with poorer focusing/shaping properties. Example TEM modes are shown (Fig. 1.14).

Mode hopping occurs when a laser operating on one particular resonator mode suddenly switches to some other mode resulting in power-sharing between the two modes with a reduction in the overall output power of the device. Often mode hopping is caused by a drift in the temperature of the gain medium which disturbs laser output. This is why lasers should be operated in facilities with stable ambient room temperature and humidity and the reason some laser

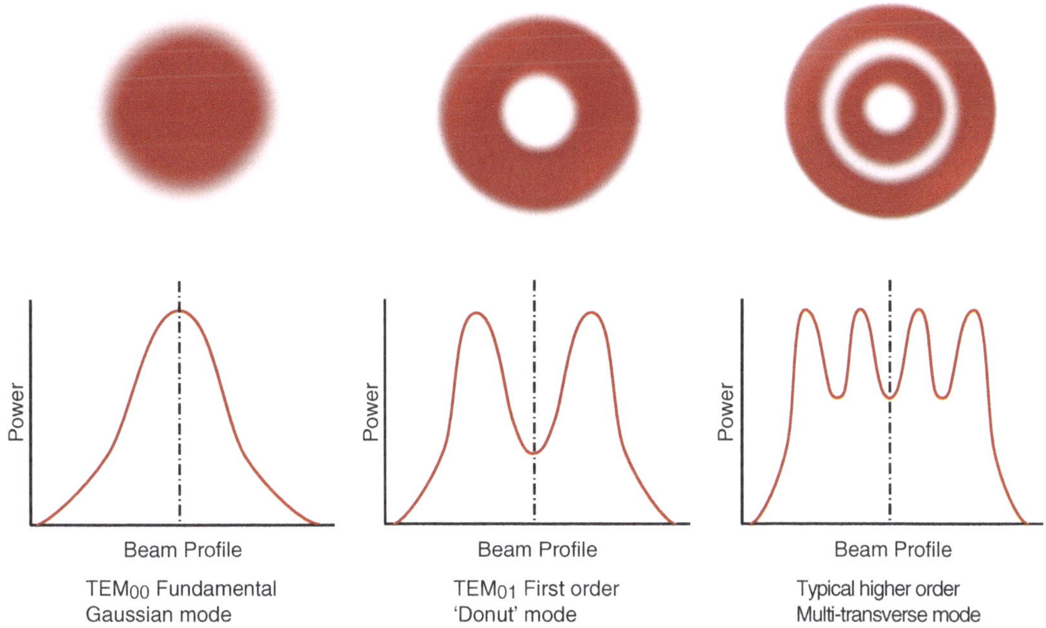

Fig. 1.14 Illustration of laser transverse electromagnetic modes (TEM)

types, e.g. dye lasers, should be left to stabilise and reach ambient operating temperature before taking output readings or delivering treatment. Lister and Brewin have reported variation in beam outputs between initial and subsequent laser pulses during the course of normal operation [25].

Monochromaticity (Linewidth)

A laser beam is often described as consisting of one pure colour or single wavelength, which is the definition of monochromatic light. As laser light is generated by stimulated emission, the ideal case would suggest that all emitted photons would have identical energy and accordingly identical wavelength (Eq. 1.1). However, due to physical and optical effects within the cavity, the output beam is more accurately described as *quasi-monochromatic* due to having a very narrow spectral output or line width compared with other sources and laser designs.

Some laser types, particularly the early dye lasers were described as *tunable lasers* since the output wavelength could be *tuned* or *adjusted* to select from a range of wavelengths generated within the cavity. In the majority of current medical laser systems, the wavelength tends to be *factory set* to an optimal output according to treatment indication, e.g., 595 nm, yellow/orange light.

Coherence

Stimulated emission results in two identical photons of the same frequency said to be *in phase,* indicating the wave crest of one photon occurs at the same time as the wave crest associated with the second photon. An avalanche of similar photons is created within the gain medium with a fixed phase relationship between them, i.e. they are highly ordered in space and time, referred to as *coherence*.

Coherence is the essential requirement for the strong directionality of laser beams and the ability to focus to extremely small spot sizes. Some applications require high degrees of coherence such as interferometry and holography, but for dermatology applications beam coherence is less critical than a stable output, larger beam sizes, variable pulse durations and an appropriate power range.

Directionality or Collimated Output

One consequence of a linear optical resonator consisting of parallel mirrors that reflect waves back and forth through the gain medium is the beam is constrained on a path perpendicular to the surfaces of the mirrors. The multiple reflections produce a well-collimated beam because only photons travelling parallel to the cavity walls are reflected from both mirrors. A perfectly collimated beam would never expand at all. However, the cavity design, output aperture size and diffraction effects will cause the beam to divergence slowly as it exits the laser aperture. Compared with incoherent light sources, the angle of divergence is extremely small, i.e. milliradians making it ideal applications such as laser telemetry, range finding and for beam delivery via fibre optics (wavelength dependent) or articulated arms (see section "Articulated Arm"). The exception to highly collimated beam output is found with diode lasers due to their unique cavity design.

To provide a summary of the components required for lasers and the properties of laser light described above an illustration of the key differences between non-coherent sources and a coherent laser source is given (Fig. 1.15).

Medical Laser Systems

Table 1.3 presents the common medical laser systems by type of gain medium.

Beam Delivery Methods

The properties of the output beam generally dictate the method of delivering the beam to the treatment area or site. For example, ultrashort pulse durations (ps pulses) produce phenomenally high peak powers that would damage quartz fibre optics; alternatively, some wavelengths are absorbed by glass, limiting transmission through an optical fibre.

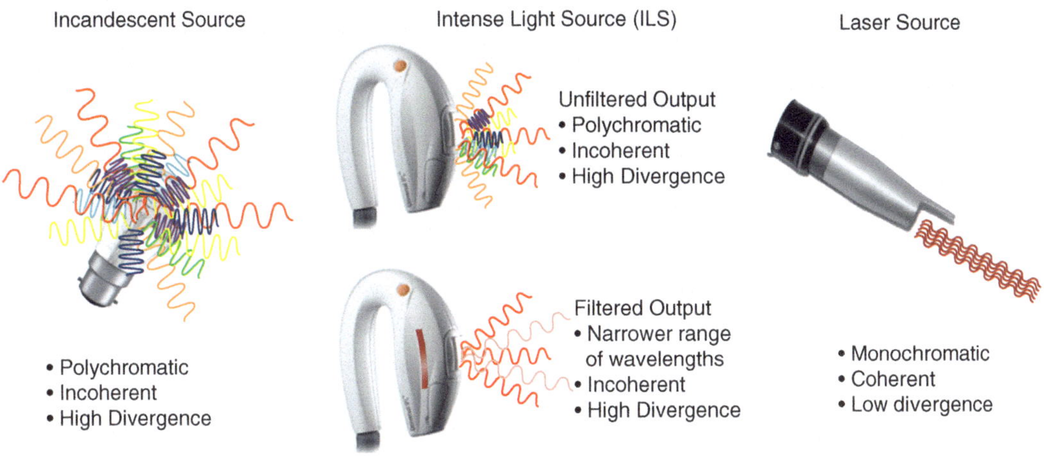

Fig. 1.15 Illustration highlighting the properties of light emitted by non-coherent sources and a coherent laser source

Table 1.3 Range of laser systems by type of gain medium

Laser type by gain medium	Typical operational wavelength (nm) and spectral region	Medical applications
Solid-state lasers with a crystalline gain medium, optically pumped by flashlamp(s) or diode laser (DPSS)		
Neodymium yttrium Aluminium garnet (Nd:YAG)	1064 nm near IR	Dermatology, ophthalmology, Gynaecology, urology, dentistry, respiratory
Frequency doubled neodymium yttrium Aluminium garnet (FD Nd:YAG)	532 nm visible green	Dermatology, ophthalmology, plastic surgery Gynaecology, dentistry, obstetrics
Ruby (Al_2O_3)	694 nm visible deep red	Dermatology, plastic surgery
Alexandrite ($Cr:BeAl_2O_4$)	755 nm near IR	Dermatology, plastic surgery
Erbium fibre/erbium glass	1550 nm/1540 nm near IR	Medical cosmetic, semi ablative skin rejuvenation
Thulium YAG (Tm:YAG)	1927 nm near IR	Medical cosmetic, semi ablative skin rejuvenation
Holmium YAG (Ho:YAG)	2100 nm mid IR	Urology, ophthalmology
Erbium YAG (Er:YAG)	2940 nm mid IR	Dermatology, plastic surgery, dentistry
Erbium yttrium scandium gallium garnet (Er:YSGG)	2790 nm mid IR	Medical cosmetic, semi/ablative skin rejuvenation
Gas lasers with a single gas or gas mixture gain medium, *electrically pumped* by pulsed or continuous electrical current		
Carbon dioxide (CO_2)	10,600 nm far IR	Dermatology, plastic surgery general surgery, neurosurgery, Gynaecology, dentistry
Excimer (excited dimer)	ArF—193 nm UV KrCl—222 nm UV KrF—248 nm UV XeCl—308 nm UV XeF—351 nm UV	Dermatology, ophthalmology
Helium Neon (HeNe)	632 nm Visible red	Aiming or pilot beam
Argon (Ar)	488 and 514 nm Visible blue and green	Ophthalmology

(continued)

Table 1.3 (continued)

Laser type by gain medium	Typical operational wavelength (nm) and spectral region	Medical applications
Organic dye in a solvent gain medium, optically pumped another flashlamp or other laser		
Dye in solvent e.g. Rhodamine 6G	Dye dependent, typically 577, 585, 595 nm. Visible yellow/ orange	Dermatology, urology
Semiconductor/diode layers gain media, electrically excited by electrical current		
Diode e.g. GaAlAs	755, 800, 810, 1064 through to 1550 nm near—mid IR	Dermatology, dentistry, physiotherapy, ophthalmology. Also used for aiming beam/pilot beam

KEY: *CW* continuous wave, *DPSS* diode pumped solid state laser

Handpiece design, ergonomics and functionality are very often overlooked when discussing laser and light technologies. The delivery of consistent and accurately placed treatment beams owes much to advances in handpiece design which has significantly increased laser applications within general surgery, dentistry, physiotherapy, podiatry and veterinary medicine. Features such as fixed or variable focusing, integrated epidermal cooling, finger switch controls, sacrificial windows, stand-off spacers, fixed or variable spot sizes, integrated plume collection, real-time imaging, beam output and alignment detection, skin temperature monitoring, pattern generation, skin vacuum/suction technology, weight and balance of a handpiece all impact the efficiency, reliability, ease of use and comfort of treatment for both practitioner and patient.

Introduced in the following sections are the most commonly used methods for delivering a beam from a laser or light device to the treatment site.

Optical Fibres

Silica-based glass fibre optics have excellent optical properties and can transmit wavelengths from >300 nm to approximately 2000 nm. This broad transmission window allows visible and near IR laser beams to be transmitted by fibre optics (ignoring beam power) making fibre optics an ideal delivery method for many surgical and medical aesthetic interventions.

Although some fibres can transmit beyond 2500 nm, they are limited to transmitting low powers due to loss mechanisms and strong absorption by silica above 2100 nm. Consequently, a different technology is required to deliver CO_2 wavelengths (10,600 nm) to the treatment site, hence the use of articulated arms (see section "Articulated Arm").

Chalcogenide-glass fibres and hollow waveguides provide an alternative to articulated arm delivery for CO_2 wavelengths. These fibres offer high laser power thresholds, low insertion loss, no end reflection and precision transmission making them for medical laser applications [26].

All fibre delivery systems should be handled with care, fibres should never over-bent or tightly coiled, and the fibre entry point into the handpiece should be robust to reduce stresses caused by frequent handling.

Lasers that deliver short (ns) and ultrashort (ps) pulse durations, e.g. for tattoos and pigmented lesion removal often use articulated arm delivery (see Fig. 1.16), even though quartz optical fibres can transmit visible and near IR beams because the high peak powers generated by such short pulses would damage silica-based fibres.

Articulated Arm

An articulated arm, as illustrated in Fig. 1.16, comprises rigid tubes of aluminium or carbon fibre with 45° mirrors mounted in rotary bearings, called knuckles, at the ends. A typical arm assembly contains six knuckles and two long beam tubes, with two additional short tubes called the input and output hubs. The knuckles are 'articulated' to allow flexible motion which

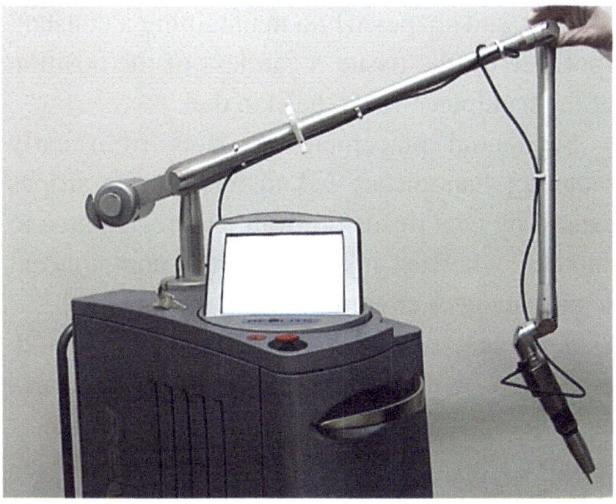

Fig. 1.16 Articulated arm beam delivery system. Courtesy of Cynosure, Inc.

when correctly aligned ensures the beam exits the arm at the same position and angle independently of the position of the freely moving tubes. Some lasers incorporate detectors that turn the laser off if a beam enters but does not simultaneously exit the arm.

As the beam path length does not change the beam remains a constant spot size and consistent output throughout the full range of articulated arm motion. The articulated arm beam path is also independent of the structural rigidity of the laser and the floor on which it is placed allowing the laser to be mounted on wheels or used on uneven surfaces.

The mirrors and hubs are factory pre-aligned and rarely require readjustment unless the arm is damaged by knocks or by incorrect storage when not in use.

Diode Arrays in Treatment Handpiece

A series of low power diodes can be arranged in clusters or 'arrays' to produce higher power outputs and arranged in different optical configurations. Diode arrays require optics to shape or focus the beam for transmission through a quartz or sapphire window or tip in direct contact with the skin. Internal cooling of the treatment tip provides a level of epidermal protection during treatment.

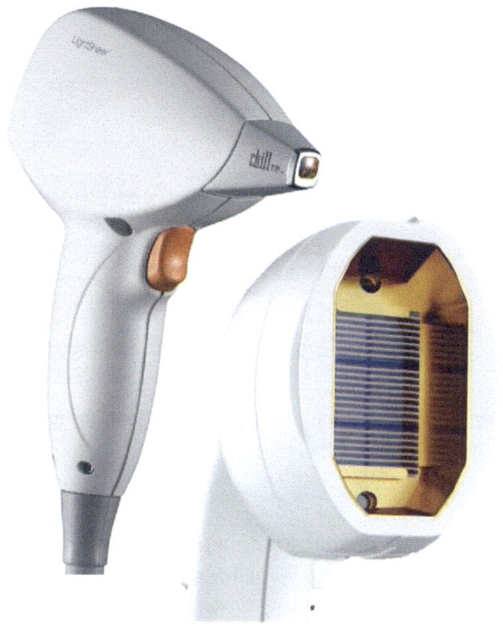

Fig. 1.17 Compact and efficient diode arrays can be incorporated directly into treatment handpieces. Courtesy of Lumenis

The compactness of laser diodes makes it possible to design handpieces that incorporate vacuum or suction technologies to reduce the depth of transmission to the intended treatment target and reduce discomfort from treatment (Fig. 1.17).

Diodes of different wavelengths can be incorporated into a single handpiece effectively extending the range of presenting conditions or skin types that can be treated without the need for multiple individual lasers. For example, diodes that emulate the laser wavelengths of 755 nm or 1064 nm for hair reduction have been found to be as efficacious as their solid-state equivalents [27].

Diode arrays in small and compact handpieces are used extensively in physiotherapy, chronic wound healing and pain management applications.

Flashlamp in Handpiece (Intense Light Source ILS/Intense Pulsed Light IPL (TM))

Intense light sources (ILS) are described more fully in section "Intense Light Sources (ILS) (Intense Pulsed Light (IPL (TM)))". A xenon

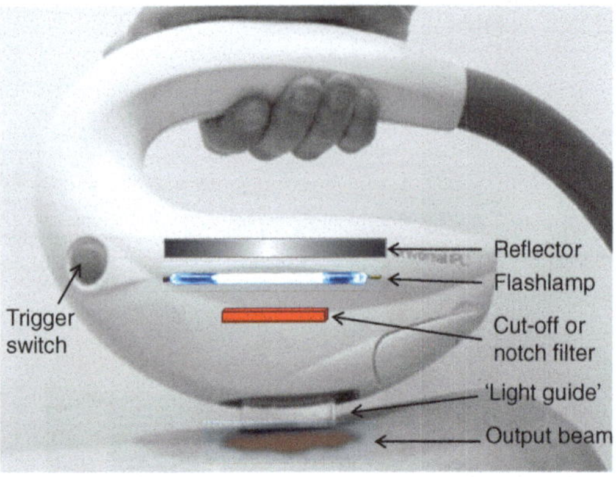

Fig. 1.18 Illustration of components within an intense light source (ILS) handpiece

flashlamp is mounted within the treatment 'head' or handpiece produces a broad-spectrum output beam. A reflector directs the beam through a quartz or sapphire treatment block or tip, which may be fixed or interchangeable. Depending upon the design of the treatment handpiece internal cooling of the treatment block or tip provides a level of epidermal protection during treatment (Fig. 1.18).

Beam Scanning Technologies

Beam scanning technology developed from the need to cover treatment areas larger than the available output treatment beam which may only be 20–30 mm maximum. Traditionally this required the treatment beam to be moved over the treatment area until the entire area had received the prescribed irradiance or fluence. The skill of manually moving a beam in this way is to avoid leaving gaps in the treatment area whilst also avoiding overlapping of the treatment beam. Overlapping can lead to overtreating sufficient to cause either patient discomfort or tissue injury.

One way to control coverage over a large area is via a hand-held *scanner* which rapidly scans a pulsed beam in a pre-programmed pattern of treatment spots. Such scanners were in use as early as 1995 for creating scalp slits for hair transplant using a CO_2 scanned laser beam. The Trost handpiece [28] included galvanometer mirrors programmed to deliver a variety of pre-set patterns and shapes while maintaining a constant spot size on the tissue regardless of the position of the handpiece from the skin due.

Sequential placement of spots from early scanning handpieces led to banding or stripes caused by heat diffusion from one treated area to another whereas non-sequential, non-adjacent scan sequences overcomes this problem [29].

Although scanners are still predominately associated with CO_2 lasers, some other lasers now incorporate scanners for hair reduction, non-ablative skin rejuvenation and treatment of vascular lesions.

Fractional Beam Technologies

While scanning beam technology was initially developed to cover treatment areas more extensive than the available output beam allowed, *fractional* or *pixelated* beams were intended to solve a different problem.

The use of conventional *Gaussian whole field* laser beams for *ablative* procedures was unquestioned in terms of clinical efficacy. (See Chap. 5 by Vishal Madan). However, the extensive thermal diffusion associated with CO_2 wavelengths often led to epidermal injury, referred to as residual thermal damage (RTD) as reported by Bernstein [30]. The associated risks and downtime of whole field ablative lasers led practitioners to investigate other devices and beam delivery methods that might achieve similar results to the CO_2 or Er:YAG wavelengths.

The first fractional devices used a *non-ablative wavelength* (Er:Fibre 1500 nm) delivered as *microscopic thermal zones* (MTZ) that caused deep dermal heating, described as fractional photothermolysis (FP) by Manstein et al. [31].

The advantages of *fractional* beam technology described by Manstein et al. [31] were quickly realised and applied to *ablative* devices for tissue *removal* rather than tissue heating and coagulation. Fractional beams from ablative lasers leave small *bridges* of healthy tissue intact, serving as reservoirs for faster tissue healing and reduced recovery times [32, 33].

Fractional handpiece design now enables multi-modal treatments using non-ablative and ablative wavelengths to create deep dermal heating independently or combined with superficial ablation increasing the range of clinical indications.

Pattern Masks/Stamping

A variation on fractional beam delivery is the use of pattern masks or pattern stamps. Rather than scanned beams or scanned fractional beams, a static *pattern mask* is generated by micro-optic lenses or holographic gratings that is *stamped* onto the tissue or skin. Pattern masks are suitable for both non-ablative and ablative wavelengths depending upon the clinical indication.

Aiming Beams

Although not specifically a beam delivery method, the majority of laser devices require a low power aiming or pilot beam to indicate the intended position of the treatment beam. Aiming beams should be available on lasers using fibre optic or articulated arm beam delivery and where there is no visible treatment beam, i.e., UV or IR wavelengths, or change in tissue when the laser is operated (Fig. 1.19). Generally, the aiming beam is produced by a low power diode (or HeNe laser on older systems) and is either red or green so is visible when wearing protective eyewear.

The aiming beam should be concentric with the therapeutic beam, with maximum allowable lateral displacement between the two centres not exceeding 50% of the diameter of the larger of the two spots. Additionally, the aiming beam spot diameter should not exceed 1.5 times the therapeutic beam's diameter.

It should not be possible to operate the laser without an operational aiming beam. Failure of the aiming beam during laser operation should prevent output of the treatment beam. Intense light devices and some diode laser systems tend not to have aiming beams as the handpiece treatment block, or tip is generally in contact with the skin.

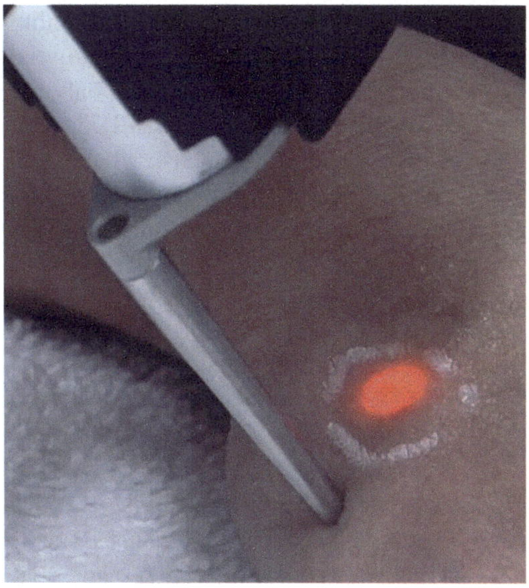

Fig. 1.19 Visible red aiming beam (pilot beam) to indicate position of the invisible infrared (1064 nm) treatment beam

Light Emitting Diodes (LEDs)

Chapter 8 discusses in detail the device technologies and treatment indications for *light emitting diodes* (LEDs) and *low-level laser therapy* (LLLT). This short section serves to introduce LED technology rather than treatment indications.

Light emitting diodes or LEDs are used in many medical and aesthetic devices particularly for interventions intended to stimulate the skin repair and wound healing processes. LED therapy is used to accelerate cell renewal and resolve a range of skin concerns such as reducing inflammation, acne therapy, enhancement of wound healing, sports injuries and joint pain. Other applications include prevention of mouth sores in cancer patients undergoing chemotherapy [34] and research into cognitive and memory disorders due to traumatic brain injury [35].

Laser practitioners may be familiar with *diode lasers* but they are not the same as light emitting diodes and are often thought of being 'new' technology. However, LEDs were developed in the 1960s in parallel with the first lasers specifically for the amplification of signals due to their ability to pass current in one direction only. Not only can LEDs transmit current in one direction only but they emit light as a consequence. LED devices use semiconductor materials such as silicon, gallium arsenide and germanium. New organic materials are available for the manufacture of *Organic Light Emitting Diodes* (OLEDs) providing the thin, flexible, white light emitting substrates used on phone screens, media devices, TV displays and computer monitors.

Early LEDs were widely used as indicator lamps on electronic devices but were expensive to produce with limited wavelengths and output brightness. Reduced manufacturing costs, improved stability and output brightness make LED devices the technology of choice for solar cells, displays and sensors, communications, aviation and domestic lighting, car and street lights, advertising displays, traffic lights, camera flashes and medical devices. They offer many advantages over incandescent light sources, including lower energy consumption, longer lifetime, improved physical robustness, smaller size, and faster switching. They are significantly more energy efficient and, arguably, have fewer environmental concerns regarding disposal than other light sources.

LEDs are electronic, *semiconducting* devices that emit light when charged with electrical voltage by the process of *electroluminescence* (EL), as opposed to incandescence from sources such as halogen or tungsten lights. The light emitting section is the junction between *n-type* and *p-type* semiconductors.

Silicon crystal has *mobile electrons* or *holes* depending upon the doping materials, e.g. boron or phosphorus, that create and control the number of electron holes allowing two separate types of semiconductors in the same crystal. Electrons and holes each have an electric charge, therefore, are affected by electric fields and diffusion (the random thermal motion of electrons and holes). When electrons in the n side are excited by an electrical current, they move across the *pn junction* to the p side where they combine with electron holes within the device. Combination results in a release of energy in the form of photons (light). The *pn junction* is typically encased in a phosphor coated epoxy shell to diffuse light and enhance brightness (Fig. 1.20).

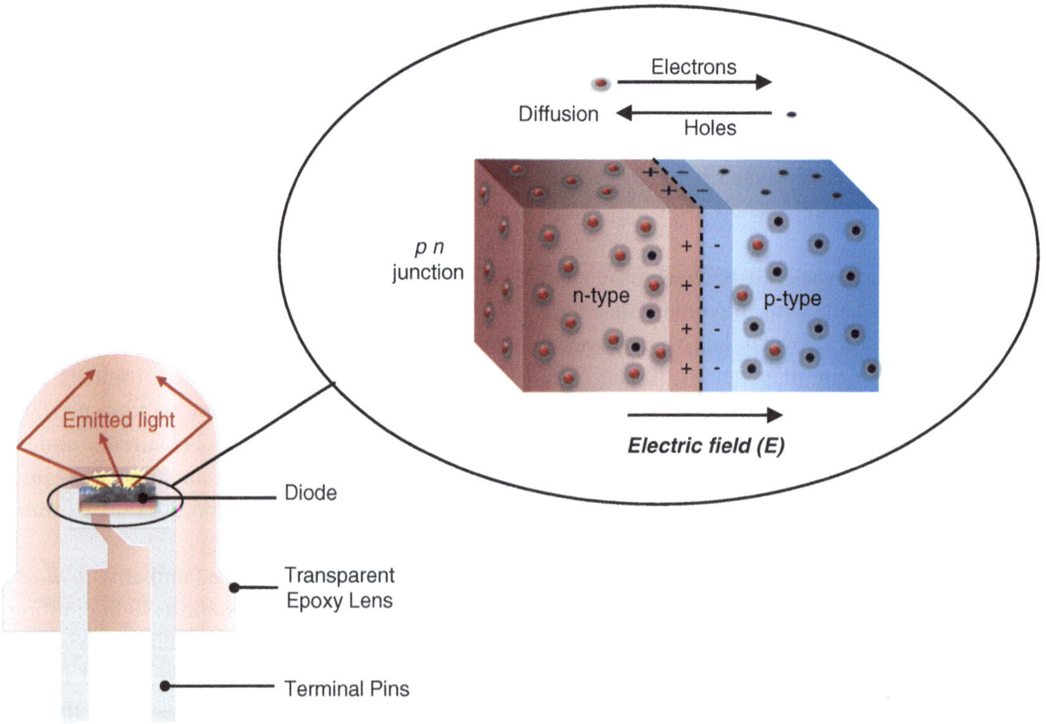

Fig. 1.20 Schematic a light emitting diode (LED)

Adding reflective surfaces to an LED effectively allows it to operate as a small diode laser.

LEDs emit narrow band, incoherent, diffuse light in a forward direction that has significantly higher divergence than laser radiation. Output wavelengths depend on the conducting medium with high output emission possible across the visible, ultraviolet, and infrared spectrum. LED output power is often quoted in *photometric,* e.g. illuminance (lumens per m^2 = Lux) versus radiometric terms, e.g. irradiance (W m^2), making it difficult to compare equivalency between sources for some applications such as diode laser phototherapy versus LED phototherapy.

It is appropriate at this point to compare lasers and LEDs with the more recently developed devices known as Intense Light Sources (ILS) or Intense pulsed light (IPL) systems.

Intense Light Sources (ILS) (Intense Pulsed Light (IPL))

In 1976 Mühlbauer et al. [36] described treatment of vascular malformations with polychromatic infrared radiation commenting on the thermo-coagulation properties of the light. Between 1976 and 1990 there were further reports of treatment of tattoos, superficial vascular lesions, warts and myxoid cysts using a tungsten halogen bulb emitting incoherent light at 400–2700 nm (VIS—N-IR), described as an *infrared coagulator* [37].

However, the majority of clinical studies and research from 1970 onwards were reporting medical laser applications rather than incoherent broadband sources applications. One such study was that by Goldman and Fitzpatrick in 1990 [38] who reported that a pulsed dye laser (585 nm, pulse duration 0.45 ms) caused thermal coagulation of blood vessels (< 0.4 mm diameter). Adverse treatment events included prolonged purpura and hypopigmentation which Goldman and Fitzpatrick hypothesised were due to the relatively 'short' pulse durations emitted by the laser.

According to the foreword by Dr. Goldberg in Fodor et al. [39] it was a fortuitous meeting between himself and Dr. Shimon Eckhouse, an aerospace engineer that led to the development and receipt of a prototype device consisting of a *filtered flashlamp* with varying pulse durations and output energy. The device was designed by Eckhouse and colleagues with the explicit intention of thermo-coagulating vessels and reducing epidermal injury [39]. Just 2 years later the prototype device used by Goldberg in 1992 was refined and brought to market by ESC Medical Systems/ Sharplan, Israel, as the *PhotoDerm VL.*

According to Goldberg [39] there were several reasons he and colleagues pursued use of incoherent, polychromatic light sources over laser devices for treatment of vascular lesions, and later for hair reduction. Goldberg et al. did this despite the early controversies that described intense pulsed light as a harmful and useless technology [40].

Firstly, Goldberg and colleagues recognised the benefits of being able to manipulate a broadband output to take advantage of the different absorption characteristic of oxygenated and deoxygenated haemoglobin. Secondly, they had successfully demonstrated that *multiple pulse trains* with variable pulse durations could achieve effective clinical coagulation while minimising epidermal injury [41].

Goldman reports that by August 1995, when the Food and Drug Administration (FDA) granted clearance for treatment of lower extremity telangiectasia, over 20 PhotoDerm VL systems were in clinical trials in the USA with a further 20 in use through Europe and Canada [39].

More recently trials and studies using intense light sources for dermatological applications have recognised the clinical significance of multiple sequential pulsing in combination with epidermal cooling/skin coupling gels. Intense light source systems that are well engineered and designed are extremely versatile and effective devices in the treatment of benign vascular and pigmented lesions, hair reduction, generalised skin 'rejuvenation', photodynamic therapy, photobiomodulation (PBM) and low-level laser therapy (LLLT) [42].

Intense Light Source Components

The central unit of an intense light source typically contains a computer, pulse-generating network and an ancillary cooling system either for the component cooling or handpiece cooling. Various treatment handpieces or treatment heads are available either fixed or detachable from the main body.

The handpiece comprises the flashlamp, selective filter (either built-in or interchangeable) and a quartz or sapphire *light guide* with either a flat or cylindrical radius along the full length of the surface that comes into contact with the skin (see Fig. 1.18). Faces, bevels and chamfers on the light guide should be polished to reduce the likelihood of skin damage during treatment.

If the handpiece does not have integral cooling of the treatment light guide, then some form of *epidermal cooling* (contact or dynamic cooling) should be employed during treatment. Water-based, clear cold gel (e.g., ultrasound gel) is often used to improve patient comfort and assists light coupling into the skin by reducing refractive index changes.

Flashlamp Characteristics

Flashlamps or arc lamps are widely used in medical and industrial applications (including for optical pumping of lasers). The majority of intense light source devices use Xenon flashlamps due to their characteristics of:

- Broadband spectral output
- Relatively low thermal conductivity
- Reliable spectral output over lamp lifetime

Flashlamps consist of a tungsten electrode contained within a cylindrical transparent silica (borosilicate or quartz) glass tube. Flashlamps may be linear or 'U' shaped depending upon the application and device manufacturer can be used in single or twin arrangements.

Doped flashlamp glass envelopes prevent wavelengths <360–380 nm exiting the flashlamp wall leaving a typical spectral output from a Xenon flashlamp between 400–1800 nm, although spectral *distribution* varies according to the gas pressure, input energy of the lamp and other factors (Fig. 1.21). Additionally, the energy distribution across the broad spectrum may vary within the duration of a pulse and between pulses, known as 'spectral jitter' [43, 44]. This variation within, and between, emitted pulses may potentially reduce the efficiency and efficacy of light-tissue interactions.

Electrode type and design and lamp ignition/discharge technology determine the mechanical, electrical and optical characteristics of the flashlamp and output measurements to traceable national standards are essential factors for establishing safe clinical treatment parameters. Town et al. [45] reported on variation between spectral widths, output power and pulse shape from flashlamps, with discrepancies between measured and

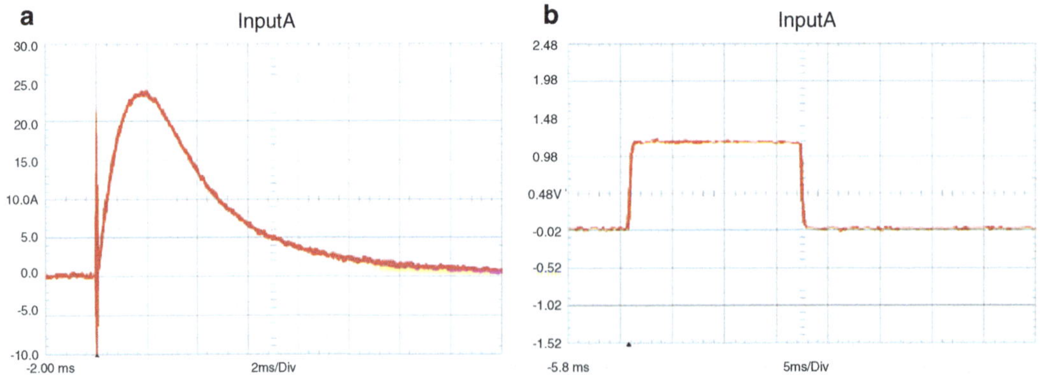

Fig. 1.21 (**a**) Example standardised lamp discharge profile measurement of a free-discharge IPL (**b**) Example standardized lamp discharge profile measurement of a 'square pulse' constant current discharge system. Reproduced from [45]

manufacturer reported figures. These variations may affect tissue heating properties and clinical outcomes (Fig. 1.21).

One key point should be emphasised to the reader regarding intense light sources. While intense lights have been shown to remove superficial pigmentation [46] it is not possible, due to flashlamp design, to produce the short (ns) or ultrashort (ps) pulse durations required for safe tattoo removal.

Flashlamp Filtering

The broad spectral output of an intense light flashlamp is *selectively filtered* to a specific wavelength range tailored to the treatment indication, e.g. 695–1200 nm for hair reduction, 515–1200 nm for superficial pigmented lesions.

One of the challenges with early intense light devices was how to achieve adequate and reliable selective filtering. Coloured glass filters intended to absorb unwanted wavelengths would crack due to thermal stresses. It is likely that patients received higher levels than expected of blue light from early devices due to poor spectral filtering, perhaps accounting for reports of epidermal injury associated with early devices [39]. Thus, the quality and accuracy of intense light filters are critical to safe and effective treatment.

Dye Filters

An alternative to coloured glass filters is organic dye filters or dye impregnated polymers that produce very narrow band outputs. For example, a dye filter can be used to narrow an intense light output to 500–660 nm to mimic a pulse dye laser spectral output targeting the absorption spectra of oxy- and deoxyhemoglobin (see Fig. 1.6). Interestingly, this narrow selective filtering was one of the original design requests that Goldman made in 1992 [39]. Treatment on cutaneous vasculature using this technology has been reported by Moy et al. [47].

The majority of intense light devices achieve selective filtering by two primary methods; dichroic mirrors/filters and absorption filtration.

Cut-off Filters

Dichroic mirrors are optical surfaces coated with multilayer *dielectric* (absorbing) coatings on a polished glass substrate, which has excellent environmental durability, the very characteristics sought by early intense light developers.

They are highly efficient reflectors, tolerating incident high power densities therefore used as laser resonator mirrors and turning mirrors in articulated arms. Dichroic mirrors are very angle-dependent so are suitable for *deviating unwanted* wavelengths from a laser or flashlamp and transmitting only the desired therapeutic wavelengths. Consequently, dichroic filters are commonly described as *cut-off or edge pass* filters because they can transmit a required spectral region and cut-off other spectral regions. However *cut-off* suggests a sharp boundary between wanted and unwanted wavelengths, which in practice is not strictly accurate in some intense light source devices [45].

Notch Filters

A variation of dichroic *cut-off* filters referred to as *notch filters* are employed on some intense light devices. *Notch filters* (band-stop filters) transmit most wavelengths with little intensity loss while attenuating light within a *specific wavelength range* (the stop band) to a very low level. Transmission is dependent on the angle of incidence with the central wavelength of the blocking region shifting to shorter wavelengths as angle of incidence increases.

Transmitted wavelengths are chosen to correspond with peak absorption by a given chromophore or multiple chromophores. For example, a *dual-band* output spectrum of 500–670 nm and 870–1220 nm will target the absorption peaks of haemoglobin and preferentially transfer heat to vascular structures by thermal diffusion from absorption by melanin. Similarly, a spectrum of 400–600 nm and 800–1200 nm for treatment of acne.

Varughese [48] has compared treatment outcomes using single band and dual-band filtered intense light devices for the treatment of photodamaged skin.

To conclude this section, it is important to mention the advances in *multi-application 'platforms'* systems that typically combine laser and intense light source devices operating from one modular unit. Platform systems allow practitioners to treat multiple indications without the need for individual lasers or intense light sources, increasing treatment flexibility, reducing floor space requirements and for some systems reducing initial capital outlay.

Laser and Light Beam Parameters

When clinicians discuss treatment settings or outcomes from different laser and light devices it is vital that variables and units are clearly defined. This short section defines laser and light beam parameters and terms intended to lead the reader to a better understanding of the light-tissue interactions discussed in section "Producing Pulsed Outputs".

Radiometric units apply to the entire EM spectrum of sources whereas *photometric* units commonly apply only to visible light. Radiometric units include; *power*, *irradiance*, *radiant intensity* and *radiance* and provide information about the *absolute* brightness of a source. *Photometric* units such as *lumens, candelas and luminance* provide information about the perceived *brightness* of a source. Unfortunately, Light Emitting Diode (LED) devices (see section "Light Emitting Diodes (LEDs)") often use photometric terms, e.g. luminance making it challenging to compare laser and LED outputs without using factoring calculations.

Radiometric units for laser and light applications, based on SI units are:

- *Energy* expressed in Joules (J)
- *Power* expressed in watts (W)
- *Distance* expressed in meters (m)
- *Time* expressed in seconds (s)

These terms are seen in context when examining the different beam types emitted from a laser or intense light source. For example; a beam might travel as a *continuous wave* (CW) (> 0.25 s duration) [49], it might be emitted as a single pulse or a series of multiple pulses (e.g., a *pulse train*). Pulses may be of different energy, duration or repetition rates (Fig. 1.22).

Radiant Energy (Q) and Radiant Power (P)

Concerning the clinical outcome, energy and power are very different concepts. Therefore, it is essential to understand the difference and relationship between them together with the related concepts that arise from each.

- *ENERGY* is described in textbooks as the ability to do work, such as moving an object, heating water or illuminating the tungsten filament of a light bulb

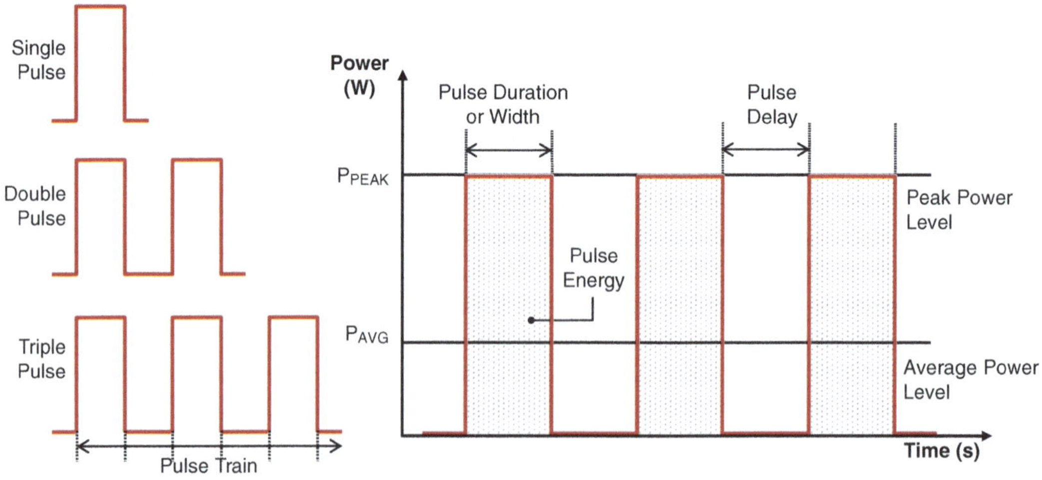

Fig. 1.22 Anatomy of laser and light pulsed outputs

- *RADIANT ENERGY* (*Q*) is the quantity of energy travelling through space in the form of light waves, expressed in *Joules* (*J*)
- As a laser pulse, *radiant energy* is expressed in *Joules (J)* and is usually fixed by the optical components and design of the system, e.g., 60 J per pulse from a diode array.
- *Radiant energy* is the product of power and time, sometimes referred to as watt second *(W s)*
- *RADIANT POWER (P)* is the amount radiant energy transferred in a given unit of time
- As the output power of a laser, *radiant power* is expressed in *watts* (*W*)
- *Radiant power* is expressed in joules per second, $(J\ s^{-1})$

The distinction between the two concepts is subtle and, in many cases, confusing. In simple terms, the tendency is to associate the specific units of either energy of power with the nature of light emitted, e.g., either pulsed or *continuous wave* (CW).

- Pulsed output
  - The energy of each pulse is expressed in *Joules (J)*.
- CW output
  - The power of the beam is expressed in *watts (W)*.

While the expression of energy describes the *quantity* of energy contained within, for example, one laser pulse, it does not describe the *rate* of delivery of that energy. For interventions involving an increase in temperature, it is the *rate* of energy delivered to the tissues that determine the type of tissue interaction, e.g. *photothermal* versus *photomechanical* effects.

The relationship between radiant energy and radiant power is

$$\text{Power}(\text{W}) = \text{Energy}(\text{J}) / \text{Time}(\text{s}) \quad (1.3)$$

Alternatively:

$$\text{Energy}(\text{J}) = \text{Power}(\text{W}) \times \text{Time}(\text{s}) \quad (1.4)$$

When converting between power and energy, it is essential to use the use time value of the light pulse otherwise a significant error can result.

Radiant Exposure (H) and Irradiance (E)

Two essential terms describing the application of laser and light beams are *radiant exposure* and *irradiance* often referred to as *energy density* and respectively (Fig. 1.23).

Radiant exposure of a beam is the amount of light *energy* passing through a given area, expressed as joules per square metre (J m^{-2}).

$$\text{Radiant exposure}\ H\left(\text{J m}^{-2}\right) = \text{Radiant Energy}\ Q(\text{J}) / \text{Beam area}\ A\left(\text{m}^2\right) \quad (1.5)$$

Clinicians and practitioners may be more familiar with the term *fluence (J cm^{-2})* rather than

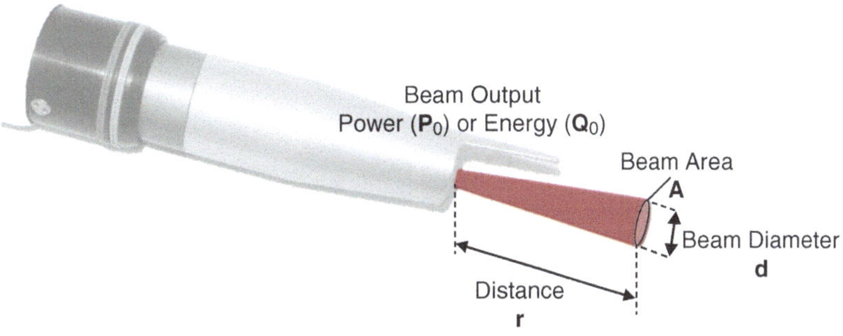

Fig. 1.23 Illustration of beam parameters that define radiant exSposure and irradiance

radiant exposure (J m^{-2}). Fluence and its significance to treatment will be explored shortly.

Irradiance is defined as the *radiant power* of a beam given through a given area, expressed as watts per square metre (W m^{-2}).

$$\text{Irradiance}\ E\left(\text{W m}^{-2}\right) = \text{Radiant Power}\ P\left(\text{W}\right) / \text{Beam area}\ A\left(\text{m}^{2}\right) \quad (1.6)$$

Note: *radiant exposure* and *irradiance* are often used interchangeably together with *intensity* and *radiant intensity* when describing the optics of laser beams, but there are subtle differences particularly for laser safety calculations and safe exposure limits which deal with irradiance.

Beam Area and Profile

Calculation of radiant exposure and irradiance rely upon measurement of *beam area* often referred to as *spot size* in clinical applications (see Fig. 1.24). Laser beams are typically illustrated as narrow collimated 'pencil' beams of light with sharply delineated edges, in which case irradiance would genuinely be the output power divided by beam area. However beam size and width measurement can vary due to; beam mode, quality of focusing optics, measurement distance from the laser aperture and to how the beam is measured. Beam imaging reveals that output is usually brightest at the centre and fades gradually towards the edges described as a *Gaussian distribution* (Fig. 1.24). This has implications for clinicians, regarding efficacy and treatment spot placement (overlapping), and for laser safety professionals concerning laser beam hazard assessments.

However, for most clinical laser and light interventions it is acceptable to assume the beam has a circular cross-section and uniform light distribution making beam area calculation area more straightforward using Pythagoras theorem for a circle.

$$\text{Beam area} = \pi \times \left(\text{beam radius}\left(r\right)\right)^{2} \quad (1.7)$$

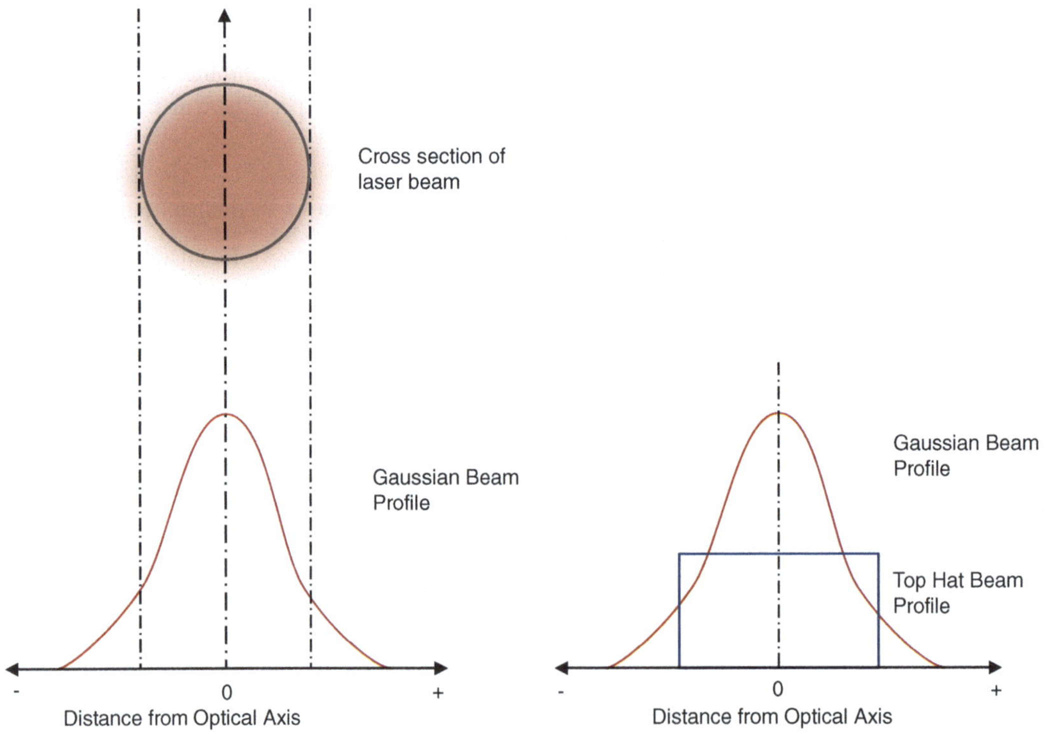

Fig. 1.24 Illustration of a Gaussian beam profile

Note: supplied data for many laser devices quotes *overall* beam diameter (d) rather than the radius (r) and usually in mm. Clinicians undertaking laser safety calculations should be mindful to convert from *beam diameter* to *radius* as appropriate.

$$\text{Beam area} = \pi r^2 = \pi d^2 / 4 \quad (1.8)$$

If we look again at "Eq. 1.6" for irradiance, irradiance is related to the inverse square of the beam diameter by:

$$\text{Irradiance}\left(\text{W m}^{-2}\right) = \text{Radiant Power} / \text{Beam area} = 4P / \pi d^2 \quad (1.9)$$

where
P laser beam radiant power
d beam diameter

Similarly, it is possible to rearrange "Eq. 1.5" (radiant exposure) in relation to beam diameter.

$$\text{Radiant Exposure}\left(\text{J m}^{-2}\right) = \text{Radiant Energy} / \text{Beam area} = 4Q / \pi d^2 \quad (1.10)$$

where
Q laser beam radiant energy
d beam diameter

"Equations (1.9)" and "(1.10)" have significant consequences for laser interventions if the laser handpiece does not detect a change in beam area or spot size, e.g. the so-called smart or intelligent technology handpieces. The consequences for treatment can be significant and illustrates the importance of maintaining a consistent beam area (spot size) during treatment.

Fluence, expressed in J cm^{-2}, is the term most frequently used when describing pulsed laser treatments. Fluence involves three factors; power, time and beam area.

Rearranging "Eq. 1.5" allows fluence to be expressed as follows:

$$\text{Fluence}\left(\text{J cm}^{-2}\right) = \text{Power}\left(\text{W}\right) \times \text{Time}\left(\text{s}\right) / \text{Beam area} \quad (1.11)$$

Where time (s) is taken to be laser *pulse duration.*

This concept is explored further when discussing light-tissue interactions (see section "Light Tissue Interactions").

Pulsed Laser Output

The majority of medical laser and light devices deliver the output beam as a pulse of light because fluence ("Eq. 1.11") is not the only treatment variable for laser and light-based interventions. *Pulse duration* and *pulse energy* impact the degree to which laser energy diffuses into surrounding tissues. Thermal diffusion is generally linked with undesired localised tissue injury, and early interventions for the treatment of vascular lesions sought to limit and reduce thermal diffusion. One approach to minimise heat spread and achieve optimal target *damage* has been to match the beam *pulse duration* with the so-called *Thermal Relaxation time (TRT)* of the target. This logic suggests that a smaller target (e.g. vellus hair) requires a shorter pulse duration than a more substantial target (e.g. terminal hair). Consequently, medical aesthetic lasers and intense light devices are typically designed to emit pulsed beams with variable duration pulses according to clinical intervention. Before describing how devices produce different pulsed outputs, there are some definitions explicitly describing pulsed beams that clinicians should understand.

Pulse Duration (PD in s)

There are different definitions of pulse duration depending upon the application, e.g. optical communications signal pulse duration versus laser pulse duration. The most common definition uses *full width at half maximum* (FWHM) of optical power versus time (Fig. 1.25). Hence the term *pulse width* (PW) as opposed to *pulse duration* (PD). For laser and light interactions, pulse duration may be more appropriate term given that output pulses are quoted in fractions of seconds (s). Hence pulse duration is taken to be how long the pulse of light lasts, or the length of time over which tissues are exposed.

It should be remembered that the laser or lamp design dictate pulse duration and not all lasers or intense lights can emit particular pulses, e.g. an intense light source cannot emit nanosecond pulses.

Pulse durations may include:

- Millisecond pulses (ms, 10^{-3} s) commonly described as *long* pulses
- Microsecond pulses (μs, 10^{-6} s)
- Nanosecond pulses (ns, 10^{-9} s) commonly described as *short* pulses
- Picosecond pulses (ps, 10^{-12} s)
- Femtoseconds (fs, 10^{-15} s) commonly described as *ultrashort* pulses.

The later chapters report specific treatment settings for a given presenting condition and discuss different pulse durations.

Pulse Repetition Frequency (PRF) (Hertz, Hz)

Pulse repetition frequency or rate (in Hz) defines the *number of pulses emitted every second.*

Number of Pulses Emitted

The number of pulses emitted within a given exposure time (T seconds) is given by

$$\text{Number of Pulses} = \text{Exposure Time}(\text{T}) \times \text{Repetition Frequency}(\text{Hz}) \tag{1.12}$$

Average Power (P_{AVG}, in watts)

The average power of a pulsed source is a measurement of average power over a period of several seconds and is a standard specification for laser output.

$$\text{Average Power}(\text{W}) = \text{Pulse Energy}(\text{J}) \times \text{Repetition Frequency}(\text{Hz}) \tag{1.13}$$

Note: peak power is a more appropriate parameter than average power when assessing potential for injury to tissues.

Peak Power (P_{PEAK}, in Watts)

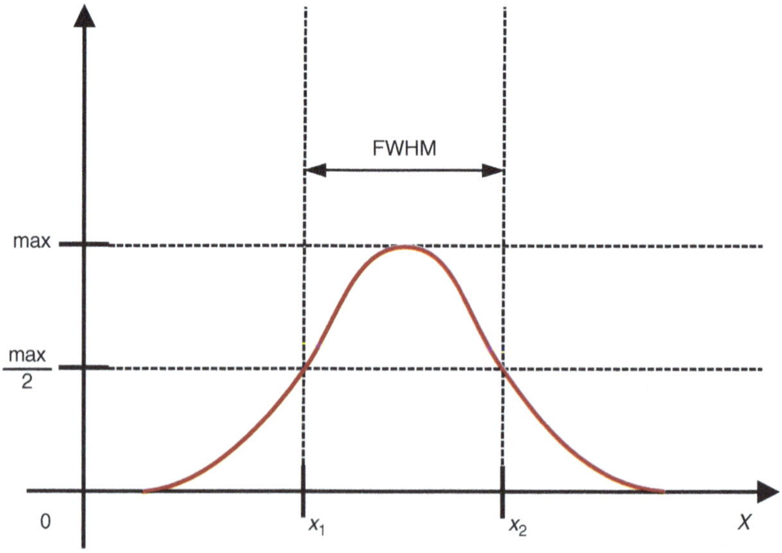

Fig. 1.25 Illustration of full width at half maximum (FWHM) to define pulse duration

Peak power is the ***maximum instantaneous power*** produced during the emission of a pulse of light. The peak power produced by nanosecond (ns), picosecond (ps) or femtosecond (fs) lasers is extremely high even for relatively small pulse energies. The ability to produce phenomenally high peak powers and the resulting specific light-tissue interactions have driven the commercial development of picosecond and femtosecond laser systems.

$$\text{Peak Power}(\text{W}) = \text{Pulse Energy}(\text{J}) / \text{Pulse Duration}(\text{s}) \quad (1.14)$$

Producing Pulsed Outputs

Many medical applications including dermatology, ophthalmology and urology require high radiant powers (W) or high peak power (P_{PEAK}) to induce specific light-tissue interactions and pulsed laser beams can provide such outputs.

There are different ways to produce pulses of light, for example, a fast shutter or modulator could be used to turn a continuous wave beam rapidly on-and-off, effectively *chopping* the beam into discrete pulses. While a *gated* or *chopped pulse* gives a visual sensation of a pulsed beam and is ideal for strobe lighting or range finding applications, *gated pulse* generation does not change the output *radiant power* (W) However, *modulating* the beam in some way, e.g. by 'Q' switching, mode locking, cavity dumping or gain switching *does* change radiant power and is an efficient way to produce very high power outputs (Fig. 1.26) and it is interesting to note that the first experimental demonstration of 'Q' switching was in 1961 at the Hughes Aircraft Company shortly after the Maiman's demonstration of the first laser in the same facility [50]. The methods of 'Q' switching and mode locking for producing short and ultrashort pulses are outlined in the following sections with complete descriptions of pulse generation available in the publication by Paschotta [51].

'Q' Switched Lasers

The letter 'Q' is short for *quality* factor and is the term used to measure the loss or gain of energy in a laser cavity defined as:

$$\text{Quality factor}(Q) = \text{energy stored per pass} / \text{energy dissipated per pass} \quad (1.15)$$

Modulating the intracavity losses, i.e. the 'Q' factor of the resonator produces very high peak

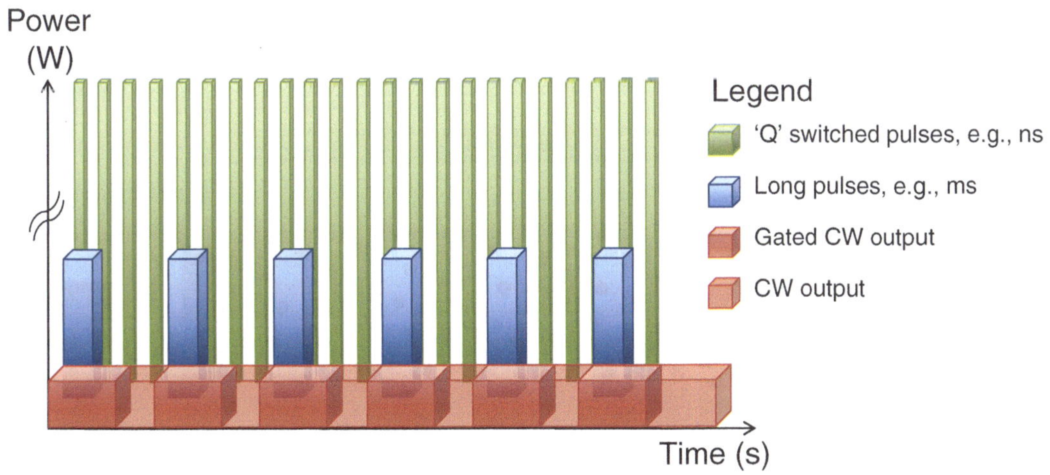

Fig. 1.26 Illustration of different beam output modes

power *short* pulses (not ultrashort) sometimes called *giant pulses*. 'Q' switching is commonly used on solid-state lasers such as Nd:YAG, alexandrite and ruby lasers, typically producing nanosecond pulses (10^{-9} s).

To generate 'Q' switched pulses the initial resonator losses are kept high, i.e., 'Q' switch is on, the quality factor is low and output lasing is prevented. This *accumulates* or *builds* energy within the gain medium, a process limited by the spontaneous emission of the gain medium. Suddenly reducing the cavity losses by switching off the 'Q' switch, allows emission of a short pulse with very high peak power. As the resonator gain is substantially higher than resonator losses, intracavity power rises exponentially (usually starting with noise from spontaneous emission of the gain medium) until the gain medium becomes saturated and the power decays. Rapidly and regularly switching between these high and low loss conditions generates a regular pulse train, typically from 1–100 Hz. A compromise must be made at very high pulse repetition frequencies as the available time for the gain medium to accumulate energy is reduced, and therefore peak power output may be lower.

Gain medium properties such as metastable lifetime, the density of active ions or atoms and saturation energy determine the percentage of stored energy in the output which is why rare-earth-doped crystals and glasses are most suitable for 'Q' switched lasers. Fibre lasers can also be 'Q' switched and when combined with fibre amplifiers to produce very high output powers.

'Q' switching is described as *active* or *passive* according to the method used to achieve the pulsed output (Fig. 1.27).

Active 'Q' Switching

Active 'Q' switching is achieved by modulating cavity losses with an *active* control element such as an acousto-optic, or electro-optic modulator, e.g. Pockels cell. Active 'Q' produces a pulse shortly after an electrical trigger signal arrives and pulse energy and duration are a function of

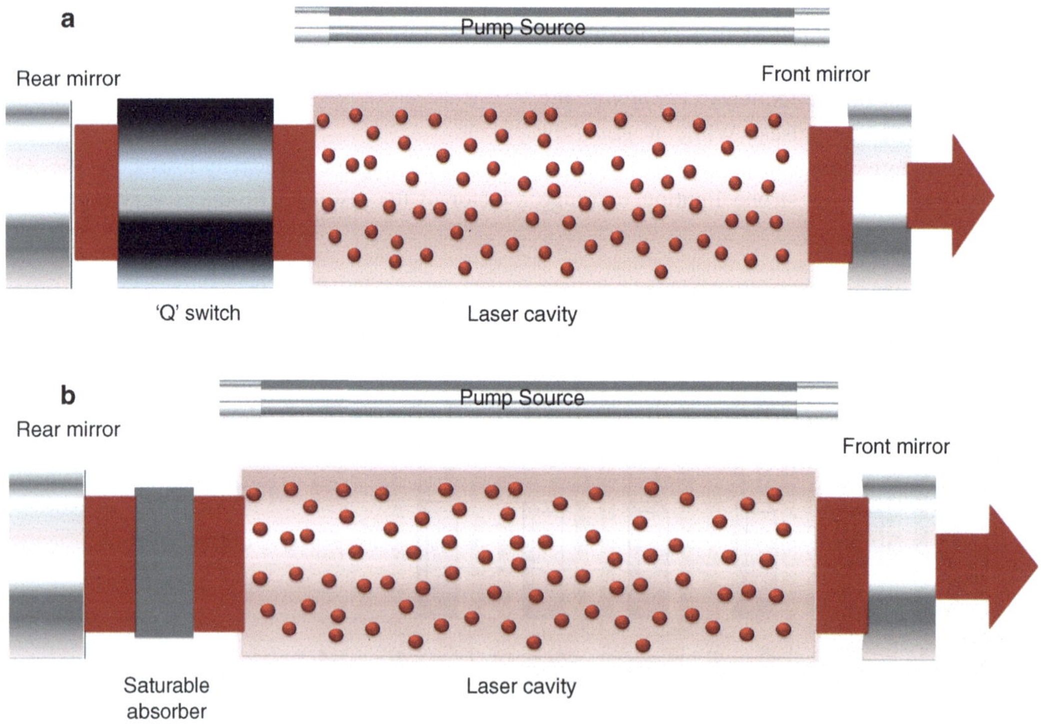

Fig. 1.27 Illustration of 'Q' switching. (**a**) Active 'Q' switching. (**b**) Passive 'Q' switching using a saturable absorber

the energy stored in the active media. Pulse repetition rates of actively 'Q' switched lasers can be externally controlled unlike *passive* 'Q' switched devices.

Passive Q Switching

Passive 'Q' switching, sometimes called self-'Q' switching is achieved by modulating cavity losses with a saturable absorber such as a dye cell or crystal, e.g. Cr:YAG is typically used in Nd:YAG lasers. The absorber introduces a high optical loss initially by absorbing the beam which briefly stops lasing output. When the absorber is saturated, cavity quality abruptly increases releasing producing a short duration pulse as a consequence. Passively 'Q' switched lasers are generally smaller, more portable and more affordable than active 'Q' switched laser because the absorbers are more cost-effective and more straightforward in operation. They are suited to very high pulse repetition frequencies, therefore tend to have lower power outputs but less control over energy or pulse duration. Passive 'Q' switch devices typically do not require articulated beam delivery.

The beam in a 'Q' switched laser generally requires several round trips within the resonator to depopulate the upper energy level completely and then several more round trips to empty the optical cavity. Consequently, the duration of the pulse is greater than one round trip. For optical cavities shorter than a metre (one round trip less than 6 ns) it is possible to generate short pulses of only a few nanoseconds. 'Q' switched lasers never reach a steady state as they stop functioning after several round trips of the light in the cavity. This is in contrast to the operation of a mode-locked output described below.

Mode-Locked Lasers

Recent developments in commercially available medical lasers have seen the introduction of picosecond (10^{-12} ps) pulses for tattoo removal and treatment of pigmented lesions and femtosecond pulses (10^{-15}, fs) for ophthalmological applications. Sub-nanosecond pulse durations generally take advantage of lower pulse energies delivered in *ultrashort* pulse durations. Pulses of this duration deliver a combination of thermal and mechanical forces that shatter a target within the skin or dermis before any substantial thermal energy diffuses to surrounding tissue.

The rationale of sub-nanosecond pulses for tattoo removal is an assumption that tattoo pigment particles of ≤1 μm diameter are cleared from the body via the immune system processes given that stable tattoos contain pigment particles in the order of 1–10 μm diameter or greater. The acoustic transit time of a sound wave in a tattoo pigment particle is calculated by dividing the radius of the particle by the speed of sound in the particle (approximately 3000 meters/second). Therefore, the acoustic transit time across such particles, and consequently the laser pulse duration required to achieve the photomechanical destruction of tattoo pigment is as short as hundreds of picoseconds [52]. Some clinical results of medical cosmetic applications of picosecond lasers show a higher percentage of tattoo clearance achieved in fewer treatments, with improved recovery time [53].

In a similar way to 'Q' switched devices, *mode locking* can be by *active* or *passive* methods either electro-optic modulators or saturable absorbers respectively. However, the operating technique for a mode-locked laser is quite different.

The laser resonator is allowed to reach steady-state, but oscillation is restricted it to a limited *packet* of photons propagating in the cavity. Each time a pulse hits the output coupler mirror part of its energy is emitted to produce a regular pulse train with pulse durations shorter than a *round trip* of the cavity. The gain medium replenishes the pulse energy in each round trip (Fig. 1.28).

In this arrangement, the resonator round-trip time and the number of pulses determine the pulse repetition frequency (PRF). For example, a 10-ns round-trip time for a single pulse leads to a PRF of 100 MHz. In steady-state operation, the pulse duration is determined by various effects on the pulse during each resonator round-trip, typically resulting in pulse durations between 30 fs and 30 ps depending upon gain medium.

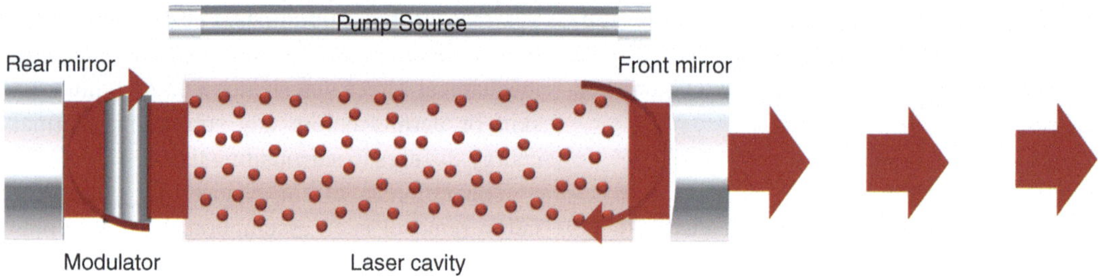

Fig. 1.28 Concept of mode-locking to produce ultrashort pulses

Pulse energy is restricted to typically a few pJ to mJ due to the high pulse repetition rates of mode-locked lasers.

Advances in the optomechanical design of medical laser devices mean that clinicians rarely need be concerned with the intricacies of laser resonators, gain pumping, beam modes, spectral bandwidth or pulse generation, allowing them instead to concentrate instead upon device functionality and application from systems capable of delivering reliable, stable and consistent outputs.

Light Tissue Interactions

Understanding light interactions and in particular light-tissue interactions, is essential for safe practice as it enables clinicians to select appropriate treatment parameters, predict the depth to which tissues are irradiated and identify tissue response, e.g. photothermal versus photomechanical interactions. It also allows identification of appropriate personal protective equipment (PPE) such as protective eyewear. This section describes key light-tissue interactions and introduces the concept of *Selective Photothermolysis* first proposed in 1983 by Anderson and Parish [16].

Selective or *preferential* absorption of light energy by targeted tissue(s) is the goal of laser and light tissue therapies. Crucially the target needs to undergo tissue or cellular changes, but surrounding areas should not, i.e. be subject to minimal *collateral* damage. This process relies on a significant number of variables coming together to achieve a safe and efficacious clinical outcome.

When light strikes biological tissue various effects are observed as a result of photon interactions with chromophores on, or within tissue. Chromophores have highly wavelength dependent *scattering coefficients* (μs) and *absorption coefficients* (μa). According to Young (1996), *chromophore* relates only to the conjugated multiple bonded (unsaturated) atoms of the molecule in question since they are responsible for its absorption properties. But in clinical practice, the term *chromophore* is loosely used to describe a whole molecule [54].

In addition to device and treatment variables tissue, *optical* and *thermal* properties of tissue influence beam interactions. *Optical* properties determine the distribution of light in the therapeutic volume of tissue while *thermal* properties deal with the conversion of light energy to heat as well as heat transport via thermal conduction.

Optical Properties of Tissues

A thorough review of optical properties of biological tissues is given by Jacques [55]. Outline explanations are given in the following sections for the purpose of leading the reader to an understanding the principles of selective photothermolysis [16].

When photons strike biological tissue, it displays a specific distribution of light including; reflection, scattering, transmission, absorption and re-emission. Typically, a combination of one or more types of interactions dominates depending on the incident energy and tissue properties (Fig. 1.29).

The measurable quantities of re-emission, reflection and transmission are often called *macroscopic optical* properties and are wavelength,

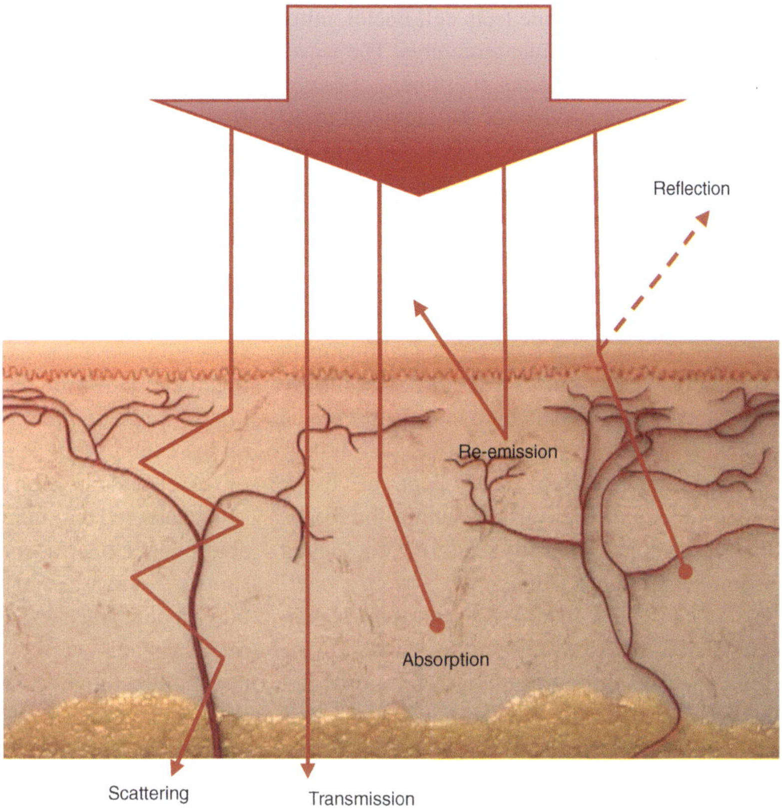

Fig. 1.29 Stylised illustration of possible light-tissue interactions from photons striking biological tissue

tissue type and layer thickness dependent. The distribution of photons and the resulting macroscopic optical properties are determined by:

- Refraction
- Scattering
- Absorption

Refraction

When photons strike the surface of biological tissue a small percentage (4–11%) is reflected due to a refractive index change from air to skin depending on angle of incidence [56]. Approximately 89–96% of photons from a beam at normal incidence to the skin are forward scattered by the epidermis but also refracted, in accordance with Snell's Law which states that photons entering from a lower (air) to higher refractive index medium (skin) are refracted towards the vertical axis of the surface depending upon the angle of incidence of the beam [57].

Refraction only plays a significant role when photons irradiate transparent media, for example corneal tissue during corrective laser eye surgery, and requires index matching gels to reduce beam direction changes at the surface boundaries.

Although clinical effects of refraction in the skin are difficult to measure, clear water based gel is often applied to laser or intense light handpieces used in direct contact with the skin which may reduce reflection and refraction at the air/skin or handpiece/skin interface. Gel also provides a level of epidermal cooling and assists with handpiece *gliding* or travel across the skin improving patient comfort during treatment.

Only photons that continue forward into the tissue can contribute to treatment efficacy, but they are subject to further interactions such as scattering.

Scattering

Scattering in tissue occurs where there is inhomogeneity of the refractive index, e.g. on a macroscopic scale from muscle fibres or skin layers, or on a microscopic scale from cell nuclei, mitochrondria and intracellular structures. The wavelength dependent scattering coefficient of tissue, μs (λ) (cm^{-1}) is a measure of the ability of particles to scatter photons out of a beam of light and is a complex phenomenon not completely described by either Rayleigh scattering or Mie scattering [57]. Scattering is significant because it is the dominant interaction for visible and near IR radiation thus determining the volume distribution of photons within the tissue and treatment efficacy. Scattering causes photons to lose energy and disperse as they penetrate into denser media becoming collectively less effective.

The scattering (μs) coefficient of tissue decreases with increasing wavelength and for the majority of skin tissues the scattering coefficient is significantly greater than the absorption coefficient (μa). Consequently a proportion of incident photons are able to penetrate deeply into the skin ignoring absorption by chromophores. Photons interact with structures within the skin such as collagen bundles and do so repeatedly until the beam either exits from the skin surface (reemission) or is absorbed by a given chromophore.

An important point for clinicians to appreciate is that photon scattering, and therefore depth of penetration, is affected by the treatment area or beam width of the incident beam [58] (Fig. 1.30).

Ash et al. [58] describes how a larger spot size (beam width) reduces the amount of lateral scattering allowing greater forward photon projection that results in a high cumulative photon energy and deeper penetration of the incident beam (ignoring absorption by chromophores). Theoretically it would be possible to use lower energy densities in combination with larger spot sizes to achieve the same penetration depth for treatment. However, for devices offering a selection of beam spot sizes, choice is usually based on the extent of the area to be treated or the size of vessel, and rarely on consideration of the depth of the targeted chromophore. Furthermore, available fluence or irradiance typically decreases as spot size increases and clinicians should take this into account when treating deeper chromophores. Some devices employ compression or vacuum handpieces to effectively shorten the distance from skin surface to target chromophore to improve penetration of the beam.

There is a limit to the depth of penetration possible through change of beam width which is estimated to be in the region of 5–12 mm for laser devices. Limited data is available for intense light sources [58, 59]. Evidence suggests that a beam

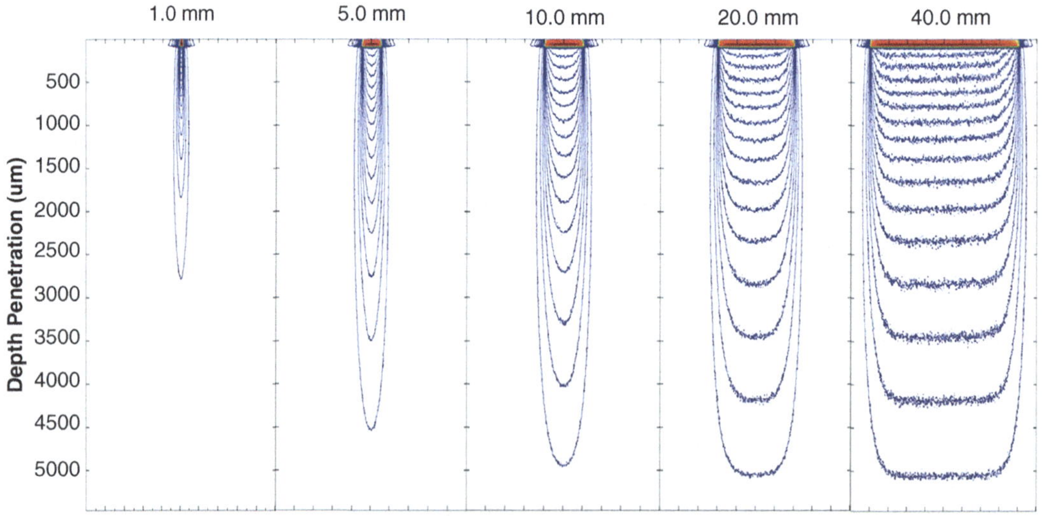

Fig. 1.30 Calculated penetration profiles for uniform 1, 5, 10, 20 and 40 mm width beam, of equal incident fluence obtained by Monte Carlo simulation using typical skin parameters for wavelengths of 525–1100 nm. Reproduced with permission [58]. Note: Figure derived from 2D Monte Carlo model and intense light source used

width of 10 mm is the point at which increasing beam width will *not* increase depth of light penetration due to the tissue becoming saturated with scattering and limiting forward photon propagation.

In practice, laser and intense light source systems are designed with fixed or variable beam spot sizes according to treatment indication and whilst it is understood a beam width of 4–6 mm may penetrate to mid dermis and deeper layers, these figures are wavelength, beam profile shape, fluence/irradiance and tissue dependent.

Absorption

Absorption of photon energy is critical to efficacious clinical outcomes. Absorption relies upon suitable endogenous chromophores within the targeted tissue that can be selectively targeted with incident photon energy. A perfectly *transparent* medium allows light to pass through without absorption whereas an *opaque* medium is one in which the incident light is strongly or completely absorbed. The terms *transparent* and *opaque* are relative since they are highly wavelength dependent. For example, the cornea and lens of the eye are *transparent* to visible light but have specific electron transitions in the UV and far IR spectrum due to these tissues consisting primarily of protein and water. Consequently the cornea and lens would appear opaque at such wavelengths.

Absorption of photon energy produces a number of effects such as PhotoBioModulation (PBM), conversion to heat (non-radiatively, i.e. without luminescence) or mechanical/acoustic effects.

Absorption of photon energy in biological tissue is mainly due to the presence of free water molecules, proteins and pigments and other macromolecules. Absorption by tissue chromophores such as; porphyrin, haemoglobin, melanin, water, flavin, retinol, nuclear acids, deoxyribonucleic acid (DNA)/ribonucleic acid (RNA) is characterised by their respective wavelength dependent *absorption coefficients*, expressed as a number proportional to the amount of photons absorbed per distance, μa (λ) (cm^{-1}). For example the dense concentration of keratinous material in the epidermis is responsible for marked short wave UV absorption (<240–277 nm). In the dermis, haemoglobin and oxyhaemoglobin have strong absorption in the blue-green-yellow region of the visible spectrum. Melanin has extensive, conjugated, double bonds within its polymer structures and demonstrates *broad* or general absorption in the UV to near IR regions of the EM spectrum.

Given that energy states of molecules are quantised, photon absorption by a chromophore only occurs when its photon energy corresponds to the energy difference between such quantised states. Photon absorption causes either a quantised change in the *distance* between charges (*electron* transition caused by absorption of UV or visible radiation), or a quantised change of *vibrational modes* of the molecule (*vibration* transition caused by absorption of IR radiation). Consequently chromophores display discrete and intense *wavelength-dependent* absorption bands.

In loose terms, chromophores may be described as:

- **General absorbers** describe a chromophore that absorbs approximately all wavelengths in a given spectrum by equal or similar amounts. Melanin demonstrates this type of absorption spectra.
- **Selective absorbers** describe a chromophore that preferentially absorbs certain wavelengths over others. Water demonstrates this type of absorption spectra.

The absorption spectra of various chromophores can be represented graphically [60]. For example, absorption by bound water at 25 °C with corresponding percentage tissue depth showing illustrates minimal selective absorption in the visible spectrum, rising to maximum absorption at approximately 3000 nm.

Water as a Chromophore

The peak absorption by water, approximately 3000 nm, is significant to many laser and light therapies and is due to the symmetric and asymmetric vibrational modes of water molecules. It is estimated that the *resonant frequency* of water is approximately 1.08×10^{14} = 100 THz [61]. When the *frequency of vibration* of incident radiation (e.g.

a laser beam) closely matches the *natural resonant frequency* of a material, (e.g. water), a greater degree of interaction occurs, including *absorption.*

Rearranging "Eq. 1.2" allows resonant frequency to be calculated as a wavelength (nm) and the resonant frequency of water equates to a wavelength of 3000 nm (3.0 μm) which closely matches the output wavelength of a family of Er^{3+} doped laser outputs, namely Er:YAG at 2940 nm and Er:YSGG at 2790 nm. As illustrated in Fig. 1.33, the closely matching *resonant frequency* of water and *frequency of vibration* of the Er:YAG laser coincide at the peak of the water absorption spectra produced by Hale and Querry [60].

By contrast, the CO_2 laser wavelength (10,600 nm, 10.6 μm) equates to a *frequency of vibration* of approximately 280 THz which is greater than the *resonant frequency* of water (100 THz), thus reducing the degree of interaction between the CO_2 laser wavelength and water. Consequently absorption by water at 10600 nm is lower than absorption by water at 2940 nm.

Haemoglobin as a Chromophore

Jacques [55] presents complied data from studies of the absorption coefficient of *whole blood* for comparison of the spectral absorption by fully *oxygenated* and fully *deoxygenated* blood. The absorption spectrum of oxyhemoglobin peaks between 400 nm and 600 nm, whereas deoxyhemoglobin peaks between 400 nm and 850 nm, revealing a shift in the absorption peak of deoxygenated blood and the characteristic '*M*' double peak around 575 nm for oxygenated blood. These different absorption spectra are significant given the interest in dual wavelength and broad-band sources for treatment of vascular lesions although Jacques [55] reports that reliable data above 1000 nm is difficult to find.

Melanin as a Chromophore

The absorption spectra for *melanin* can be represented in a similar way as water and haemoglobin. Two types of melanin, namely eumelanin and phaeomelanin are both found in the skin, hair and eyes of animal species. Eumelanin is brown black in colour, whilst phaeomelanin (a sulphur containing macromolecule) is red to yellow in colour and responsible for the red colour of human hair and chicken feathers. The broadband absorption spectrum of melanin may be due to its photoprotective role, but the optical processes responsible for its appearance are disputed, e.g. amorphous semiconduction, scattering or electronic absorbance. Melanin is a significant chromophore in laser and light based therapies, acting as a target chromophore for interventions such as hair reduction, but also as a competing chromophore for interventions such as non-ablative skin rejuvenation.

A combined absorption spectrum of the chromophores of water, haemoglobin and melanin is frequently presented, and all laser and light clinicians should be familiar with the concepts that underpin this graphical illustration (Fig. 1.31).

Depth of Penetration

By combining an understanding of chromophore absorption spectra and the relationship between scattering and absorption, it is possible to identify the appropriate wavelength(s) to selectively target and maximise absorption by the presenting chromophore, and whether the depth of light penetration is likely to be capable of reaching the targeted chromophore.

Zhao and Fairchild [62] examined the transmission of coherent radiation (532–1064 nm) through tissues over a range of skin types and showed that 1064 nm light penetrated deepest into tissue.

Incident wavelength is a critical factor in determining not only the extent to which photons are absorbed by the intended chromophore, but also likely depth of penetration of the incident beam (ignoring other variables such as beam width) [63]. An appreciation of this phenomenon should help clinicians select optimal treatment variables according to the presenting condition as will be explored in the chapters ahead.

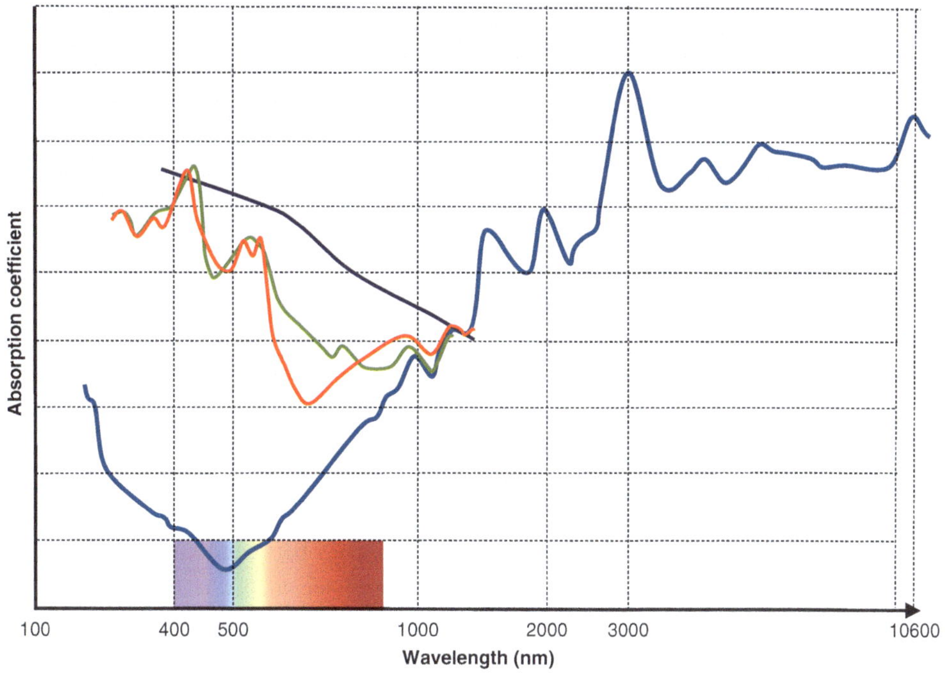

Fig. 1.31 Combined absorption spectra showing melanin, water and blood (oxygenated and deoxygenated)

Interaction Mechanisms

It is beyond the scope of this section to discuss theories that describe the transport of light energy through absorbing and scattering media such as; photon transport theory, Monte Carlo simulations or Arrhenius theory. Therefore, an overview of interaction *mechanisms* is presented, and readers can find specific detail included within each of the treatment indication chapters.

Laser and light-based therapies rely on the absorption of photon energy resulting in localised *thermodynamic changes* in the target structure(s), the exception being PhotobioModulation (PBM). The selectivity and efficacy of this process are determined by the optical properties of the tissue (coefficients of reflection, scattering and absorption) that collectively determine the *total transmission of energy* into the tissue at any given wavelength. Additionally, the properties of the optical radiation itself (wavelength, fluence, irradiance, spot size and pulse duration) affect absorption of photon energy and resultant tissue. The critical variable in determining the interaction *mechanism* is reported to be *pulse duration* [57].

The interaction *mechanisms* for clinical interventions and those that cause adverse effects such as injury to the eye or skin tissues are generally classified as photochemical, photothermal, and non-linear effects, broadly described as photomechanical interactions which include photodisruption, photoacoustic, photoablation, plasma-induced ablation. Each shall be briefly described.

The interactions described above were presented as a *medical laser interaction map* by Boulnois [64] indicating that distinct interactions mechanisms share a single common datum: a total specific energy dose (fluence) between 10 and 1000 J cm^{-2}. A single variable distinguishes these processes, namely the *exposure time* sufficient for delivery of the given fluence.

Boulnois [63] showed irradiance (power density) in W cm^{-2} against interaction time (s) (or exposure duration) plotted on a logarithmic scale with diagonal lines illustrating a constant fluence (J cm^{-2}). Hence interaction time could be roughly divided into sections:

1. *Photochemical* interaction at low power densities, long exposure durations, e.g., continuous wave (CW).
2. *Photothermal* interactions (hyperthermia, coagulation and welding) at higher power densities at shorter exposures, approx. 1 min to 1 μs.
3. *Photoablative* (1 μs –1 ns) and *photodisruptive* effects (<1 ns) at very high power densities, very short exposure times.

The reciprocal correlation between irradiance (W cm^{-2}) and exposure time (s) demonstrates that approximately the same fluence (energy density) in J cm^{-2} is required for any intended type of interaction. Thus, the exposure time (pulse duration) appears to be the primary determinant of interaction mechanisms.

Interaction effects are unlikely to occur in isolation. For example, thermal effects may play a role in photochemical interactions and even ultrashort pulses that individually might have little or no thermal effect may produce measurable temperature rises in tissue when delivered at very high repetition rates.

Photochemical Interactions

Photochemical interactions and injury are described by changes in the biochemical properties of tissue, either temporary or permanent. Photochemical effects are evidence of the *particle* or *photonic* nature of light whereby photon energy is responsible for initiating changes in tissue chemistry, for example, Photodynamic Therapy (PDT). PDT uses a photosensitising agent exposed to red to N-IR radiation to initiate several simultaneous or sequential decays resulting in intramolecular transfer reactions. The reactions release highly cytotoxic species that produce irreversible oxidation of essential cell structures. Widely used for the treatment of skin tumours and photodamaged skin, photochemical interactions require only low irradiance W cm^{-2} (power density), typically 1 Wcm^{-2} with exposure duration in the order of seconds or longer. Diode lasers and LEDs are ideal sources for such treatments.

Direct photochemical interactions result from exposure to short wavelengths (high photon energy), specifically UV and blue light (200–400 nm) and is a cumulative process. The risk of eye or skin injury is proportional to the total dose, i.e. the number of sufficiently energetic photons incident upon exposed tissue (irradiance and exposure time). Chronic exposure to scattered UV radiation may have the same deleterious effect as a short duration exposure to a direct UV laser beam.

Photothermal Interactions

Photothermal interactions and injury are characterised by an increase in local tissue temperature induced by longer wavelengths and CW or long-pulsed exposures. Absorption of photon energy produces an increase in the vibrational energy and collisions between tissue molecules. Part of the vibrational energy is transferred as kinetic energy, seen on a macroscopic scale as an increase in tissue temperature. The extent of injury to the tissue depends on the temperature reached and the duration held at that temperature, established from the early work of Moritz and Henriques [65]. If natural heat diffusion or epidermal cooling cannot mitigate skin or tissue temperature increase, the damage may be irreparable depending upon the tissue damage thresholds and incident beam characteristics. At the immediate impact site there may be a zone of vaporisation leading to zones of necrosis or carbonisation caused by thermal diffusion. Farther from the exposed site is a zone of coagulation and further still, an area of hyperthermia.

Photomechanical Interactions

The pulses emitted by nanosecond (ns) and picosecond (ps) lasers induce a number of *photomechanical interactions* in soft tissue or fluids depending upon incident wavelength and pulse characteristics.

Photoablation involves the direct breaking of molecular bonds by high-energy UV radiation causing molecular dissociation and material ejection or *spatter*. Photoablation is a clean and precise way to remove material with no thermal damage in surrounding areas. Material or tissue is effectively etched from the surface with depth and geometry of the etch dependent on the pulse energy and shape of the incident laser beam. Corrective eye surgery by high power excimer (UV) lasers is achieved via photoablation.

Plasma-induced ablation occurs when solids and liquids are exposed to very high irradiance (power density) (>10^{11} W cm^{-2}) [57] causing *optical breakdown* (OB). The physical effects associated with optical breakdown are *plasma formation* and *shock wave generation* through an avalanche effect of free electrons and ions. A significant secondary effect of plasma formation within soft tissues or fluids is *cavitation and jet formation.* Interventions such as tattoo removal utilise these *mechanical* side effects of plasma formation to rupture tissues giving an additional category of interactions described as *photodisruption.*

Photodisruption damages tissue via mechanical shock waves that result from plasma generation. In nanosecond pulse durations this mechanical effect is in order of millimetres even at the threshold of breakdown, meaning it is possible to damage adjacent tissues with these disruptive forces. However, the ultrashort pulse durations achieve optical breakdown with reduced plasma energy and therefore have less disruptive effects on surrounding tissue. Spatial confinement and predictability of tissue interaction is an additional benefit of such ultrashort pulses. Laser-induced optical breakdown (LIOB) is claimed to offer significantly faster clearance of tattoos and pigments from the skin and achieve skin rejuvenation with reduced downtime and epidermal healing [66].

In practice it is difficult to distinguish between the mechanism of plasma-induced ablation and photodisruption since both interactions rely upon the production of plasma. However, photodisruption is often regarded as a multi-cause mechanical effect starting with optical breakdown (the interaction of plasma-induced ablation).

Each of these mechanisms is discussed further in the individual chapters that follow. This overview has shown that the critical parameter in determining *type* of interaction is *pulse duration,* leading to the concept of thermal damage *confinement* and *selective* damage or injury to tissues, in other words, the *Theory of Selective Photothermolysis.*

The Theory of Selective Photothermolysis

A significant advancement in clinical laser practice therapy came with the Anderson and Parish 1983 publication [16] which drew together much of the published data on optical properties of tissue, light-tissue interactions, depth of penetration and selective absorption. Anderson and Parish proposed a method for confining thermal diffusion to an intended chromophore, namely pigmented targets and supported their theory with experimental data for treatment of blood vessels and melanocytes. They described a treatment methodology intended to cause *selective* damage to a target, with limited thermal damage to overlying or neighbouring structures by confining light energy within the targeted tissue through judicious choice of incident wavelength, pulse duration and incident energy. Anderson and Parish called this theory *Selective Photothermolysis* (SP). Note: this original work applied only to *photothermal interactions* and not those associated with PhotoBioModulation (PBM).

The absolute requirement to ensure specificity of a treatment is that the intended target has a greater absorption coefficient (α_{target}) at the incident wavelength than the absorption coefficient of the surrounding tissue (α_{tissue}). Anderson and Parish [16] suggested the ratio of $(\alpha_{target})/(\alpha_{tissue})$ should be in order of 10 or greater, but reported that selective photothermolysis may be achievable with ratios as low as 2. Clinically this explains the importance of appropriate patient selection whereby the chromophore has a high contrast compared with the surrounding tissue/skin, e.g. dark hair against pale skin.

During treatment, photon energy may be converted to thermal energy within a given chromophore (assuming photothermal interaction mechanisms) and over the period of exposure to the incident beam, the peak tissue temperature may well exceed the threshold for thermal denaturation of the intended target. In that same period of exposure the surrounding tissue would initially be expected to be below the damage threshold. After exposure thermal diffusion from the target transfers heat to the surrounding tissue and may cause a rise in ambient tissue temperature. The *rate* at which a target and its surrounding tissue heats and cools (or relaxes) varies according to the optical and thermal properties of the tissue.

Concept of Thermal Relaxation Time (TRT)

One means to reduce thermal diffusion from the intended target to surrounding tissue is by judicious choice of wavelength, i.e. selective absorption. However, Anderson and Parish [16] argued that undesirable thermal diffusion could still occur if the incident *pulse duration* was too long, indicating that photon energy is not sufficiently confined to the intended target.

Using predictive modelling, Anderson and Parish [16] suggested that between the extremes of long and short pulse durations, e.g. ms and ns, a continuum exists with varying degrees of thermal damage confinement. They hypothesised that the transition from *specific* to *nonspecific* damage (e.g. photothermal to photomechanical interactions) occurs as the pulse duration equals, and then exceeds the thermal relaxation time (TRT) for the target. Hence they constructed a link between selective absorption by a target and pulse duration.

Thermal relaxation time (TRT) is a theoretically constructed parameter reported as early as 1968 by Hayes and Wolbarsht using spheres and cylinders to model chromophores within human tissue [67]. TRT provides an indication of the *thermal susceptibility of tissues*, i.e. the ability to damage tissue with electromagnetic radiation.

The original theory of *selective photothermolysis* [16] provided a quantitative description of interventions intended to damage targeted structures while sparing surrounding tissue and for this to occur, it was suggested that the *pulse duration* must be short compared to the thermal relaxation time (TRT) of the whole target.

TRT was defined as the time taken 'for the central temperature of a Gaussian temperature distribution with a width equal to the target's diameter to decrease by 50 %'.

TRT is calculated (in cylinders as a first approximation).

$$\mathrm{TRT} = \mathrm{d}2 / 16\alpha \qquad (1.16)$$

where

d the target diameter (mm)

α issue diffusivity (mm^2 per second)

Hence TRT is approximated as the square of the diameter of the target structure and the theory of selective photothermolysis proposes that minimal *collateral* thermal damage is achievable if the photon energy is delivered within this time.

The work by Anderson and Parish [16] suggested treatment of targets on the subcellular organelle scale required nanosecond-domain or shorter pulses, whereas non-capillary vessels and other small structures required millisecond-domain or shorter pulses. Estimates of TRT for typical chromophores vary considerably between sources, but may be summarised;

- TRT of epidermis ≈ 1–10 ms
- TRT of terminal hair ≈ 40–100 ms (assuming 200–300 μm diameter)
- TRT of blood vessels ≈ 1–50 ms
- TRT of melanosomes ≈ 250–1000 ns (assuming 1.0 μm diameter)
- TRT of cellular water ≈ 1000 ns

However, if the condition of matching pulse duration to target TRT were fully met it would limit thermal diffusion entirely until the intended target was completed coagulated or damaged. Furthermore, the original model has limitations in that blood vessels were modeled as long cylinders which could not allow for spatial separation between absorbing chromophore and the target. Consequently, the significance and relevance of TRT gives rise to much debate.

For thermal interactions TRT is a useful construct as it can be used as a measure of the *thermal susceptibility* of tissue (see section "The Extended Theory of Selective Photothermolysis"). For example, if pulse duration < target TRT, there is limited or no thermal energy diffusion from the target (due to optical penetration depth constraints). Conversely, if pulse duration > target TRT, diffusion of thermal energy to tissue adjacent *may* induce injury.

Neimz [57] calculated the TRT of water and reported the shortest TRT is approximately 1 μs (1000 ns). Plotting the TRT of water against wavelength reveals that the shortest TRT (1 μs) corresponds with the absorption peak of water at approximately 3000 nm. It was concluded that pulse durations <1 μs are *not* normally associated with thermal damage (ignoring high repetition rates) a finding exploited in clinical practice by the ultrashort laser pulses (ps) for removal of tattoos and pigmented lesion and skin rejuvenation therapies.

The Extended Theory of Selective Photothermolysis

In 2001 [68] a new theory of selective damage was explicitly presented to address the treatment of *non-uniformly pigmented structures* targets that are *spatially separated* within biological tissue. Altshuler et al. [68] argued such targets could *not* be effectively treated with pulse durations ≤ the estimated TRT of the target, using in-vitro geometries of hair follicles and telangiectasia to support the need for a different approach to that of *containment* and *confinement* of thermal energy.

Altshuler et al. [68] presented the concept of *Thermal Damage Time* (TDT) rather than *relaxation* (cooling) time and defined it as 'the time when the outermost part of the target reaches the target damage temperature through heat diffusion from the heater (tissue)'.

The extended theory of selective photothermolysis distinguishes between an *absorber* or *heater* chromophore (e.g. melanin in the hair shaft having a high absorption coefficient in the UV and visible spectrum) and a distant target (e.g. the stem cells of isthmus with a low absorption coefficient with unknown absorption spectra). The *absorber* can be used to transfer photon energy to a distant target and cause injury or damage as a result. This process relies upon thermal *diffusion* rather than thermal *confinement*, and therefore a different consideration of pulse duration concerning TRT is required (Fig. 1.32).

In the extended theory of selective photothermolysis, thermal diffusion is no longer considered an adverse outcome but one that can be used to promote and enhance treatment indications that rely on heat spread to a greater or lesser extent (Table 1.4).

However, there are limiting factors to the extended theory of selective photothermolysis, for example, insufficient photon energy absorbed by the heater chromophore may limit diffusion with little or no therapeutic effect on target chromophore. Conversely, high absorption by the heater chromophore may reduce selectivity and damage non-target tissue, e.g., the epidermis. Altshuler et al. [68] acknowledge these critical

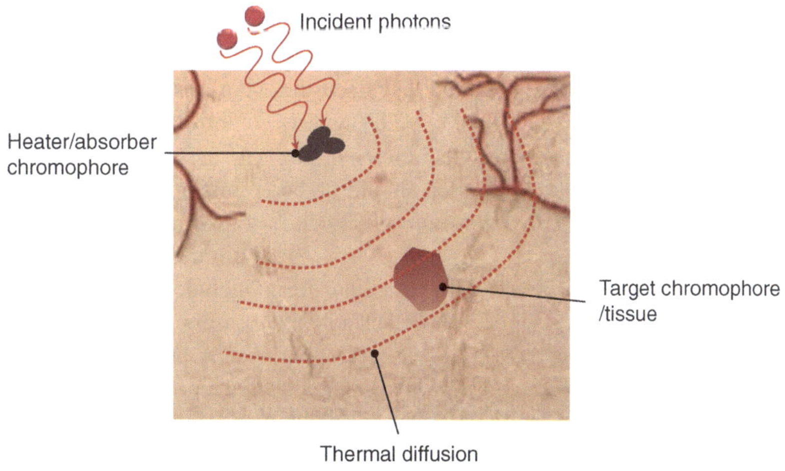

Fig. 1.32 Illustration of the extended theory of selective photothermolysis and the concept of absorber or heater chromophores

Table 1.4 Clinical indications that may take benefit from longer pulse durations according to the extended theory of selective photothermolysis [67]

Clinical indication	Heater/absorber chromophore	Target chromophore/ tissue
Hair reduction	Melanin in the hair shaft	Isthmus/stem cells in bulge and capillaries in dermal papilla
Vascular lesions and vascular malformations	Haemoglobin within vessel	Protein in the inner vessel wall
Non-ablative skin rejuvenation	Haemoglobin in capillaries, water in cells, and most existing tissue pigmentation	Collagen and fibres

factors in their research regarding pulse geometry and target-chromophore geometry that affect thermal diffusion, particularly in uniform targets when the heater and target geometry are similar. Specifically, the epidermis (a planar target) exposed to a rectangular or square optical pulse at a wavelength strongly absorbed by melanin, produces a continuous rise in temperature during a long pulse, whereas a spherical target, such as the hair bulb matrix and a cylindrical shape target such as a vessel, stabilise to a steady-state temperature during long pulse exposure. Beam pulse shape may be critical to the different heating rates of targets and ideally should display a leading edge high power output with decaying amplitude over the pulse duration.

In 2001, Ross [69] questioned the range of longer pulse durations for hair reduction proposed by Altshuler et al. [68] and discussed the concept of *Tissue Damage Time (TDT),* suggesting it required a more rigorous definition hypothesizing that optimal pulse duration should lie be between the thermal relaxation time (TRT) and the TDT.

Murphy and Torstensson [70] also question the TRT approach of selective photothermolysis arguing that the critical parameter of time required to induce *irreversible protein denaturation* within the target and a complete temporal, transient temperature history of the target tissue volume has to be considered and calculated using the general expression of the Arrhenius. The time to induce irreversible protein denaturation is determined by the tissue's intrinsic structure, not its physical dimensions. Murphy [70] suggests that a constant temperature profile in the absorbing tissue is more important than *cooling time*, particularly for smaller vessel diameters.

Early theories of selective photothermolysis and the extended theory of selective photothermolysis utilised computer modelling, in-vitro, animal and cadaver studies looking mainly at vascular treatments. The laser and light sources available at the time had a limited range of variables compared with those available now, and new device features such as epidermal cooling are known to impact the theory of selective photothermolysis [71].

In clinical practice, the choice of wavelength, pulse duration and fluence for any given presenting condition-skin type combination are often dictated by device default treatment settings or treatment protocols and whilst the theory of selective photothermolysis is well researched, the number of published high-level evidence studies is more limited and consequently there is much still to learn about the choice of treatment parameters in order to achieve selective, safe and efficacious clinical outcomes as is explored in the chapters that follow.

Safety Management of Laser and Light Sources

Lasers, intense light sources (ILS) and LED devices are subject to standards and regulatory controls due to the potential hazard they present to tissues of the eye and skin. Although lasers emit non-ionising radiation and do not induce the tissue changes associated with ionising radiation, injury from medical laser devices can include blindness and significant skin burns. Lasers are classified as *medical devices* and as such are subject to the requirements of the European Medical Device Regulation (MDR) [72] and have the correct Conformité Européenne (CE mark) applied.

The safety management requirements, including appointment of key staff, training provision, methods for controlling hazards, requirements for a Laser Controlled Area (LCA) and safe working practice are described in the MHRA *Guidance* document for laser, light and LED safety [49].

The key *standard* for medical lasers is EN 60601-2-22:2013 'Medical electrical equipment: Particular requirements for basic safety and essential performance of surgical, cosmetic, therapeutic and diagnostic laser equipment' [73] and those responsible for management of a laser clinic/facility should be aware of this document and the MHRA guidance document [49].

Classification of Lasers

Lasers are grouped into 'classes' according to the potential for harm from the laser beam (Table 1.5). Classification of lasers and LEDs is given in IEC 60825–1;2014 [17]. In 2001, the classification system was revised and three new laser classes of

Table 1.5 Laser classification system [17]

Laser class	Laser type	Potential eye or skin hazard
Class 1	Very low power	Class 1 laser products are safe under reasonably foreseeable conditions of operation, including long-term direct intrabeam viewing, even when using optical viewing instruments, e.g., eye loupes or binoculars
Class 1 (embedded)	Laser completely enclosed	Generally eye-safe during use. Hazards arise from the output of the enclosed laser if interlocks are overridden
Class 1 M	Low power. Collimated large beam diameter or divergent	Eye-safe for long-term intrabeam viewing, but potentially hazardous with magnifiers (divergent beams) or binoculars (large diameter collimated beams)
Class 1C	Laser products designed explicitly for contact application to the skin or non-ocular tissue. Examples include home use hair reduce devices. The irradiance or radiant exposure levels may exceed the skin maximum permissible exposure (MPE) that is necessary for the intended treatment procedure. During operation ocular hazards are prevented by engineering means, e.g. the device can only emit a beam while contacting the skin or tissue. The accessible emission is stopped or reduced to below the AEL of class 1 when the applicator is removed from the skin or non-ocular tissue. No requirement for eye protection	
Class 2	Low power Visible wavelengths only	Eye-safe for brief (accidental) direct exposure with the naked eye and optical instruments. Prolonged staring into beam may injure the eye, especially blue wavelengths
Class 2 M	Low power visible. Collimated large beam diameter or divergent Visible outputs	Eye-safe for brief exposure with the naked eye, but potentially hazardous when exposure occurs with magnifiers (divergent beams) or binoculars (large diameter collimated beams)
Class 3R (visible radiation)	Low power Typically alignment lasers	Accidental exposure usually not hazardous, but eye injury possible for intentional intrabeam viewing
Class 3R (invisible radiation)	Low power	Accidental exposure usually not hazardous, but eye injury possible for intentional intrabeam viewing
Class 3B	Medium power	Exposure (including brief accidental exposure) of the eye to the direct beam may cause serious eye injuries. Very limited skin hazard. Diffuse reflection viewing is normally eye safe
Class 4	High power	Exposure (including brief accidental exposure) of the eye to the direct beam and close viewing of diffuse reflections may lead to serious eye injuries. May cause serious skin hazard. Presents a fire hazard

Note: Use of the term 'eye-safe' in this context applies to wavelengths from 180 nm to 1 mm, not just the retinal hazard range of 400–1400 nm. Outside the retinal hazard range there is the potential hazard to the cornea and therefore wavelengths outside the retinal hazard range are not automatically eye-safe

1 M, 2 M and 3R were introduced with the abolition of Class 3A. The 2001 revised standard also included a letter appended to particular laser classifications as follows:

- 'M' as in Class 1 M and Class 2 M, derived from magnifying: optical viewing instruments.
- 'R' as in Class 3R derived from *reduced* or *relaxed* requirements. The 'R' relates to certain equipment and user requirements e.g. *manufacturer requirement*; no key switch and interlock connector required; *user requirement*: no eye protection is usually required.

The letter 'B' in Class 3B is historical and the previous classification scheme (Class 1, 2, 3A, 3B and 4) applies to older lasers still in use. Lasers already classified and labelled as Class 3B may not have to be re-classified depending upon the clinic or facility laser safety policy.

The majority of medical laser systems are Class 4 laser and therefore carry an inherent hazard of risk of injury to the eyes and skin, together with a risk to the environment from fire and laser-generated *plume*. Consequently, users of Class 4 devices are expected to have completed manufacturer, procedural and safety training ('Core of Knowledge') as per the MHRA guidance [49].

Practitioners should also be aware that the photopic visual response for human eyes is in the yellow-green region, indicating human eyes are most sensitive to the colour green, at wavelengths between 500 and 550 nm. This explains why a green laser beam appears visually brighter than a red laser beam, even if the green beam is of lower power output than the red beam. Consequently, a visual judgement of whether a beam is safe or not safe is never acceptable.

BSEN 60825–1 [17] applies equally to lasers and LEDs but generally speaking LED devices fall into the lower Classes of 1, 1 M, 2, 2 M, 3R, and very exceptionally Class 3B. This arises from beam geometry and the fact that LEDs are *extended sources,* whereas lasers are *point sources* and have higher power limits for a given laser Class. For example, an LED emitting 10 mW of visible radiation may be Class 2 whereas a laser pointer of the same output power and visible radiation would be Class 3B.

Laser *equipment* of a given class may contain an embedded laser *system* at a higher classification than the class assigned to the product, e.g. a CD player may be a Class 1 product but contain a Class 3B laser system. In these cases safety and engineering controls are required to ensure that access to the beam in excess of the laser system class is not possible. It is the responsibility of the laser/LED manufacturer to implement all appropriate safety and engineering controls as applicable for example, Class 3B and Class 4 lasers must have remote interlocks, a key switch, a beam stop and an emission warning.

Labelling to the British and European standards requires black text and black border against a yellow background [17] with specific wording according to the class of laser and type of label, e.g. laser output Table 1.6.

Intense Light Source Classification Scheme

BSEN 62471:2008 Photobiological safety of lamps and lamp systems, [74] provides *lamp classification* which includes lamps and lamp systems from electrically powered sources of optical radiation, including LEDs and intense light sources. Such devices are not classified in the same way as lasers as the lamp classification scheme indicates only the *potential* risk and depending upon lamp use these potential hazards may or may not become actual hazards. The pulsed lamp criteria apply to a single pulse and any group of pulses within 0.25 seconds. The hazard values are at a distance of 200 mm. The risk group determination of the lamp being tested is detailed in the standard.

In practice, clinicians using intense light sources are encouraged to apply the same level of safety controls for both lasers and intense light sources.

Table 1.6 Example BS EN laser labels

	*Laser Starburst symbol*
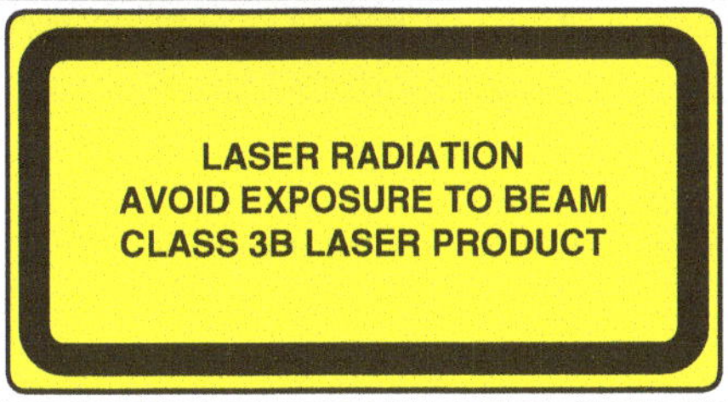	*Label showing requirements for layout and colours. Class 3B device wording*
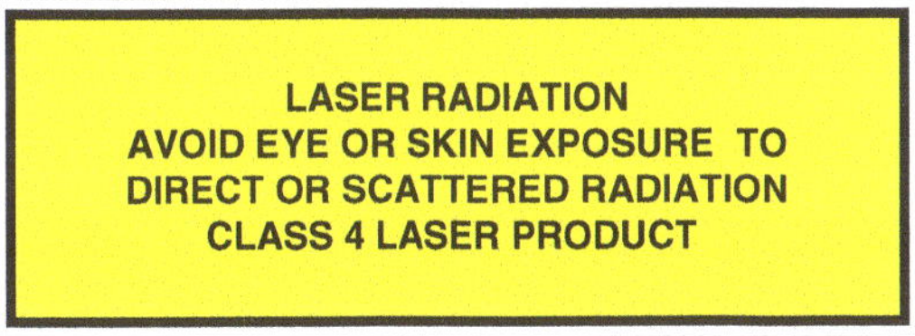	*Label showing requirements for layout and colours. Class 4 device wording*

Optical Radiation Hazards

Laser and intense light source devices are potentially hazardous to clinicians, patients and the environment depending upon classification, wavelength and output power/energy of the system. Hazards include eye injury, skin burns, fire and smoke/plume inhalation.

The mechanism for injury to eye or skin tissues may be photochemical, photothermal, and non-linear effects, broadly described as photomechanical effects which include photodisruption, photoacoustic, photoablation, plasma-induced ablation, depending upon the output characteristics of the device and absorption coefficient of the exposed tissue. A further consideration is the healing properties of the exposed tissue, for example the repair mechanisms of the cornea are different from those of the retina.

Laser and Light Hazards to the Eyes

The principle of selective absorption applies to the laser and light safety insofar as the tissues and structure of the eye display specific absorption spectra (Fig. 1.33).

Laser and Light Hazards to the Skin

In a similar way that tissues of the eye are affected by different wavelengths of incident radiation, so too are the tissues and structures within the skin as illustrated in Fig. 1.34.

Non-beam and Associated Hazards

Table 1.7 lists the common potential hazards from laser and intense light devices and provides example control measures that can easily be applied in the Laser/Light Controlled Area.

Other hazards that arise from the use of laser or intense light sources should be not be overlooked as they often present a greater risk than direct beam hazard which is usually well controlled. For example:

- **Fire Hazard** Class 4 lasers and intense light systems are a potential fire hazard and care should be taken when using around drapes, patient clothing, swabs and gauze. If protective clothing is necessary it must be flame or heat resistant but must not be overly restrictive or uncomfortable as to prevent safe working.

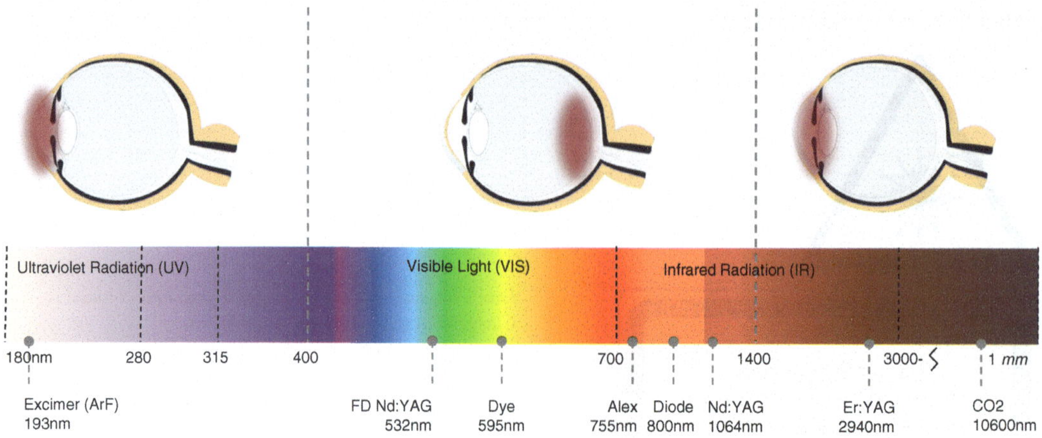

Fig. 1.33 Potential hazard to the tissues of the eye from optical radiation

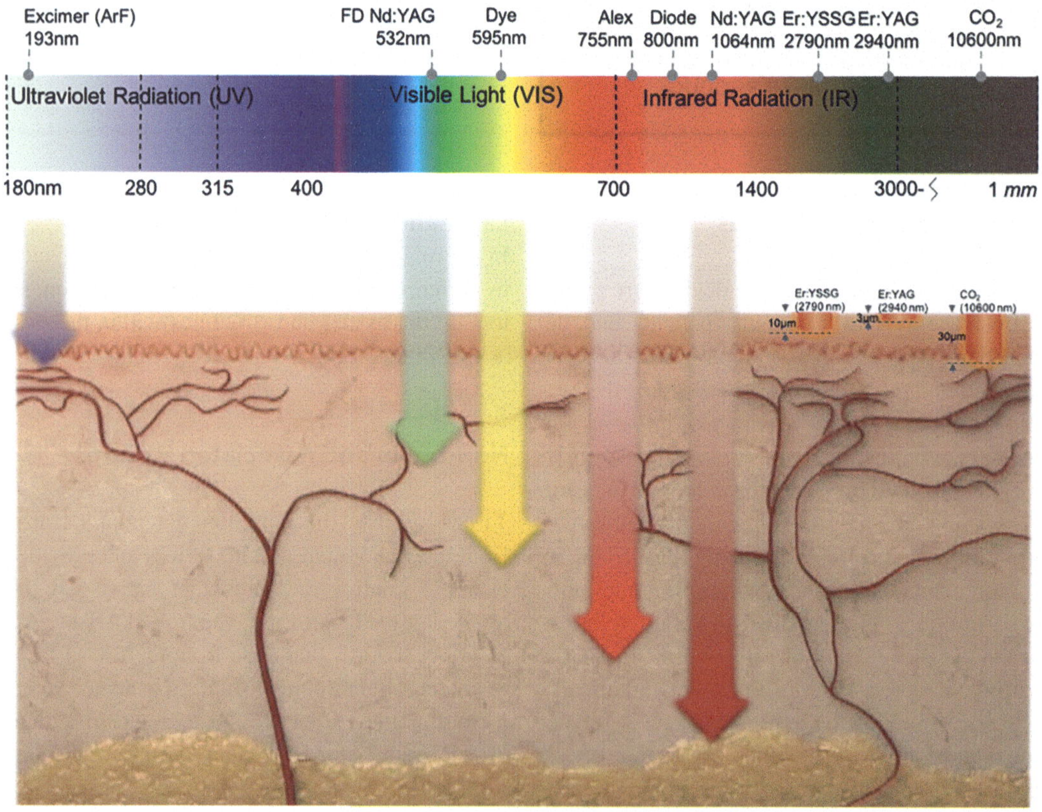

Fig. 1.34 Schematic illustration of the wavelength dependant depth of penetration into human skin. (Not to scale)

Table 1.7 Common potential hazards from laser and intense light devices with example control measure

<table>
<tr><th>Dangers to staff</th><th>Dangers to patients</th></tr>
<tr><td colspan="2">Stray optical radiation—Misdirected beams, unintentionally reflected or emitted from damaged/broken fibres may cause damage to eyes and skin:
• Review the location and orientation of reflective surfaces with respect to laser/ILS/LED beam output
• Inspect optical fibres and protective housings before each use
• Remove patient jewelry or reflective items close to the treatment area
• Ensure correct protective eyewear is available and worn by all staff in the vicinity
• While LED and intense light devices pose a slightly lower risk of eye injury due to being extended sources</td></tr>
<tr><td>Fire hazards—All instruments, tubing or other associated equipment close to the output beams should be fire or laser resistant:
• A small quantity of sterile water close to the working environment may be appropriate</td><td>Accidental exposure to laser/ILS beams can ignite flammable materials such as clothing, hair, hair styling products, couch covers, skin preparation or cleaning materials and surgical drapes:
• A small quantity of sterile water close to the working environment may be appropriate
• Keep all loose hair and clothing away from the treatment area
• Keep alcohol wipes and flammable materials away from the treatment area</td></tr>
<tr><td>Smoke/plume hazards—may pose a health risk to the operating staff:
• Effective extraction at source via plume evacuation systems and use of laser masks is recommended, particularly for ablative treatments</td><td>The smoke/plume may be unpleasant for the patient but has not been reported to pose health risks</td></tr>
<tr><td></td><td>Skin burns—Scratched or damaged output windows, lenses or filters on ILS systems can result in skin injury by causing 'hot spots' or absorption at the skin surface:
• Thoroughly clean all filters, lenses and output windows are before each treatment session
• Remove loose or stray hairs from the skin surface
• Cover pigmented lesions or tattoos (assuming they are not being treated) within the treatment area to avoid skin burns</td></tr>
<tr><td colspan="2">Unexpected adverse events—No more than one laser or ILS device should be switched on during patient treatment</td></tr>
</table>

- **Smoke/Plume Inhalation** Clinicians may suffer from the inhalation effects of smoke and plume caused by tissue ablation. There is some evidence of the possibility of disease transmission through liberated plus from virally infected tissue, particularly with the use of CO_2 lasers [75]. The facility Laser Safety Policy should detail laser hazard control measures such as plume extraction.
- **Electrical hazards** All laser and intense light equipment must be regularly serviced and maintained to ensure electrical safety and compliance.
- **Mechanical hazards** Slip, trip, trap, noise, repetitive strain and work-related musculature disorders are described as mechanical hazards. Good facility design and staff training are essential to reduce mechanical hazards in the clinical environment.
- **Chemical hazards** Cleaning solvents, dye laser solutions, smoke/plume emission can pose chemical hazards. Risk assessment, issue of datasheets and staff training will reduce or control chemical hazards.

Training for Laser and Intense Light Practitioners

There are standards and guidance documents relating to the *use* of laser and light devices, but international or national standards for the *training* of practitioners are less widely available [76]. The MHRA Guidance document [49] contains the 'Core of Knowledge' syllabus (Appendix C) which in the UK remains a fundamental component of laser and light-related education and training in both the private and public sectors.

Laser and Light 'Core of Knowledge' Syllabus

MHRA Guidance [49] stipulates the training requirements and expected 'competencies' of key personnel in a laser or intense light facility. Specifically it identifies three areas that training should address;

1. Equipment-based training, typically provided by the device supplier/manufacturer.
2. Safety training, defined as the 'Core of Knowledge'.
3. Procedural training provided either by the device supplier or clinical experts.

The 'Core of Knowledge' [49] is regarded as the minimum level of safety-orientated training for all laser and light practitioners. The syllabus lists 20 topics including risk assessment, characteristics of optical radiation, hazards and safety controls, and the document states that course lectures should generally total between 2 and 3 hours depending on the course and content depth. The MHRA guidance suggests that to achieve the minimum competency level and as part of safety training, staff should attend an initial and subsequent refresher 'Core of Knowledge' courses. It is good practice for staff to periodically re-attend a core of knowledge course (e.g. at least every 5 years) to maintain their awareness levels.

The 'Core of Knowledge' course should be delivered by persons who have a high level of knowledge and understanding of different optical radiation devices systems, optical radiation safety and the hazards associated with the equipment. (i.e., a certified Laser Protection Adviser (LPA).

Summary

This chapter has introduced the range of lasers, intense light sources (ILS) and LED devices that may be found in clinical practice. The indications for use and specific case studies will be found in the following chapters.

References

1. Einstein E. Zur Quantentheorie der Strahlung (on the quantum theory of radiation). Phys Z. 1917;18:121–8.
2. Hecht J. Beam: the race to make the laser. Oxford: Oxford University Press; 2005. p. 7.
3. Maiman T. Stimulated optical radiation in ruby. Nature. 1960;187(4736):493–4.
4. Nobelprize.org. Nobel Media AB 2014. The Nobel Prize in Physics 1918. http://www.nobelprize.org/nobel_prizes/physics/laureates/1918. Accessed 18 Feb 2018.
5. Einstein A. Concerning an heuristic point of view toward the emission and transformation of light. Ann Phys. 1905;17:132–48.
6. Edison Tech Centre. 2016. http://www.edisontechcenter.org/GordonGould.html. Accessed 10 Jan 2018.
7. Schawlow AL, Townes CH. Infrared and optical masers. Phys Rev. 1958;112:1829.
8. Javan A. Possibility of production of negative temperature in gas discharges. Phys Rev Lett. 1959;3:87.
9. Alferov Z, Kazarinov RF. Semiconductor laser with electric pumping. Inventor's Certificate No. 181737 [in Russian]. Application No. 950840, priority as of March 30, 1963.
10. Kroemer H. A proposed class of heterojunction injection lasers. Proc IEEE. 1963;51(12):1782.
11. Bridges WB. Laser oscillation in singly ionized argon in the visible spectrum. Appl Phys Lett. 1964;4:128–30. Erratum Appl. Phys. Lett 1964;5:39
12. Patel KN. Continuous-wave laser action on vibrational-rotational transitions of CO_2. Phys Rev. 1964;136(5A):1187–93. https://doi.org/10.1103/PhysRev.136.A1187.
13. Geusic JE, Marcos HM, Van Uitert LG. Laser oscillations in Nd-doped yttrium aluminum, yttrium gallium and gadolinium garnets. Appl PhysLetters. 1964;4(10):182.
14. Sorokin PP, Lankard JR, Moruzzi VL, Hammond EC. Flashlamp-pumped organic-dye lasers. J Chem Phys. 1968;48:4726. https://doi.org/10.1063/1.1668055.
15. Basov NG, Danilychev VA, Popov Y. Zh Eksp Fiz i Tekh. Pis'ma Red. 1970;12:473.
16. Anderson RR, Parish JA. Selective photothermolysis: precise microsurgery by selective absorption of pulsed radiation. Science. 1983;220:524–7.
17. International Electrotechnical Commission. IEC60825–1:2014. Safety of laser products: Part 1: Equipment classification, requirements and user's guide.
18. Allen CW. Astrophysical quantities. 3rd ed. London: The Athlone Press; 1973.
19. Nauenberg M. Max Planck and the birth of the quantum hypothesis. Am J Phy. 2016;84:709. https://doi.org/10.1119/1.4955146.
20. Ottaviani J. Suspended in language: Niels Bohr's life, discoveries, and the century he shaped. 2nd ed. Ann Arbor, MI: G.T. Labs; 2009.

21. Hess RA. Blast from the past. Highlights of a vintage laser collection; 2010. https://www.photonics.com. Accessed 10 Jan 2018.
22. Sennaroglu A. Photonics and laser engineering: principles, devices, and applications. 1st ed. New York: McGraw-Hill Education; 2010.
23. Paschott R. Beam quality deterioration of lasers caused by intracavity beam distortions. Opt Express. 2006;14(13):6069–74.
24. Foz A, Tingye L. Resonant modes in a maser interferometer. Bell Syst Tech J. 1961;40(2):453–88. https://doi.org/10.1002/j.1538-7305.1961.tb01625.x.
25. Lister TS, Brewin MP. Variations in laser energy outputs over a series of simulated treatments. Derm Surg Lasers. 2014;171(4):806–12. https://doi.org/10.1111/bjd.13228.
26. Wei C, Menyuk CR, Hu J. Geometry of chalcogenide negative curvature fibers for CO_2 laser transmission. Preprints. 2018;6:74. https://doi.org/10.20944/preprints201807.0263.v1.
27. Royo J, Moreno-Moraga J, Trelles M. Clinical assessment of a new 755 nm diode laser for hair removal: efficacy, safety and practicality in 56 patients. Lasers Surg Med. 2016;49:355–60. https://doi.org/10.1002/lsm.22618.
28. Trost David. U.S. Patent 5743902A; 1995.
29. Berlin A, Hussain M, Phelps R, Goldberg A A prospective study of fractional scanned nonsequential carbon dioxide laser resurfacing: a clinical and histopathologic evaluation. Dermatol Surg [Serial Online]. 2009;35(2):222–228. Available from: Academic Search Complete, Ipswich, MA.
30. Bernstein L, Kauvar A, Grossman M, Geronemus R. The short- and long-term side effects of carbon dioxide laser resurfacing. Dermatol Surg. 1997;23(7):519–25. Accessed 20 July 2018
31. Manstein D, Herron GS, Sink RK, Tanner H, Anderson RR. Fractional photothermolysis: a new concept for cutaneous remodeling using microscopic patterns of thermal injury. Lasers Surg Med. 2004;34:426–38.
32. Clementoni M, Gilardino P, Muti G, Beretta D, Schianchi R Non-sequential fractional ultrapulsed CO_2 resurfacing of photoaged facial skin: preliminary clinical report. J Cosmet Laser Ther. [Serial Online]. December 2007;9(4):218–225. Available from: Academic Search Complete, Ipswich, MA.
33. Clementoni MT, Lavagno R, Munavalli G. A new multi-modal fractional ablative CO_2 laser for wrinkle reduction and skin resurfacing. J Cosmet Laser Ther. 2012;14(6):244–52. https://doi.org/10.3109/14764172.2012.738918.
34. Bensadoun RJ. Photobiomodulation or low-level laser therapy in the management of cancer therapy-induced mucositis, dermatitis and lymphedema. Curr Opin Oncol. 2018;30(4):226–32. https://doi.org/10.1097/CCO.0000000000000452.
35. Poiani G d CR, Zaninotto AL, AMC C, Zangaro R, ASI S, Parreira RB, Paiva WS. Photobiomodulation using low-level laser therapy (LLLT) for patients with chronic traumatic brain injury: a randomized controlled trial study protocol. Trials. 2018:19–7. https://doi.org/10.1186/s13063-017-2414-5.
36. Mühlbauer W, Nath G, Kreitmair A. Treatment of capillary hemangiomas and nevi flammei with light (in German). Langenbecks Arch Chir. 1976;(Suppl):91–4.
37. Colver G. The infrared coagulator in dermatology. Dermatol Clin. 1989;7(1):155–67.
38. Goldman MP, Fitzpatrick RE. Pulsed-dye laser treatment of leg telangiectasia: with and without simultaneous sclerotherapy. J Dermatol Surg Oncol. 1990;16:338–44.
39. Goldman M. Foreword II. In: Fodor L, Ullmann Y, Elman M, editors. Aesthetic applications of intense pulsed light. 1st ed. Berlin: Springer; 2011.
40. Goldman M, Weiss RA, Weiss MA. Intense pulsed light as a non-ablative approach to photoaging. Dermatol Surg. 2005;31:1179–87.
41. Weiss RA, Weiss MA, Marwaha S, Harrington AC. Hair removal with a non-coherent filtered flashlamp intense pulsed light source. Lasers Surg Med. 1999;24:128–32.
42. Clement M, Daniel G, Trelles M. Optimising the design of a broad-band light source for the treatment of skin. J Cosmet Laser Ther. 2005;7:177–89.
43. Ash C, Town G, Clement M. Confirmation of spectral jitter: a measured shift in the spectral distribution of intense pulsed light systems using a time-resolved spectrometer during exposure and increased fluence. J Med Eng Tech. 2010;34(2):97–107.
44. Ash C, Town G, Bjerring P. Relevance of the structure of time-resolved spectral output to light-tissue interaction using intense pulsed light (IPL). Laser Surg Med. 2008;40:83–92. https://doi.org/10.1002/lsm.20596.
45. Town G, Ash C, Eadie E, Moseley H. Measuring key parameters of intense pulsed light (IPL) devices. J Cosmet Laser Ther. 2007;9(3):148–60.
46. Emerson R, Ash C, Town G, Donne K, Omi T, Daniel G. Pigmentation: selective photothermolysis or non-specific skin necrosis using different intense pulsed light systems? J Cosmet Laser Ther. 2013;15:133–42.
47. Moy WJ, Yakel JD, Osorio OC, Salvador J, Hayakaw C, Kelly KM, Choi B. Targeted narrowband intense pulsed light on cutaneous vasculature. Lasers Surg Med. 2015;47:8,651–7. https://doi.org/10.1002/lsm.22393.
48. Varughese N, Keller L, Goldberg D. Split-face comparison between single-band and dual-band pulsed light technology for treatment of photodamage. J Cosmet Laser Ther. 2016;18(4):213–6. https://doi.org/10.1080/14764172.2016.1177188.
49. Medicines and Healthcare products Regulatory Agency. Lasers, intense light source systems and LEDs – guidance for safe use in medical, surgical, dental and aesthetic practices. London: MHRA; 2015.
50. Smith G. The early laser years at Hughes aircraft company. IEEE J Quantum Electron. 1984;20(6):577–84.
51. Paschotta R. Field guide to laser pulse generation. Bellingham: SPIE Press; 2008.

52. Cynosure Inc. Picosecond laser apparatus and methods for treating dermal tissues with same. U.S. Patent Application No. 61/625,961 filed Apr. 18, 2012 and Picosecond laser apparatus and methods for treating target tissues with same filed Mar 15, 2013.
53. Brauer JA, Reddy KK, Anolik R, Weiss ET, Karen JK, Hale EK, et al. Successful and rapid treatment of blue and green tattoo pigment with a novel picosecond laser. Arch Dermatol. 2012;148(7):820–3. https://doi.org/10.1001/archdermatol.2012.901.
54. Young A. Chromophores in human skin. Phys Med Bio. 1997;42(5):789–802, https://doi.org/10.1088/0031-9155/42/5/004. https://www.researchgate.net/publication/14047002_Chromophores_in_human_skin. Accessed 20 May 2018.
55. Jacques S. Optical properties of biological tissues: a review. Phys Med Biol. 1997;58:R37. http://iopscience.iop.org/0031-9155/58/11/R37
56. Randall V, Lanigan S, Hamzavi I, Chamberlain J. New dimensions in hirsutism. Lasers Med Sci. 2006;21(3):126–33. https://doi.org/10.1007/s10103-006-0387-9.
57. Niemz MH. Laser-tissue interactions: fundamentals and applications. 3rd ed. Berlin: Springer; 2003.
58. Ash C, Dubec M, Donne K, Bashford T. Effect of wavelength and beam width on penetration in light-tissue interaction using computational methods. Lasers Med Sci. 2017;32(8):1909–18. https://doi.org/10.1007/s10103-017-2317-4.
59. Klavuhn K. Illumination geometry: the importance of laser beam spatial characteristics. Laser Hair Removal Technical Note No. 2: Lumenis; 2000. http://www.dermathoslaser.com.br.
60. Hale GM, Querry MR. Optical constants of water in the 200 nm to 200 μm wavelength region. Appl Opt. 1973;12:555–63.
61. Pohl RW. Optik und Atomphysik. Berlin: Springer; 1976. Cited by Niemz MH (58)
62. Zhao Z, Fairchild P. Dependence of light transmission through human skin on incident beam diameter at different wavelengths. SPIE Proc Laser-Tissue Interaction IX. 1998;3254:354–60.
63. Cheong WF, Prahl SA, Welch AJ. A review of the optical properties of biological tissues. IEEE J Quant El. 1990;26:2166–85.
64. Boulnois JL. Photophysical processes in recent medical laser developments: a review. Laser Med Sci. 1986;1:47. https://doi.org/10.1007/BF02030737.
65. Moritz AR, Henriques FC. Studies of thermal injury: II. The relative importance of time and surface temperature in the causation of cutaneous burns. Am. J Pathology. 1947;23(5):695–720.
66. Habbema L, Verhagen R, Liu Y, Varghese B. Minimally invasive non-thermal laser technology using laser-induced optical breakdown for skin rejuvenation. J Biophotonics. 2012;5(2):194–9.
67. Hayes JR, Wolbarsht ML. Thermal model for retinal damage induced by pulsed lasers. Aerosp Med. 1968;39(5):474–80.
68. Altshuler GB, Anderson RR, Manstein D, Zenzie HH, Smirnov MZ. Extended theory of selective photothermolysis. Lasers Surg Med. 2001;29: 416–32.
69. Ross EV. Extended theory of selective photothermolysis: a new recipe for hair cooking? Lasers Surg Med. 2011;29:413–5. https://doi.org/10.1002/lsm.1135.
70. Murphy MJ, Torstensson PA. Thermal relaxation times: an outdated concept in photothermal treatments. Lasers Med Sci. 2014;29:973. https://doi.org/10.1007/s10103-013-1445-8.
71. Seo MJ, Lee JH, Park SR, Park SY, Kim SM. Effects of the various cooling conditions on 1,064-nm Nd:YAG laser treatment for selective photothermolysis. Exp Heat Transfer. 2014;27(5):488–500. https://doi.org/10.1080/08916152.2013.803177.
72. Regulation (EU) 2017/745 of the European Parliament. Medical Device Regulation (MDR). https://www.gov.uk/guidance/medical-devices-eu-regulations-for-mdr-and-ivdr.
73. British Standards Institution. BS EN 60601–2022:2013. Medical electrical equipment. Particular requirements for basic safety and essential performance of surgical, cosmetic, therapeutic and diagnostic laser equipment. London: BSI; 2013.
74. British Standards Institution. BS EN 62471:2008 Photobiological safety of lamps and lamp systems. London: BSI; 2008.
75. Garden JM, O'Banion MK, Bakus AD, Olson C. Viral disease transmitted by laser-generated plume (aerosol). Arch Dermatol. 2002;138(10):1303–7. https://doi.org/10.1001/archderm.138.10.1303.
76. Raymond Brown E, Town G. Laser and light intervention standards; 2017. https://aestheticsjournal.com/cpd/module/laser-and-light-intervention-standards.

Lasers for Vascular Indications

2

Giulia Rinaldi, Samira Batul Syed, and Vishal Madan

Introduction

In the last three decades there have been major advances in the use of lasers for cutaneous vascular anomalies.

This chapter will focus on the practical experience, standardized practice, practical applications and the suitability of lasers for different cutaneous vascular indications.

Lasers emit powerful beams Chap. 1 of light that can be directed to target certain tissues or vessels on the surface of the skin. The light from laser is monochromatic and collimated, meaning it is directed to travel in a precise straight line [1]. Lasers can be used for desired medical purposes in various clinical specialties through their photothermal, photoablative, photodisruptive and photochemical properties.

Lasers are highly variable and can differ by wavelength, pulse width, fluence, spot size and cooling methods. Cutaneous lasers are most often categorized by their wavelength as this varies their absorption by different tissues and the depth with which a laser can penetrate the skin. Lasers with shorter wavelengths, for example pulse dye laser (PDL) with a wavelength of 585 nm, is well absorbed by blood and pigment and is not able to penetrate deeply into the skin. On the other hand, lasers with longer wavelengths, for example Nd:YAG with a wavelength of 1064 nm, is poorly absorbed by blood and pigment, therefore, is able to penetrate deeper into tissues [2]. The main chromophore targeted during the treatment of vascular lesions is blood and these vessels are often located at or deep to the dermo-epidermal junction. Therefore, darker skin with larger amounts of melanin absorbing the laser, often requires longer wave lengths to target deep sited vessels.

Altering pulse duration alters the absorption mechanism of the laser onto the tissue. Lengthening the pulse duration decreases the intensity of the laser shot and allows for a gentler approach to laser treatment. A balance is always required between maximizing epidermal absorption in order to allow laser to penetrate the skin and reach our desired target and avoiding excessive epidermal absorption by melanin which can cause photothermal damage leading to blisters, scars or pigmentary changes. Increased melanin allows for greater epidermal absorption of laser energy, therefore, longer pulse durations and

G. Rinaldi
Guys & St. Thomas' Hospital NHS Trust, London, UK
e-mail: giulia.rinaldi@nhs.net

S. B. Syed (✉)
Pediatric Dermatology, Great Ormond Street Hospital, London, UK
e-mail: SamiraBatul.Syed@gosh.nhs.uk

V. Madan
Consultant Dermatologist, Laser and Mohs Surgeon, Salford Royal NHS Foundation Trust, Stott Lane, Salford, UK
e-mail: vishal.madan@srft.nhs.uk

V. Madan (ed.), *Practical Introduction to Laser Dermatology*,
https://doi.org/10.1007/978-3-030-46451-6_2

wavelengths are often used for darker skin types as it reduces adverse effects to the skin.

The fluence is the energy in joules (j) delivered per unit area in centimetres (cm) which is measured as j/cm^2 on laser devices [3]. Optimal fluence, one that gives the desired clinical response, varies for every patient and must be established using assessment shots. The power density of a laser can also be varied by changing the spot size used. Using a smaller spot with the same fluence will concentrate the photon over a smaller surface area creating a greater clinical effect. However, the smaller spot will not penetrate as deeply into the skin tissue due to a rapid scatter of photons causing a more powerful, albeit, superficial treatment.

Cooling methods are of upmost importance to minimize epidermal damage when using lasers. Integrated cooling methods can be categorized into contact and non-contact technologies such as air cooling, cryotherapy spray or contact with ice water [4]. Different vascular lasers and their advantages and disadvantages are summarized in Table 2.1.

Table 2.1 Vascular laser/light based de characteristics [5–7]

Laser settings	Characteristics	Advantages	Disadvantages
Argon			
Wavelength: 488–514 nm Pulse duration: 20–100 millisecond Fluence: 0–240 j/cm^2 Spot size: 0.1–1 mm	An argon quasi continuous wave laser emitting blue-green light	• Very successful in treating telangiectases • Good for small treatment areas	• Not safe in darker skin types • Penetrates only superficially • Small spot sizes • Limited scope of conditions that can be treated • No longer used due to high rates of side effects • Bulky machine
KTP (frequency doubled Nd:YAG)			
Wavelength: 532 nm Pulse duration: 1–150 ms Fluence: 0–240 j/cm^2 Spot size: 3–5 mm	A quasi continuous laser that uses Nd:YAG crystal and a potassium titanyl phosphate (KTP) crystal	• Long pulse duration • Small laser machine that is more portable • Small spot sizes available	• Superficial penetration which is not as effective as the other lasers • Small spot sizes only • Scarring risk
PDL (585 nm–595 nm)			
Wavelength: 585–600 nm Pulse duration: 0.45–40 ms Fluence: 0–40 j/cm^2 Spot size: 3–15 mm	Rhodamine dye dissolved into a solvent and emitted via a flash lamp emitting a pulse of yellow light	• Low side-effect profile • Targets specific chromophore (specific oxyhaemoglobin) specifically • Long standing data on safety and effectiveness • User friendly machine • Skin bruising allows you to monitor location of pulses and ensure treatment of target • Variable pulse durations • Different sized spots to allow flexible lesion • Good outcomes in most conditions Integrated cooling cryogen spray	• Machine difficult to maintain and service • Expensive laser machine with high maintenance and service costs • Only penetrates to the depth of 1.2–1.5 mm so only targets superficial lesions

(continued)

Table 2.1 (continued)

Laser settings	Characteristics	Advantages	Disadvantages
Alexandrite (755 nm)			
Wavelength: 755 nm Pulse duration: 3–40 ms Fluence: 0–40 j/cm^2 Spot size: 6–18 mm	Solid state laser using the alexandrite gemstone	• Good for deeper lesions • Less skin bruising • Useful for laser hair removal • Large spot sizes available	• Does not target haemoglobin well • Not safe in darker skin types • Very expensive machine • Needs a warmer environment temperature for ideal efficacy • More painful than lower frequency laser
Nd:YAG			
Wavelength: 1064 nm Pulse duration: 0–300 ms Fluence: 0–900 j/cm^2 Spot size: 3–10 mm	Solid laser with a crystal rod of yttrium-aluminium-garnet doped with neodymium ions	• Safe in darker skin types • Good for deeper lesions • Greater range of pulse widths • Less skin bruising • Can be used for a greater range of conditions including blue lesions, pigmented lesions and hair removal.	• More painful than lower frequency lasers • Higher risk of scarring • Expensive laser machine with high maintenance and service costs • Air flow cooling system
Carbon dioxide			
Wavelength: 10,600 nm Pulse duration: 0.2–50 ms Spot size: 0.1–2 mm	A laser that uses carbon dioxide gas as its medium and	• Can be used to tighten the skin in flabby, stretched from haemangioma remnants. • Good for the complete removal of small lesions	• Very expensive machine • Not studied well in many vascular anomalies • Cannot be used to solely target pigment or haemoglobin cells as non-selective heating of tissue occurs
Intense pulsed light			
500–1200 nm Long pulse durations Wider rectangular foot print	Not a laser. Uses wide spectrum of visible and near infrared wavelengths with cut-off filters.	• Least expensive • Versatile machine as can treat many indications • Effective for diffuse redness such as in rosacea	• Generally less effective than vascular lasers • Use in caution in patients with darker skin

Laser Technique

Ideally, patients with vascular anomalies should be referred as early as possible to allow for timely assessment and formulation of a treatment plan. This is especially true of vascular anomalies in paediatric population as early treatment is likely to improve final outcomes.

A full medical history and detailed examination of the patient and their vascular anomaly is undertaken at the first consultation. A multidisciplinary team approach involving orthopaedics, plastics, ophthalmologists, radiologists or physiotherapists may be required when treating paediatric vascular malformations. If laser is deemed an appropriate intervention, informed and written consent is obtained from the patient or parents. Clinical photographs are very beneficial to monitor progress of treatment. Patient is then invited for an initial test patch with the laser.

Assessment shots are carried out under local anaesthetic using topical Ametop (3% amethocaine gel) or EMLA cream (Eutetic Mixture of Local Anaesthetic using 2.5% lignocaine and 2.5% prilocaine) which is applied 45 min to 1 h before the session [8]. Controversy exists on whether applying topical anaesthetics which vasoconstrict vasculature to the extent that they may affect laser outcomes [9]. However, evidence that has explored this as concluded there is no overall effect on treatment outcomes [10]. Adult patients generally require no anaesthesia prior to vascular laser treatments. The cooling used with the vascular laser provides comfort and obviates the need for any topical anaesthetic in adults.

In paediatric patients, assessment shots are most often performed on a patient's normal forearm skin usually on the same side of the vascular anomaly they are being treated for. The first assessment shot uses a low fluence of 3.0 j/cm^2 and the patient's skin will be assessed for any erythema immediately after. The fluence will be increased by 0.5 j/cm^2 until the laser pulse causes visible erythema. This often takes two or three assessment pulses (Fig. 2.1). Once this fluence is established it is doubled to deliver a number of pulses, usually 3–9, on the site of the vascular anomaly to be treated (Fig. 2.2). The test patch area is cooled with an integrated cryogen spray and further cooled with ice cool gauze. This is to ensure that the treated area is cooled to minimise the risk of blisters, scabs and scars.

	Laser type (wavelength)	Energy (j/cm^2)	PW (ms)	Spot size (mm)	Cooling	Pulses used
Test patch	585 nm	6.25	0.45	7	DCD 30/20	2
		6.50	0.45	7	DCD 30/20	2
		6.75	0.45	7	DCD 30/20	3

The test patch response is assessed in 8–12 weeks. Depending on the patients' age, preferences, extent and site of their lesion it may be preferarable to treat them under general anaesthesia. This is especially true of patients under the age of 5 or those with extensive treatment sites.

When treating adults with vascular lasers, the test shots are delivered directly on the lesion and assessment is carried out in 2–4 weeks. Most laser units have standardised laser protocols for vascular lasers. The initial test patch comprises of 2–3 shots of conservative to standard fluence e.g. for facial erythema, one may use 8.0, 8.25 and 8.5 j/cm^2, 7 mm spot, 1.5 ms pulse width with cooling. Such treatment would be considered purpuagenic and needs to be altered if patient prefers non-purpuric treatments. The highest tolerable fluence resulting in a discernible improvement in the absence of post-laser

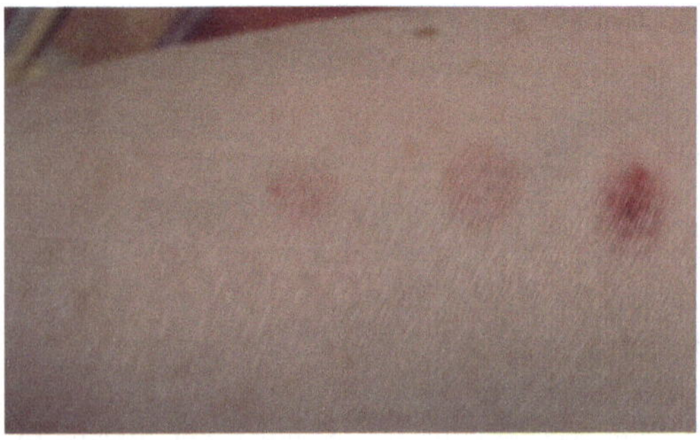

Fig. 2.1 Assessment shots on normal Skin (used with kind permission by Dr. Graham Bisset, BSc, PhD)

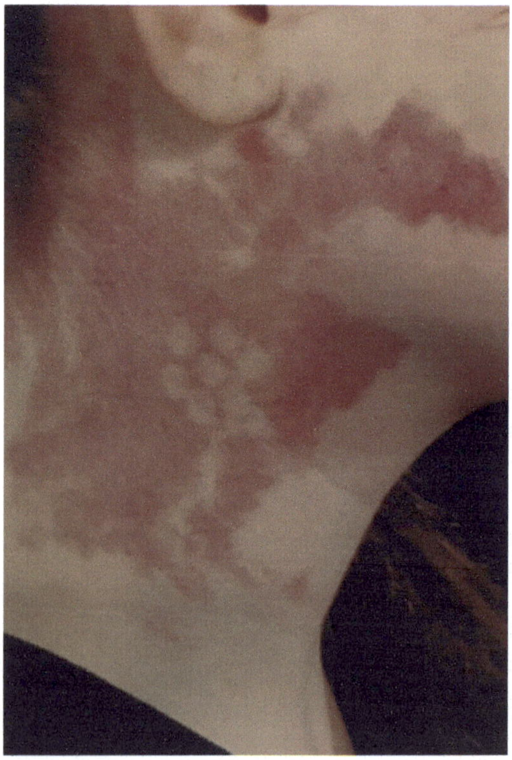

Fig. 2.2 Test patch on a port wine stain

hyperpigmentation or prolonged purpura should be used for the first session.

After care is with bland topical emollients and avoidance of irritants such as soaps, bubble bath or shampoos. Make up is permitted 3–4 days following treatment. Sun avoidance before and after treatment is mandatory and SPF 50 should be recommended.

If any blistering occurs or scabs form, then topical antibiotic ointment such as mupirocin can be prescribed.

Part 1: Lasers for Vascular Indications—Paediatric

Vascular Anomalies and Their Classification

Vascular anomalies sometimes referred to as vascular birthmarks, can be divided into two main subgroups; vascular malformations and vascular tumours (Table 2.2). Vascular malformations can either be categorised as low flow or high flow lesions. The ones with low flow are subdivided into capillary malformations, lymphatic malformations and complex vascular malformations, which include a mix of both capillary and lymphatic components. Those of high flow include arteriovenous malformations and arterial fistulas. The commonest vascular malformations are port wine stains which are present in 0.3% of the general population [11].

Vascular tumours, on the other hand, can be subdivided into benign haemangiomas and aggressive vascular tumours. Benign haemangiomas include infantile haemangiomas, and non-infantile haemangiomas. These are then classified as to their depth in the dermis and their involuting properties. Aggressive vascular tumours are rare and must be promptly treated systemically due to their invasive nature. The commonest vascular tumours are infantile haemangiomas which are present in up to 8.5% of the newborn population [12].

The majority of vascular anomalies present in childhood and can have both visually disfiguring and physically challenging difficulties. The location of the vascular anomaly is one of the main determinants of the physical and emotional disability. Port wine stains are most commonly located on the face, therefore, these often carry an emotional burden to children and their parents, especially during school age, but often throughout life [13]. Similarly, vascular tumours and complex malformations can impact both growth and physical ability of a child. The most common complaints of vascular anomalies include pain and swelling, moreover, careful monitoring for deformity in the body area is paramount [14]. Extensive vascular anomalies often require multidisciplinary care including surgical debulking from plastic surgeons to physiotherapy from specially trained therapists and consideration for laser therapy in a selected group of patients [15].

Table 2.2 Simplified classification of vascular anomalies

Vascular tumours			Vascular malformations	
Benign haemangiomas		Aggressive	High flow	Low flow
Infantile Haemangiomas • IH • HOF • CH Pyogenic granulomas Tufted Haemangioma Angiokeratoma	Congenital • RICH • PICH • NICH • TICH	• Kaposiform haemgiothelioma • Segmental Haemangioma • Angiosarcoma • Other rare ones	• Arteriovenous malformations • Arteriovenous fistulas	• Capillary malformations • Port wine Stains • RVN • VVM • CMTC • Livedo Reticularis • Venous malformations • Lymphatic malformations • Complex Vascular anomalies

Paediatric Vascular Laser Applications

Table 2.3 outlines the vascular anomalies and other conditions that can be treated with vascular lasers.

Rarer skin conditions, like Elastosis Perforans Serpiginosa which is known to be recalcitrant and commonly fails numerous topical therapies have also been successfully treated using laser with excellent outcomes [16].

The table above highlights the multitude of dermatological conditions that can be successfully treated with vascular lasers in children. Ongoing evaluation and reporting of our laser outcomes will continue to identify the most appropriate conditions and demographic of patients for which laser treatment is most beneficial.

Table 2.3 Paediatric vascular laser indications

Vascular anomalies	Other conditions
Port wine stain	Viral warts
Capillary malformation	Hirsutism/Hypertrichosis
Haemangioma	Elastosis Perforans Serpiginosa
Spider nevus/ telangiectasia	Congenital melanocytic Naevus (hairy mole)
Verrucous Vascular malformation	Epidermal Naevus
Venous malformation	Fibroadenoma of TS
Lymphatic malformation	Angiokeratoma
Keratosis Pilaris	Mollusca contagiosa
Pyogenic granuloma	Keloid scars
Phacomatosis Pigmento vascularis	Scars (post trauma, surgical)
Poikiloderma	Café au Lait marks
CMTC/RVN	Cutaneous lymphangioma circumscriptum
Complex Vascular anomaly	Ulerythema ophryogenes
NICH	Elastosis perforans serpiginosa
RICH	
CMTC/RVN	
PICH	
ILVEN	
Glomuvenous malformation	
Angioma Serpiginosum	

Capillary Malformations

Port Wine Stains

Port wine stains (PWS) represent a congenital and progressive ectasia of the vascular plexus in the dermis resulting in the red or purple appearance of one's skin in that location [17]. PWSs are one of the commonest vascular anomalies, with a prevalence of 0.3% in newborns. Almost half of these birthmarks present on the face, which results in a large proportion of these children becoming adults who suffer from negative psychological and behavioural consequences [18]. Treating these patients as children has proven to be the most beneficial in terms of their social and mental wellbeing as 75% of teenagers with port wine stains report that their life would change radically if they did not have one [19].

There are a few predictors of response to treatment with laser therapy (Table 2.4). Firstly, the

Table 2.4 Poor prognostic factors for PWS response to laser therapy [20–24]

Category	Poor prognostic factors
Port wine stain factors on examination	• Central facial V2 area • Distal limb area • Darker colour at presentation • Hypertrophic thickening at presentation
Patient characteristics	• Older age at presentation
Dermoscopy features	• Subpapillary capillaries on dermoscopy, showing deep red linear vessels • A bright red background • Thick vessels
Reflectance confocal microscopy	• Blood vessels with high blood flow, large diameter and located deeper in the skin
Video microscopy	• Deeper vessels in the superficial horizontal plexus presenting as small fine capillary dots

anatomical location of port wine stains is an important predictor of response to laser treatment. Port wine stains in the V3 lateral facial area, neck or trunk are known to respond better to laser treatment compared to those in the V2 central facial area or in the distal limbs [20]. Secondly, the colour appearance of the PWS can aid to predict the success of laser with darker purplish port wine stain known to being more stubborn and resistant to treatment with laser. Thirdly, those with hypertrophic thickening of the port wine stain at presentation also are known to be poor responders to laser therapy [25]. PWS are known to naturally progress with time, especially during pubertal change, with 65% of patients reporting hypertrophy and nodularity by the age of 50 [26]. Therefore, treating patients as children also greatly improves their chances of clearance using laser therapy.

The use of Pulsed Dye Laser (PDL) therapy on facial port wine stains has transformed the clinical outcomes for children with these birthmarks. A large cohort study has shown that treatment with PDL can improve PWS of one fourth of patients by 75% and almost one half of patients by 25–50% [27]. Similarly, the Perfecta VBeam 595 nm laser has also shown similar response rates amongst patients with PWS with an average clinical improvement rate of 70% [28]. At GOSH, 70% children treated with PDL show an overall 70% lightening in colour of their PWS with up to 43% showing a 90% improvement. The clinical outcomes are measured using a Visual Analogue Scale by comparing before and after pictures or by using a SIAscope (Astron Clinica, Cambridge, UK) to objectively measure the amount of haemoglobin present in the dermis of a PWS. The majority of our patients with PWS require 6 treatment sessions to achieve the desired clinical outcome; however, this is highly variable (Fig. 2.3).

	Laser type (wavelength)	Energy (j/cm^2)	PW (ms)	Spot size (mm)	Cooling	Pulses used
Treatment 1	585 nm	6.5 6.75	0.45	10	DCD 30/20	12
Treatment 2	585 nm	7.00	0.45	10	DCD30/20	37
Treatment 3	595 mm	8.5 8.75 9.00 9.25 9.5	0.45	10 10 10 10 10	DCD30/20	1 1 1 1 1

Laser treatment using PDL is well established for PWS, however, for a small number of patients that do not response to PDL laser therapy there are new innovative laser treatments in the pipeline (discussed later).

The practicalities of laser treatments including time interval, fluence, and starting age has been demonstrated to be highly variable amongst U.K. practices [29]. There is also a lack of consensus regarding the ideal time interval between each laser sessions. 84% of U.K paediatric laser practices recommend 8–12 week intervals between laser sessions [29]. However, other centres have demonstrated that short intervals of 2–3 weeks between each PDL session are safe and more clinical effective than longer intervals [30, 31]. Similarly, there is a large variation in the ideal starting age for laser therapy in children. At our hospital we believe that starting at 1–2 years of age is the most appropriate clinical decision when weighing up the benefits of early laser treatment against the risks of multiple general anaesthetics in an infant. Nevertheless, data has demonstrated large variability in practice amongst U.K. centress [32].

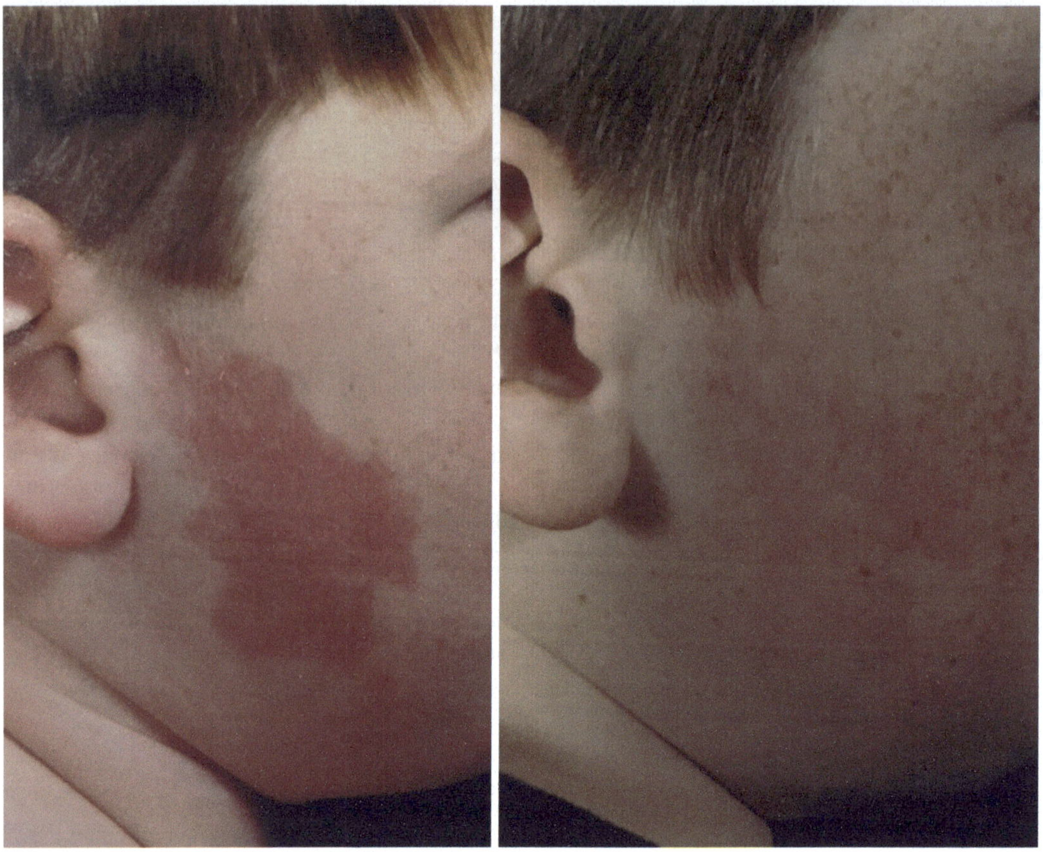

Fig. 2.3 Port wine stain before and after laser treatment

Spider Naevi

Telangiectases are enlarged blood vessels in the superficial layer of the skin and the most common subtype is often called the spider naevus. The spider naevus consists of one small feeding vessel from which smaller spider-like branches extent creating a network. The most common area for which individuals seek treatment is usual spider naevi due to their visibility. Due to the superficiality of these lesions they respond exceptionally well to laser treatment. The average clearance of a spider naevus after one to two laser treatments is around 90% and this rate can be even higher in facial spider naevi [33]. Complete resolution is accomplished for almost all patients after two to three treatments with PDL laser [34]. Laser treatment can be extremely beneficial for patients prone to numerous telangiectases, for example, those with rheumatological conditions, ataxia telangiectasia or hereditary haemorrhagic telangiectasia [35] (Fig. 2.4).

	Laser type (wavelength)	Energy (j/cm^2)	PW (ms)	Spot size (mm)	DCD/Cryo 5	Pulses used
Treatment 1	Perfecta (595)	7.5	0.45	10	30/20	1

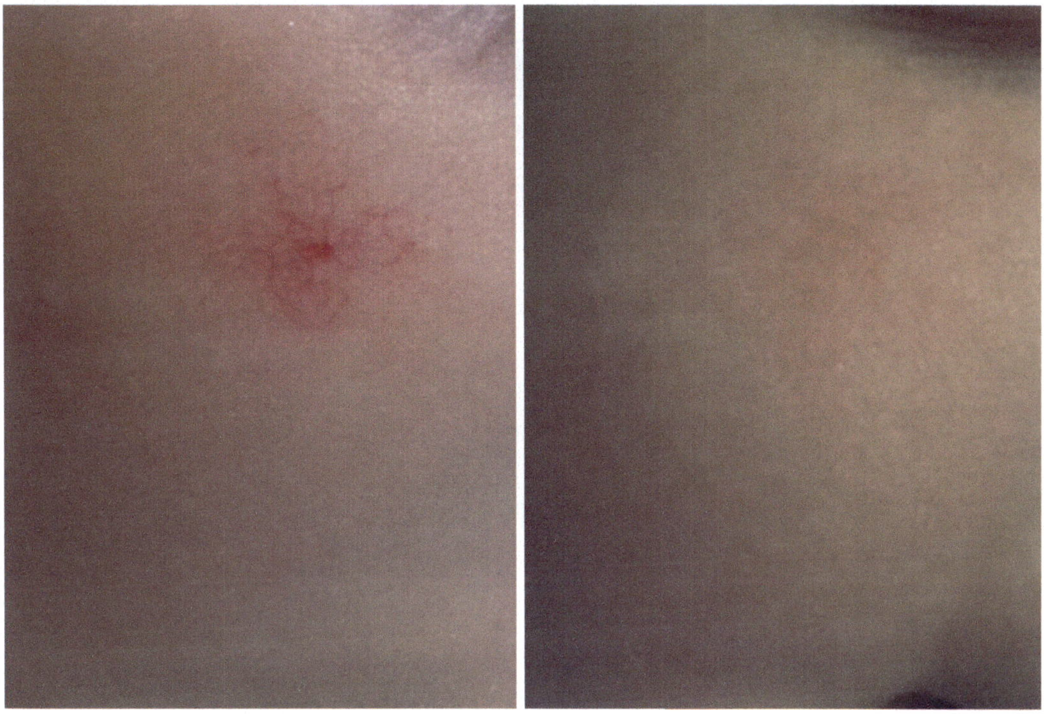

Fig. 2.4 Spider Naevus before and after laser treatment

MAT Telangiectasia

Mat telangiectases are a subset of telangiectasia most often seen in specific genetic disorders and systemic sclerosis. They appear more concentrated and widespread, arranged in a mat-like manner compared to other telangiectases [36]. Of important mention is Capillary Malformation Arteriovenous Malformation syndrome caused by an autosomal dominant mutation to the RASA1 or EPHB4 genes. Some of these lesions feel much warmer compared to the normal skin thus give you a hint to look for other pathology than clinically straight forward telangiectases. These patients present with multiple mat telangiectases as small capillary malformations, however, a number of these will have active doppler flow due to an arteriovenous malformation (AVM) or arterial fistula (AF) [37]. Laser treatment of such lesions is contraindicated as it may activate the AVM (Fig. 2.5).

	Laser type (wavelength)	Energy (j/cm^2)	PW (ms)	Spot size (mm)	Cooling	Pulses used
Treatment 1	585 nm	6.25	0.45	7	DCD 30/20	109
Treatment 2	585 nm	6.25	0.45	7	DCD30/20	59

CMTC/RVN

Cutis Marmorata Telangiectatica Congenita (CMTC) is another rare vascular disease which consists of a congenital, fixed, reticulate rash that may result in atrophy or ulceration over time [38]. Our results show variable responses for these patients and we only offer laser treatment if there are raised papules or visible lipoatrophy. Laser therapy seems to help activate the fat cells to pro-

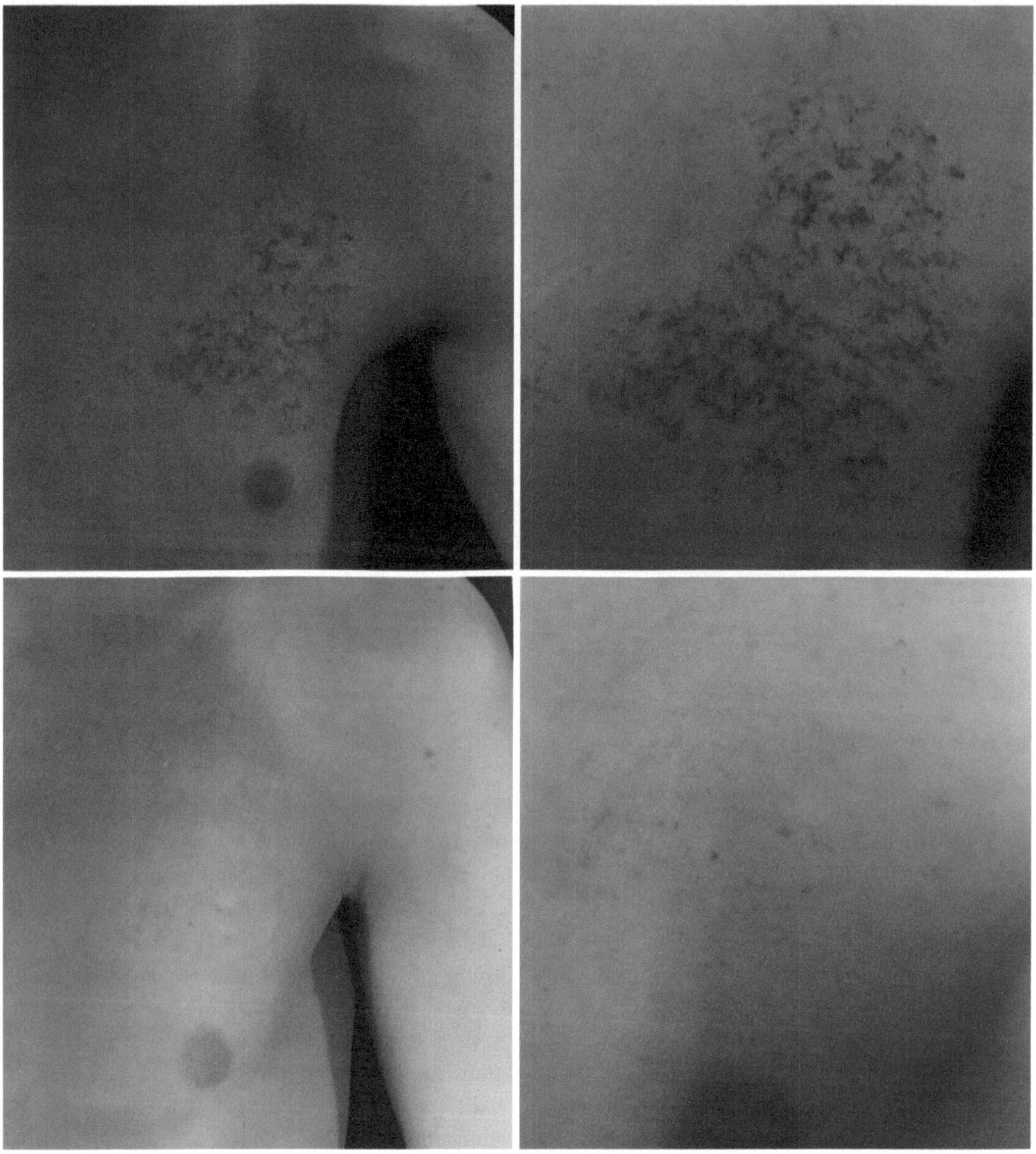

Fig. 2.5 MAT Telangiectasia before and after laser treatment

duce fat around the vessels and improves the lipoatrophic sections of the CMTC.

Reticulate vascular naevi (RVN), sometimes called reticulate capillary malformations, are closely related to PWS, however, RVNs often lighten with time. RVNs show variable responses to lasers (Figs. 2.6 and 2.7).

	Laser type (wavelength)	Energy (j/cm²)	PW (ms)	Spot size (mm)	Cooling	Pulses used
Treatment 1	585	6.50	0.45	7 7 10	DCD 30/20	72 2 18
Treatment 2	595	6.0 7.0 8.0 9.0 10.0	1.5 1.5 1.5 1.5 1.5	10 10 10 10 10	DCD 20/10 DCD 20/10 DCD 20/10 DCD 20/10 DCD 20/10	1 1 1 17 48
Treatment 3	595	11.0 12.0 12.0	3 3 1.5	7 7 7	DCD 30/20 DCD 30/20 DCD 30/20	12 23 107
Treatment 4	Cynergy	PDL 8.0	NDYAG 40	10 Group 3	Cryo 4	70
Treatment 5	Cynergy	PDL 8.5	NDYAG 45	10 Group 3	Cryo 4	104

	Laser type (wavelength)	Energy (j/cm²)	PW (ms)	Spot size (mm)	Cooling	Pulses used
Treatment 1	595	8.0	0.45	10	DCD 30/20	74
Treatment 2	595	9.0	1.5	10	DCD 30/20	139
Treatment 3	595	9.5	1.5	10	DCD 30/20	87
Treatment 4	595	10.0	1.5	10	DCD 30/20	51
Treatment 5	595	11.0	1.5	7	DCD 30/20	43

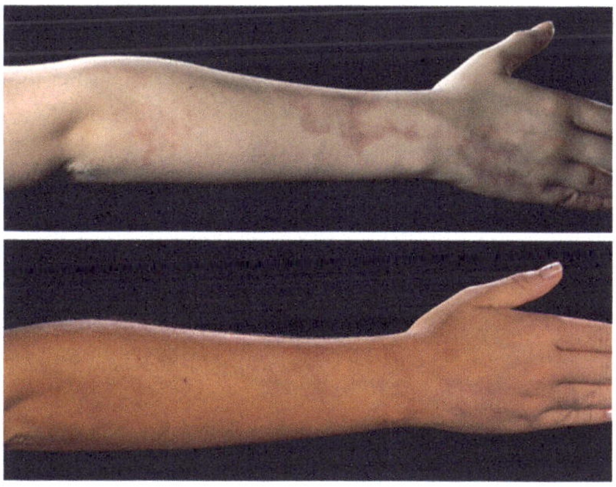

Fig. 2.6 CMTC with good outcome before and after laser

Lymphatic Malformations

Lymphatic malformations are slow flow vascular malformations involving the lymphatic system consisting of vesicles filled with lymphatic fluid. They can be classified as purely lymphatic or as complex with mixed capillary, venous and lymphatic elements. Lymphatic anomalies continue to progress throughout life and necessitate lifelong treatment [39]. As a child grows, an increased number of superficial blood or lymphatic filled vesicles appear on the area of the lymphatic anomaly. Laser treatment can be used to target these "blebs" and significantly

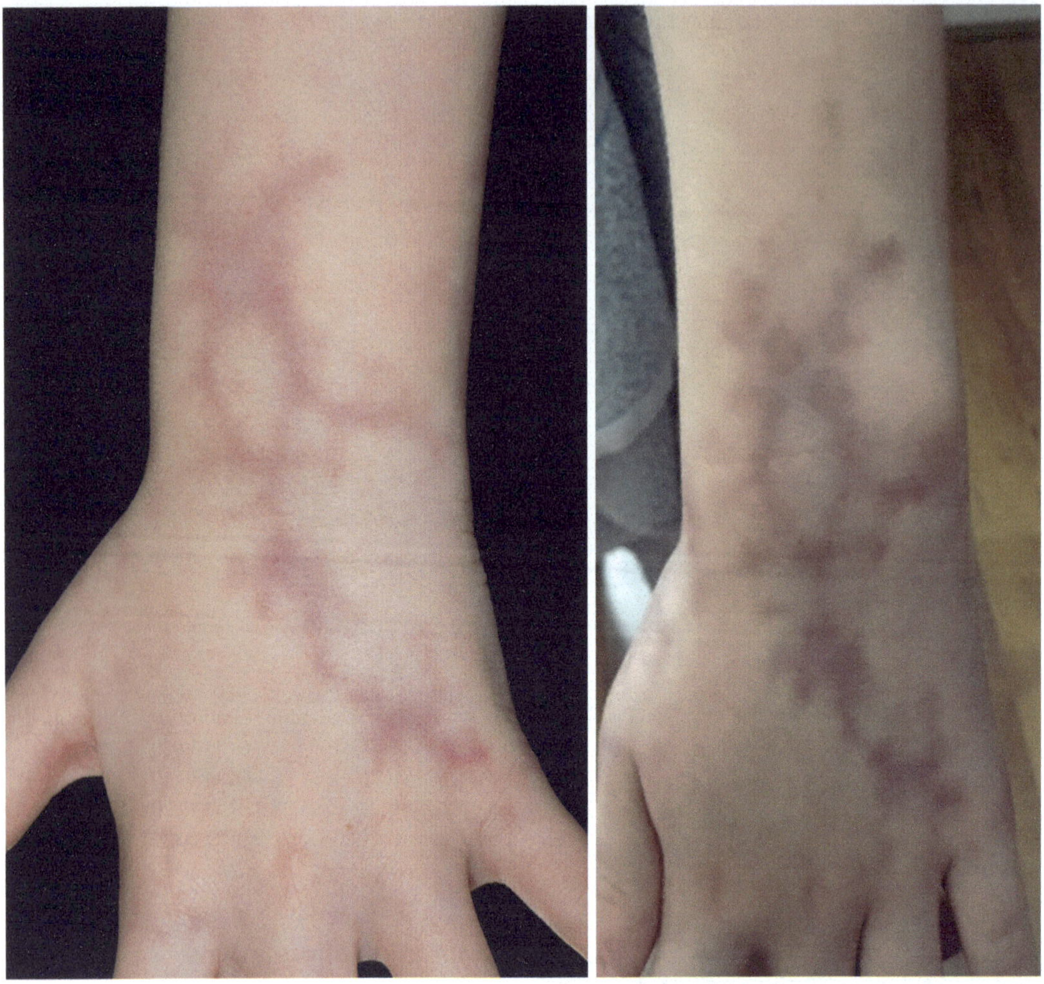

Fig. 2.7 CMTC with poor outcome before and after laser treatment (Note: Pigmentary change was transient but the outcome was a poor response to laser)

reduce the morbidity caused by the pain, leakage and appearance of the vesicles. PDL is the most common laser used to target these complex vascular anomalies as it is highly selective for vascular tissue causing a lower rate of complication from surrounding tissue damage [40]. Multiplex laser consisting of Nd:YAG (1064 nm) and PDL (585 nm) is also another successful laser for the treatment of symptomatic lymphangiomas, lymphangioma circumscriptum and complex vascular anomalies [41] (Figs. 2.8 and 2.9).

	Laser type (wavelength)	Energy (j/cm^2)		PW (ms)	Spot size (mm)	Cooling	Pulses used
Treatment 1	595	8.0		1.5	10	DCD 30/20	5
Treatment 2	595	9.0		1.5	10	DCD 30/20	10
	Cynergy	PDL 9.0	NDYAG 50	Group 3	10	Cryo 4	5

	Laser type (wavelength)	Energy (j/cm²)		PW (ms)	Spot size (mm)	Cooling	Pulses used
Treatment 3	595	10.0		1.5	7	DCD 30/20	10
	Cynergy	PDL 10.0	NDYAG 50	Group 3	10	Cryo 4	2
Treatment 4	595	8.0		1.5	10	DCD 30/20	8
	Cynergy	PDL 9.5	NDYAG 55	Group 3	10	Cryo 4	11
Treatment 5	595	9.0		1.5	10	DCD 30/20	8
	Cynergy	PDL 10.0	NDYAG 60	Group 3	10	Cryo 4	11

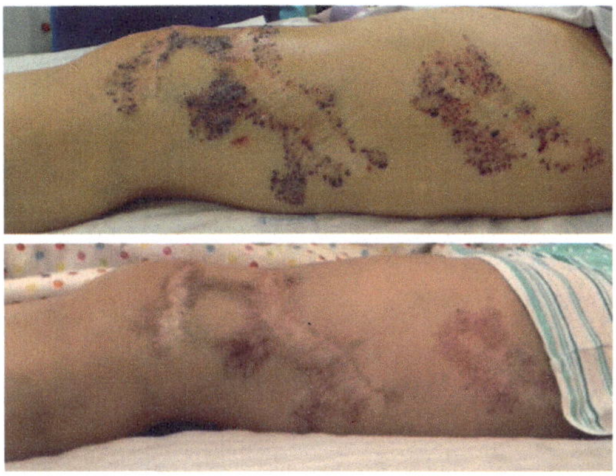

Fig. 2.8 Complex lymphovascular malformation before and after laser treatment

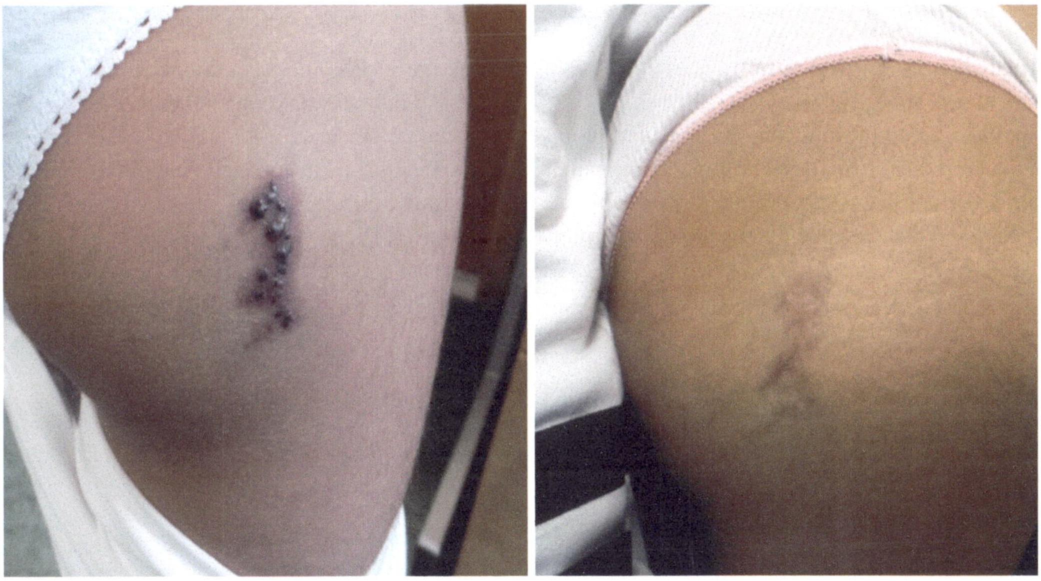

Fig. 2.9 Lymphovascular malformation before and after laser treatment

Verrucous Vascular Malformations

Verrucous vascular malformations (VVMs) present at birth, previously labelled as verrucous haemangiomas, are a superficial venous malformation with a hyperkeratotic appearance that leads to oozing, itching and infection [42]. The mainstay of treatment is surgical resection; however, laser can be helpful for patients whose specific lesions are more suited to medical treatment. Pre-laser treatment is with salicylic acid or urea cream to soften the overlying hyperkeratosis. PDL and Nd:YAG laser can be used together with the to target both superficial and deep components of these malformations. These lesions are often deeply seeded in tissues and require multiple laser sessions [43]. We advise our patients that laser therapy is usually not curative but can significantly improve the appearance of the lesion. A review study of children at GOSH demonstrated a mean of 3.9 laser sessions per patient with an average improvement of over 50% in VVM severity score. As part of our standardized practice for VVM's we also prescribe 10% Urea cream for the patients to apply onto the lesions for 8 weeks between laser treatments to soften the overlying crust (Fig. 2.10).

	Laser type (wavelength)	Energy (j/cm^2)		PW (ms)	Spot size (mm)	Cooling	Pulses used
Treatment 1	595	7.5		0.45	10	DCD 30/20	66
	Cynergy	PDL 9.0	NDYAG 50	Group 3	10	Cryo 4	10
Treatment 2	595	8.0		1.5	10	DCD 30/20	87
	Cynergy	PDL 10.0	NDYAG 50	Group 3	10	Cryo 4	52
Treatment 3	595	9.0		1.5	10	DCD 30/20	65
	Cynergy	PDL 10.0	NDYAG 60	Group 3	10	Cryo 4	71
Treatment 4	595	10.0		1.5	10	DCD 30/20	70
	Cynergy	PDL 10.0	NDYAG 50	Group 3	10	Cryo 4	72
Treatment 5	595	12.0		1.5	7	DCD 30/20	110
	Cynergy	PDL 10.0	NDYAG 60	Group 3	10	Cryo 4	85

Angioma Serpiginosum

Angioma Serpiginosum is a rare vascular anomaly comprising of small red non-blanching punctate lesions in the upper dermis due to capillary dilatation which arrange themselves in a serpiginous pattern. It is most commonly found on the limbs and buttocks of young patients. Laser treatment with PDL usually requires 4 sessions and overall results in a good clinical improvement with around 50% of lesions fully regressing [44, 45] (Fig. 2.11).

	Laser type (wavelength)	Energy (j/cm^2)	PW (ms)	Spot size (mm)	Cooling	Pulses used
Treatment 1	595	9.50	1.5	10	DCD 30/20	51
	PDL SPTL (1b)	7.50	0.45	7	DCD20/20	30
Treatment 2	595	11.0	1.5	7	DCD 30/20	94
Treatment 3	595	7.0	1.5	12	DCD 30/20	18

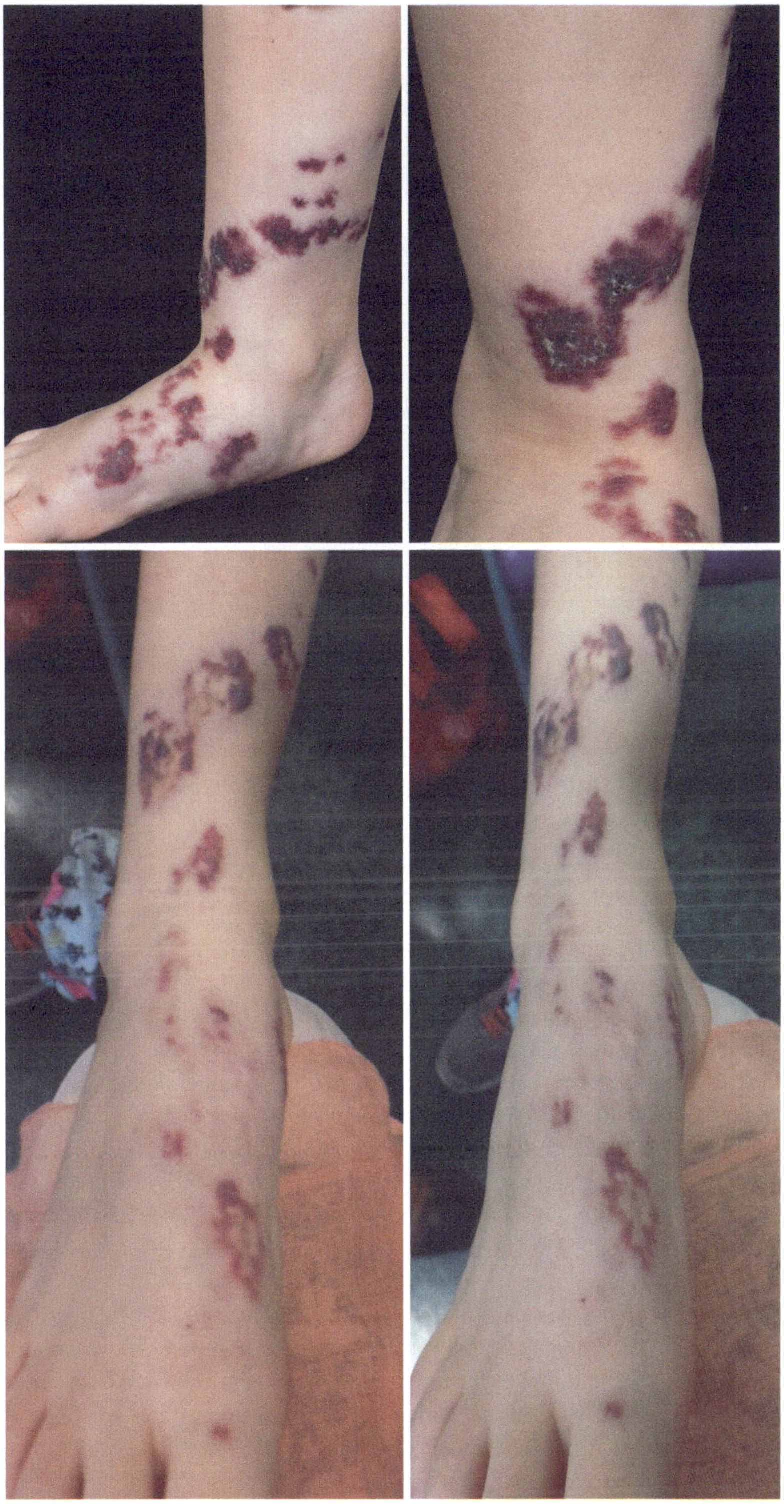

Fig. 2.10 VVM before and after laser treatment

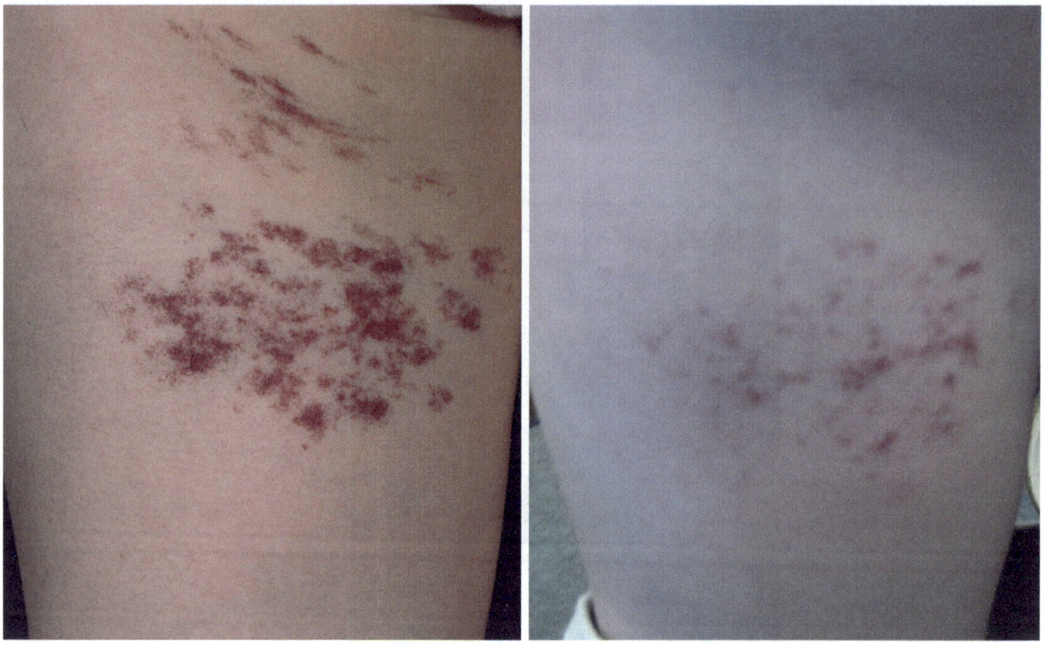

Fig. 2.11 Angioma serpiginosum before and after laser treatment

Vascular Tumours

Haemangiomas

Haemangiomas are the most common vascular tumour found amongst children and are often referred to as capillary haemangiomas, haemangiomas of infancy, infantile haemangiomas or strawberry birth marks. They are present in about 1 in 10 babies, first appear between the ages of 1 and 6 weeks of life and most commonly present on the head and neck [46]. Known risk factors for developing haemangiomas are older maternal age, twin births, pre-term birth and being of Caucasian ethnicity. The most common complications of haemangiomas include ulceration, bleeding and, if located near the orbit, threat to vision [47]. Haemangiomas have three growth phases including the rapidly proliferating phase up to the age of 1 year, the involuting phase between 1 and 5 years of age and, lastly, the involuted phase up to the age of 10 years. At the age of 5 years about 50% of haemangiomas will have fully regressed. However, up to 40% of haemangiomas never fully regress leaving residual skin changes such as telangiectasia, scarring, or epidermal atrophy [48].

The choice of treatment for infantile haemangiomas using laser is dependent on the anatomical location, size and observed natural regression of haemangioma. Most haemangiomas can be conservatively managed, however, pharmacological therapy using beta blockers such as oral propranolol, atenolol or topical timolol is the first line treatment for large haemangiomas or those that are present in compromising locations such as near the eye, airway, vital organs or joints [49]. Beta blockers have shown great outcomes with up to 84% of haemangiomas showing a 50% decrease in size after 6 months of treatment, nevertheless, using beta blockers in children must be weighed against the known side effects of this medication. In some cases, beta blocker therapy is used in combination with PDL treatment for a more rapid and successful response [50].

Laser therapy with PDL selectively photocoagulates blood vessels whilst keeping the overlying epidermis intact. There are two main clinical indicators for laser therapy for haemangiomas. Laser treatment rapidly alleviates pain and stimulates the healing of ulcers. Our outcomes demonstrate that children treated with PDL experienced a relief in their pain within 24 h and that almost all ulceration healed within 4 weeks [51]. Other centres have reported similar data with all patients experiencing pain relief within 48 h and most patients needing only one to three sessions [52, 53]. The second indication for laser treatment is to treat the remnants of haemangiomas, including residual changes like atrophic skin, fibro-fatty tissue or post-resolution telangiectasia [54]. These most often present after the involution of deep haemangiomas. Remnants of haemangiomas are often treated once the child is over 4 years of age. Treatment of remnants of haemangiomas using laser therapy is extremely successful with over half of patients experiencing a complete response to treatment [55] (Fig. 2.12).

	Laser type (wavelength)	Energy (j/cm^2)		PW (ms)		Spot size (mm)	Cooling	Pulses used
Treatment 1	595	8.0		0.45		10	DCD 30/20	12
	595	9.0		0.45		10	DCD 30/20	185
Treatment 2	595	11.0		1.5		7	DCD30/20	12
		12.0		1.5		7	DCD30/20	158
	Cynergy	PDL 9.0	NDYAG 50	Pulse grp 3		10	Cryo 4	8
		10.00	50			10	Cryo 4	33
Treatment 3	595	12		1.5		10	DCD30/20	2
	595	13		1.5		10	DCD30/20	41
	595	14		1.5		10	DCD30/20	14
	595	7		1.5		12	DCD30/20	31
	595	6.75		1.5		12	DCD30/20	63
Treatment 4	Cynergy	PDL 9.0	NDYAG 50	PDL 6.0	NDYAG 15	10	Cryo 4	16

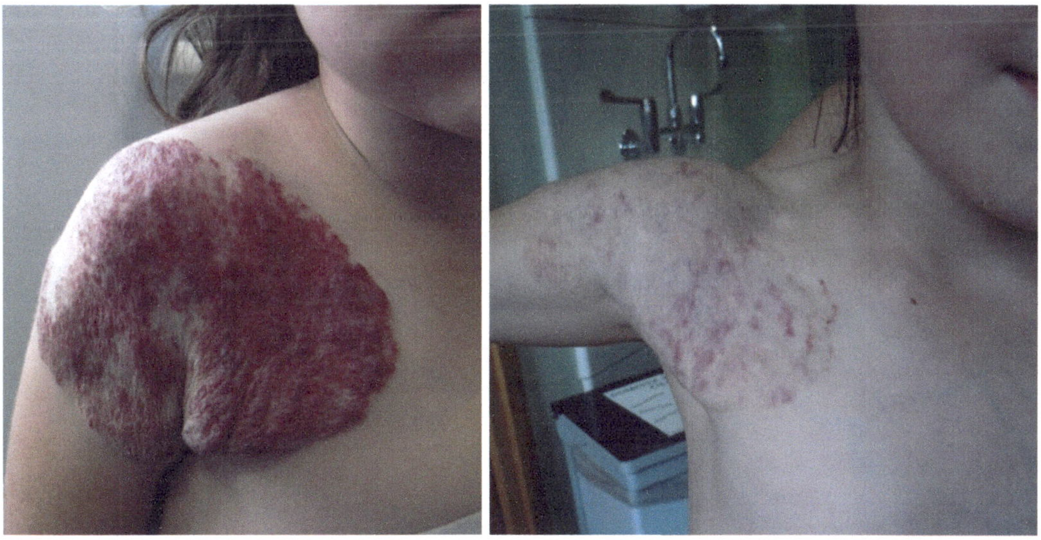

Fig. 2.12 Remnant Haemangioma before and after laser therapy

Pyogenic Granulomas

Pyogenic granulomas (PG) are a common and benign vascular growth which is often categorised as a lobular capillary haemangioma. They can be cosmetically displeasing and can also be prone to bleeding due to very minor trauma. Excisional surgery used to be considered the main treatment method, however, laser therapy is now a less invasive method to successfully treat PGs [56]. These vascular tumours have on overall good response to laser therapy. Using PDL laser therapy on twenty children with PGs the outcomes showed that 25% had complete resolution after one treatment, 40% after two treatments and 30% after three treatments [57]. However, sometimes PGs can recur and grow with time. Therefore, early treatment is recommended, and if they recur, they may need surgical excision (Fig. 2.13).

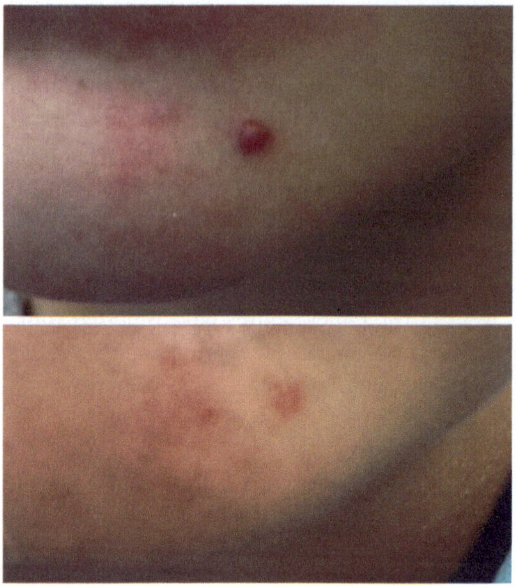

Fig. 2.13 Pyogenic granuloma before and after laser therapy

	Laser type (wavelength)	Energy (j/cm^2)	PW (ms)	Spot size (mm)	Cooling	Pulses used
Treatment 1	595	11.0	0.45	3	DCD 30/20	1

Congenital Haemangiomas

Congenital haemangiomas are vascular tumours presenting at birth at their final size because they grow throughout pregnancy with the growing foetus. There are four subtypes which are categorized by their involuting abilities. These are the non-involuting congenital haemangiomas (NICH), the partially involuting congenital haemangiomas (PICH), newly described tardive involuting congenital haemangiomas (TICH) and the rapidly involuting congenital haemangiomas (RICH) [58]. The latter often have involuted and flatted by 18 months of age, however, they can leave a remnant indentation due to lipoatrophy which can respond to laser therapy by fat cell stimulation. NICH and PICH subtypes do not involute spontaneously and may need either plastic surgery or laser therapy to help with cosmetic outcomes of remnants (Fig. 2.14).

	Laser type (wavelength)	Energy (j/cm^2)	PW (ms)	Spot size (mm)	Cooling	Pulses used
Treatment 1	595	7.25	0.45	7	DCD 30/20	9
Treatment 2	595	7.75	0.45	7	DCD 30/20	15
Treatment 3	595	8.00	0.45	10	DCD 30/20	8
Treatment 4	Cynergy	**PDL** 8.5 8.0 8.0 8	**NDYAG** 50 45 40 45	10 10 10 10	Cryo 4	1 1 1 8
Treatment 5	595	6	0.45	12	DCD 30/20	8-second pass
	Cynergy	**PDL** 8	**NDYAG** 60	10	Cryo 4	4

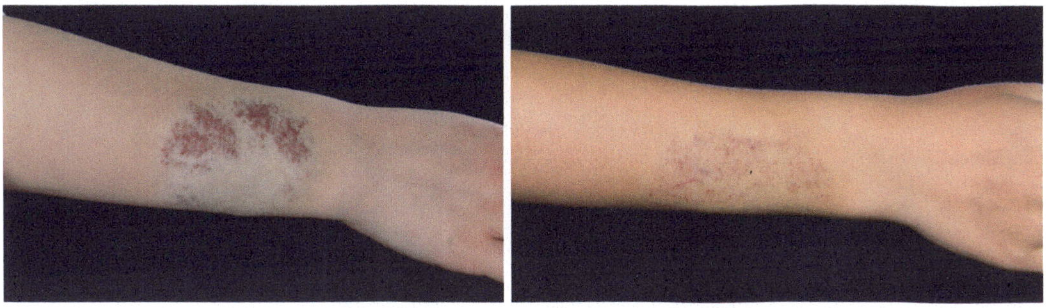

Fig. 2.14 Non involuting congenital haemangioma before and after 5 laser treatments

Tufted Angioma

Tufted angiomas are rare vascular tumours caused by vascular proliferation. They often appear in the first year of life as dark painful plaques most commonly on the trunk area [59]. These lesions can regress with time, but often are recalcitrant and persist into adulthood. Treatment for tufted angiomas includes oral rapamycin (sirolimus) and oral steroids, however, recalcitrant or remnant lesions may need surgical excision or laser treatment. Laser treatment can improve pain and cosmetic appearance of the lesion. The reports on the success of laser treatment in other centres is varied, with some reporting excellent outcomes after a single laser treatment, whilst, others reporting a slight improvement in pain, but with limited visual improvement [60] (Fig. 2.15).

	Laser type (wavelength)	Energy (j/cm^2)		PW (ms)	Spot size (mm)	Cooling	Pulses used
Treatment 1	595	7.5		0.45	10	DCD 30/20 DCD 30/20	243
Treatment 2	595	8.0		0.45	10	DCD30/20	261
Treatment 3	595	9.0 14.0		1.5 3	7 10	DCD 30/20 DCD 30/20	164 649
Treatment 4	Cynergy	PDL 8.0 9.0	NDYAG 40 50	Pulse group 3	10	Cryo 4	113 257

Recalcitrant Lesions

Most vascular lesions can have very good cosmetic outcomes with 4–6 treatment sessions using solely vascular lasers. Nevertheless, a small number of lesions are recalcitrant and require higher numbers of treatment sessions or combination therapy. Recalcitrant lesions include certain PWSs and CMTCs.

CMTCs often take a benign course with up to 50% of patients experiencing resolution of lesions by 2 years of age, however, those with persistent lesions can often experience atrophic skin changes [61]. In our experience, the response to lasers in these patients is highly variable and unfortunately, due to the rarity of this condition, strong evidence reporting laser outcomes is lacking.

On the other hand, PWS are one of the commonest vascular anomalies. It is reported that around 70% of them respond well to laser treatment, however, a minority are stubborn and do not respond well to the initial laser sessions [62]. Recalcitrant PWS can respond to innovative treatment methods. One new laser method called "triple pass therapy" involves a 'first pass' of laser using the PDL 585 nm and Nd:YAG 1064 nm. After 5 min, a 'second pass' is administered by super-

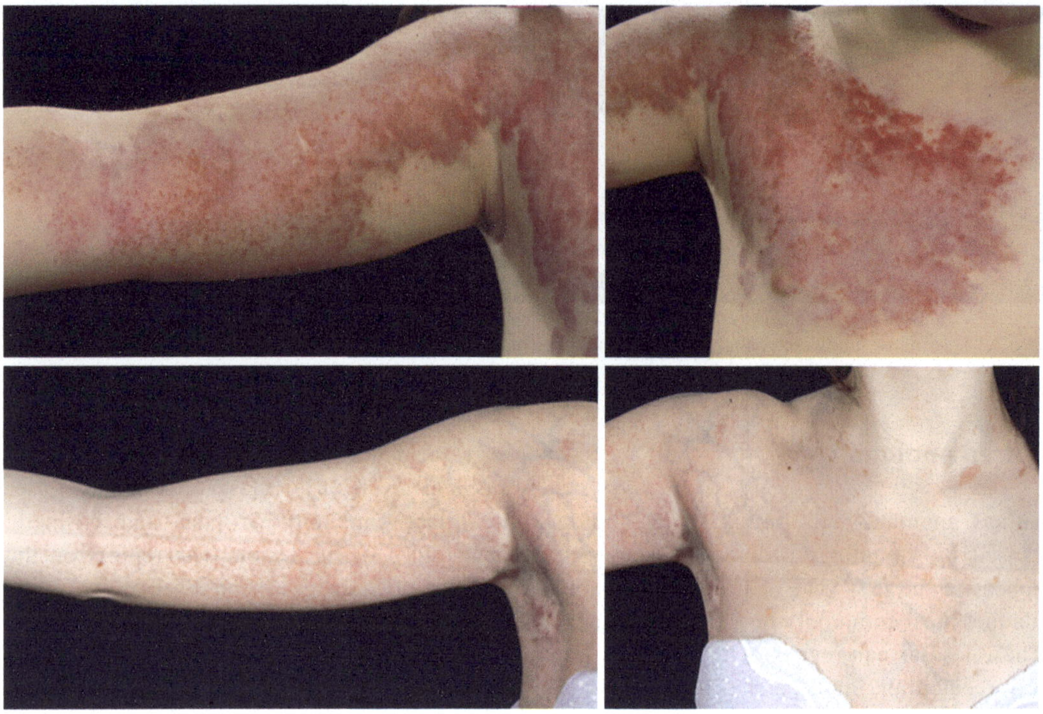

Fig. 2.15 Tufted Angioma before and after laser therapy

imposing the 595 nm laser. Due to its novelty, the outcomes by using this new treatment method have not yet been reported. However, preliminary results have shown clinically significant outcomes. Other treatment options for recalcitrant PWS include the use of topical rapamycin (sirolimus), imiquimod or systemic photodynamic therapy [63–67]. The outcomes from these method are controversial with some studies reporting up to 50% improvement in recalcitrant port wine stains that were resistant to multiple laser treatments, however, other studies report no clinical difference.

Adverse Effects

Laser complications arising from treatment of vascular anomalies are rarely reported in the literature. In China, a retrospective analysis of 100 patients reported a 14% complication rate with the most common complication being pigmentation changes [27]. This, however, may reflect the varied incidence of post-laser complication dependent on skin type. Overall, the most common complications reported after vascular laser therapy are erythema, oedema, pigmentation changes, blisters and scabs [66, 67]. Rarer known complications of lasers include retinal injury; therefore, the use of protective eye wear or eye shields is imperative during laser treatment. All patients who have laser treatment near the orbit should have corneal shields inserted just prior to the procedure. Cooling methods, such as ice, cryogen spray or cryo air cool systems, are used for each laser procedure because they are essential to reduce the complications, related to intense heat, for example, scabbing and blistering.

Part 2: Lasers for Vascular Indications—Adults

Laser treatment of vascular lesions and malformations in adults follows the same general principles as in the paediatric population. Notable differences in treatment include anaesthetic considerations and frequency of treatment. Most vascular laser treatments in adults are undertaken without infiltration or general anaesthetic. This permits more frequent treatments and consequently better outcomes. Additionally, the main indications for vascular laser treatments in adults differ from those seen in paediatric populations with most patients presenting with cosmetic or acquired vascular lesions. The devices commonly used in the treatment of vascular indications in adults are listed in Table 2.1 in the previous section. Most currently used lasers devices listed in the table are vascular specific. Intense Pulsed Light (IPL) sources are very commonly used in the treatment of vascular indications in adults and are discussed in detail in Chap. 9.

Adult Vascular Laser Applications

Commonly presenting vascular laser indications in adults are listed in Table 2.5.

Table 2.5 Adult vascular laser indications

• Mature port wine stains	• Leg telangiectases
• Facial telangiectases and erythema	• Poikiloderma of Civatte
• Cherry angiomas	• Angiokeratomas
• Verrucae/warts	• Spider naevi/angiomas
• Venous lakes	• Hypertrophic scars
• Angiofibromas	• Some inflammatory skin conditions e.g. granuloma faciale; psoriasis.

Mature Port Wine Stains

There is little doubt that early treatment of port wine stains is beneficial [17–19]. However, several patients with PWS may have not had access to lasers in their childhood or teenage years and may first present to the laser services in adult life. Additionally, many patients who have had laser treatment in younger years may notice a recurrence of their PWS.

For patients having their first treatments in adult life and for recurrent PWS, standard treatment protocols need to be employed. Mature PWS tend to be darker in colour and require more frequent treatments. Novel treatments such as topical sirolimus or systemic photodynamic therapy could be considered for recalcitrant PWS in adults [64–67].

PWS naturally progress to hypertrophy and nodularity in 65% of patients by the age of 50 years [26, 68]. Treatment options for hypertrophic PWS or those displaying nodularity incude longer wavelengths (Nd:YAG; 1064 nm) or ablative lasers such as carboin dioxide (Figs. 2.16 and 2.17).

Facial Telangiectases and Erythema

Erythemotelangiectatic rosacea (ETR) is one of the most common vascular laser indications in adult population. Isolated facial telangiectases in

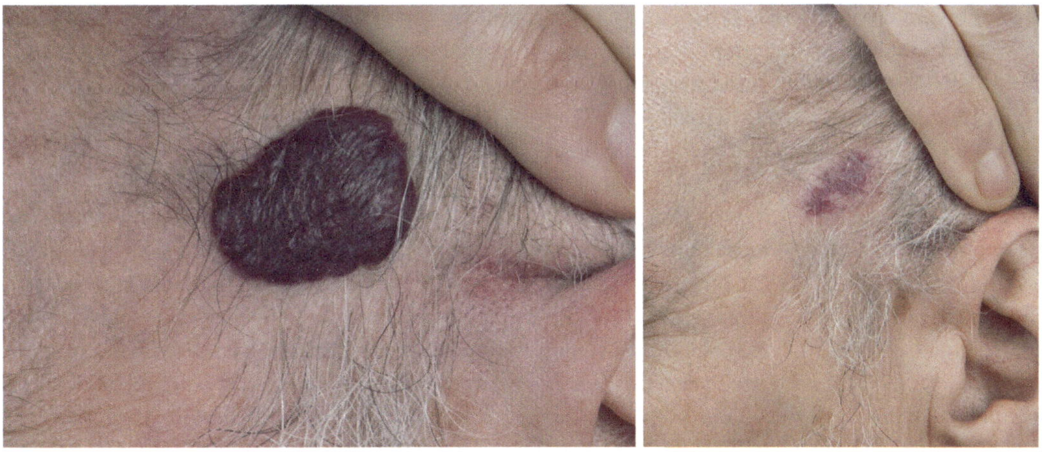

Fig. 2.16 Hypertrophic mature port wine stain. These hypertrophic element was treated with ablative carbon dioxide laser. 18 W, 6 mm spot, 10,600 nm, scanned waveform

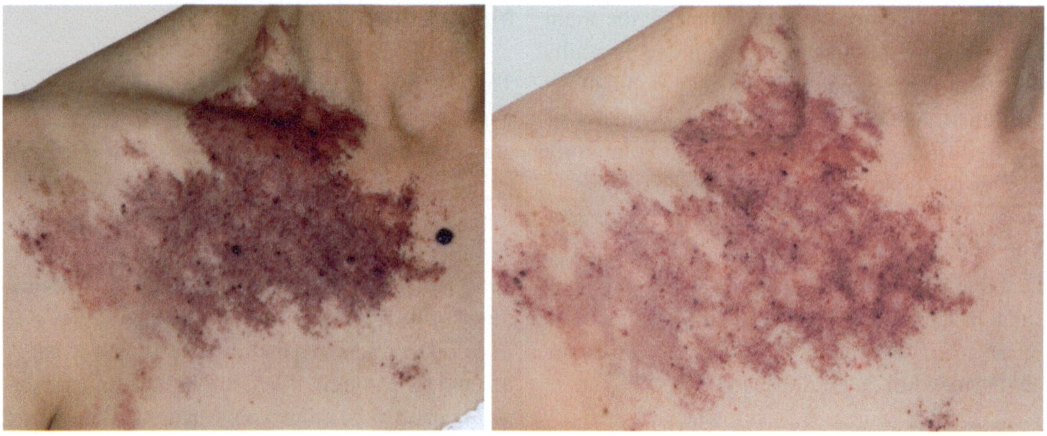

Fig. 2.17 Port wine stain on the upper chest with vascular papules and nodules and improvement after CO_2 laser treatment

the absence of flushing or inflammatory component of rosacea are also commonly treated with vascular lasers or IPL. PDL is usually considered the laser of choice for ETR (Figs. 2.18 and 2.19). Other lasers such as the KTP are useful for facial and perinasal telangectases (Fig. 2.20). Stubborn perinasal and nasal telangiectases respond well to Nd:YAG laser, however this wavelength is associated with higher risk of scarring and should be used with caution and only by experienced laser practitioners.

Results of comparative studies between PDL and IPL for diffuse facial erythema and telangiectases have been equivocal [69, 70]. Therefore, the choice of device therefore depends upon its availability and practitioner's experience.

While some patients may report an improvement in flushing symptoms, laser and light based devices are usually ineffective in treating flushing associated with rosacea. Additionally, inflammatory rosacea can worsen with laser treatment, therefore, adequate treatment with topical or oral medications is mandatory for patients presenting with inflammatory and ETR. Concerns over concomitant use of oral tetracyclines and laser or IPL and resultant phototoxicity have not been found to be true [71]. The author's standard practice is to commence an oral tetracycline such as lymecycline for papulopustular ETR before commencing laser treatment. In a recent study, oxymetazoline 1.0% cream, an α adrenergic agonist in combination with PDL was found to be effective and safe in the treatment of ETR [72].

Besides rosacea, facial telangectases can be a manifestation of photoaging and conditions such as hereditary haemorrhagic telangiectasia, scleroderma and post radiotherapy (Fig. 2.21). Such telangiectases can also be readily treated with vascular lasers or IPL.

The purpura associated with PDL can be a deterrent for most patients seeking PDL treatment for their ERT. Non-purpuragenic settings can be achieved by increasing the pulse duration however, in clinical practice results are usually unsatisfactory. In the author's experience, more than twice the number of purpuric treatments is required to achieve beneficial results, thus making non-purpuric treatments less cost effective.

Leg Telangiectases

Whenever possible, small calibre reticular lower leg veins <4 mm are best treated with sclerotherapy with sclerosants such as aethoxysclerol, hypertonic saline or polidocanol. Laser treatment is reserved for patients who are needle phobic, have allergy to certain sclerosing agents and in the presence of vessels smaller than 3 mm.

The depth of vessels and differing diameters makes laser treatment of such veins very difficult with unpredictable final results. The lasers most

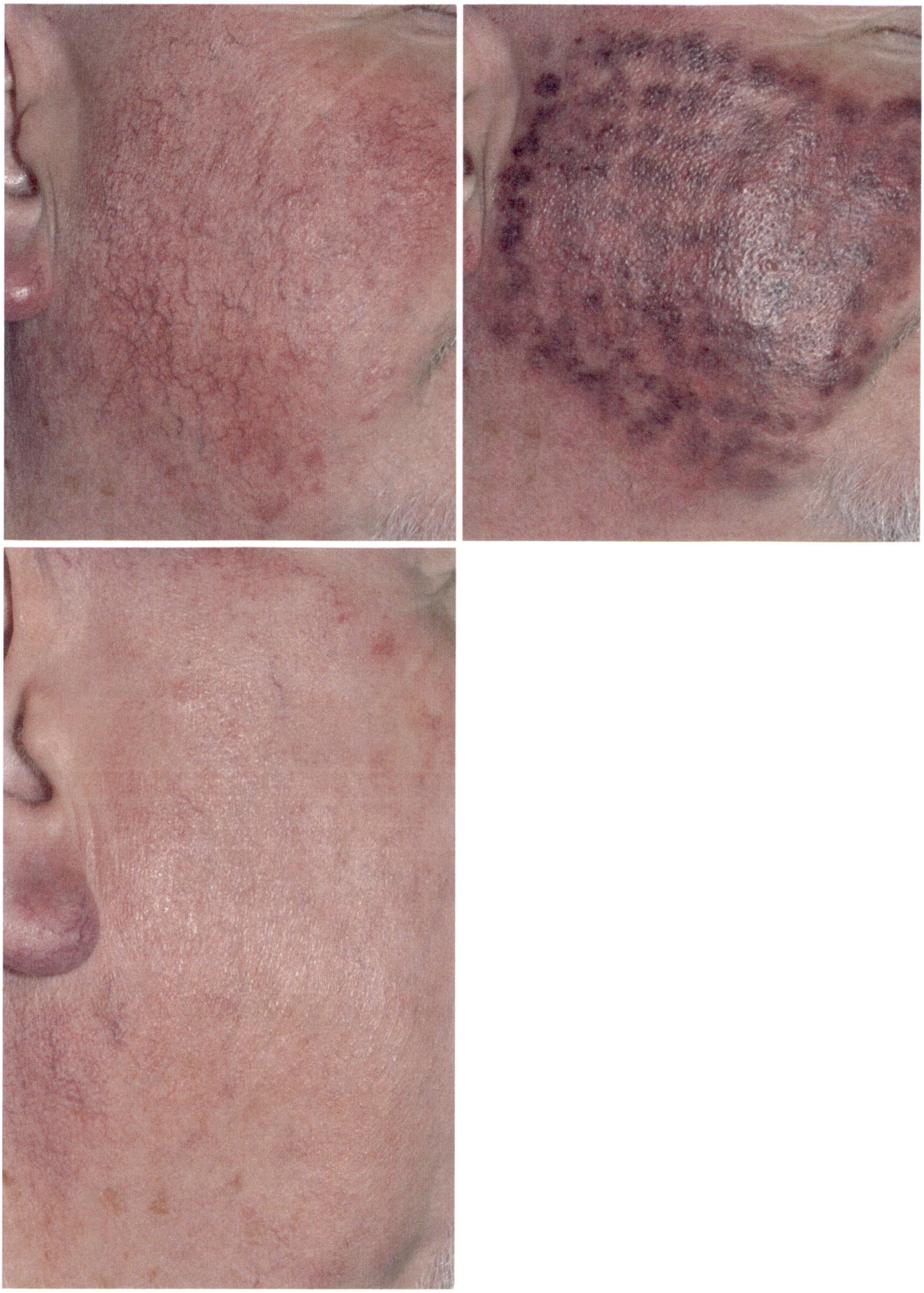

Fig. 2.18 Erythemotelangiectatic rosacea before and after 6 treatment with PDL. 5.5–6.5 j/cm^2, 10 mm spot, 1.5 ms pulse duration and DCD 30:20. Note the intense purpura immediately following treatment

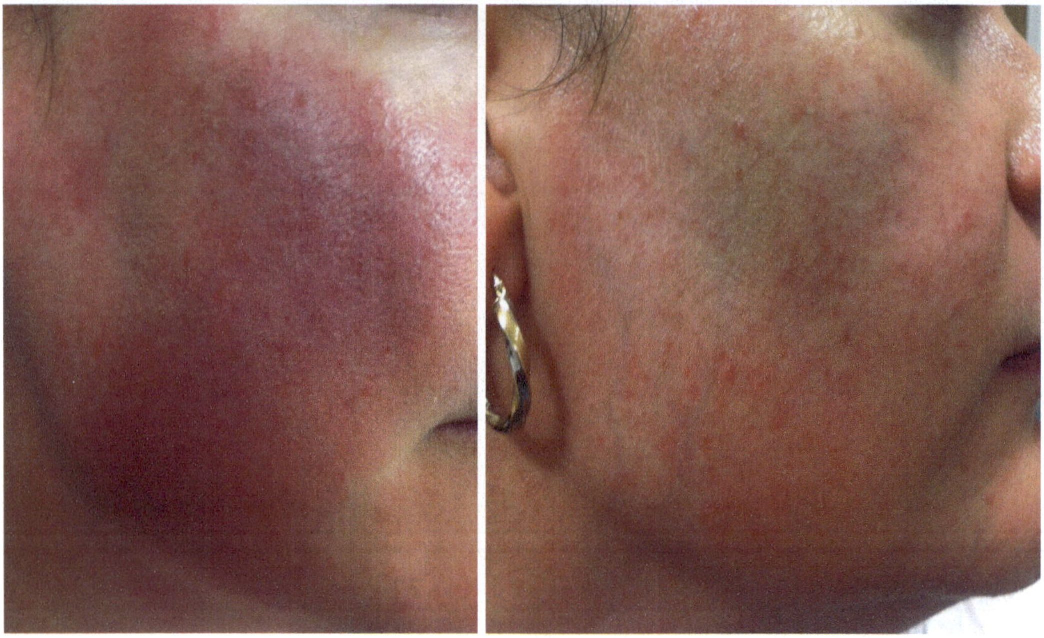

Fig. 2.19 Diffuse erythema secondary to rosacea before and after 5 sessions with PDL. 6–7.5 j/cm^2, 10 mm spot, 1.5 ms, 30:20DCD. IPL device would have also be an appropriate choice in this case

commonly employed for treatment of small calibre leg veins include long pulsed 1064 nm Nd:YAG and 800–983-nm diode lasers [73, 74]. Other lasers such as KTP, PDL can be effective for vessels measuring <1 mm, telangeictatic matting and essential telangiectases (Fig. 2.22). Combination of laser therapy with sclerotherapy or radiofrequency, and indocyanin green enhanced laser therapy have been explored but none of the methods have been universally adopted in clinical practice [75].

Cherry Angiomas (Campbell de Morgan Spots), Angiokeratomas, Acquired Haemangiomas and Angiofibromas

Small angiomas on the trunk and limbs respond readily to PDL or Nd:YAG lasers. Any other vascular laser device would also be useful for treating these lesions. (Fig. 2.23) Other similar vascular lesions such as small acquired haemangiomas (Fig. 2.24), small pyogenic granulomas, truncal (Fig. 2.25) and scrotal angiokeratomas (Fig. 2.26) can also be readily treated with vascular lasers.

Until recently, PDL was the treatment of choice for facial angiofibrmas associated with Tuberous sclerosus. This has largely been superseded by topical sirolimus.

Warts

Both PDL and long pulsed Nd:YAG lasers have been proven to be effective in the management of cutaneous warts [76, 77]. PDL is perhaps the more commonly used of the two lasers for plantar warts (Fig. 2.27). The mechanism of action of lasers in the treatment of warts is not completely understood, but the limitation of depth of penetration of laser beam would suggest that selective photothermolysis is unlikely to play a role. Good quality studies comparing the efficacy of PDL with conventional wart treatments such as cryotherapy are lacking. Nd:YAG laser has been found to be similar in efficacy to cryotherapy in the treatment of acral warts [78]. Due to the low expense and ease of administration and

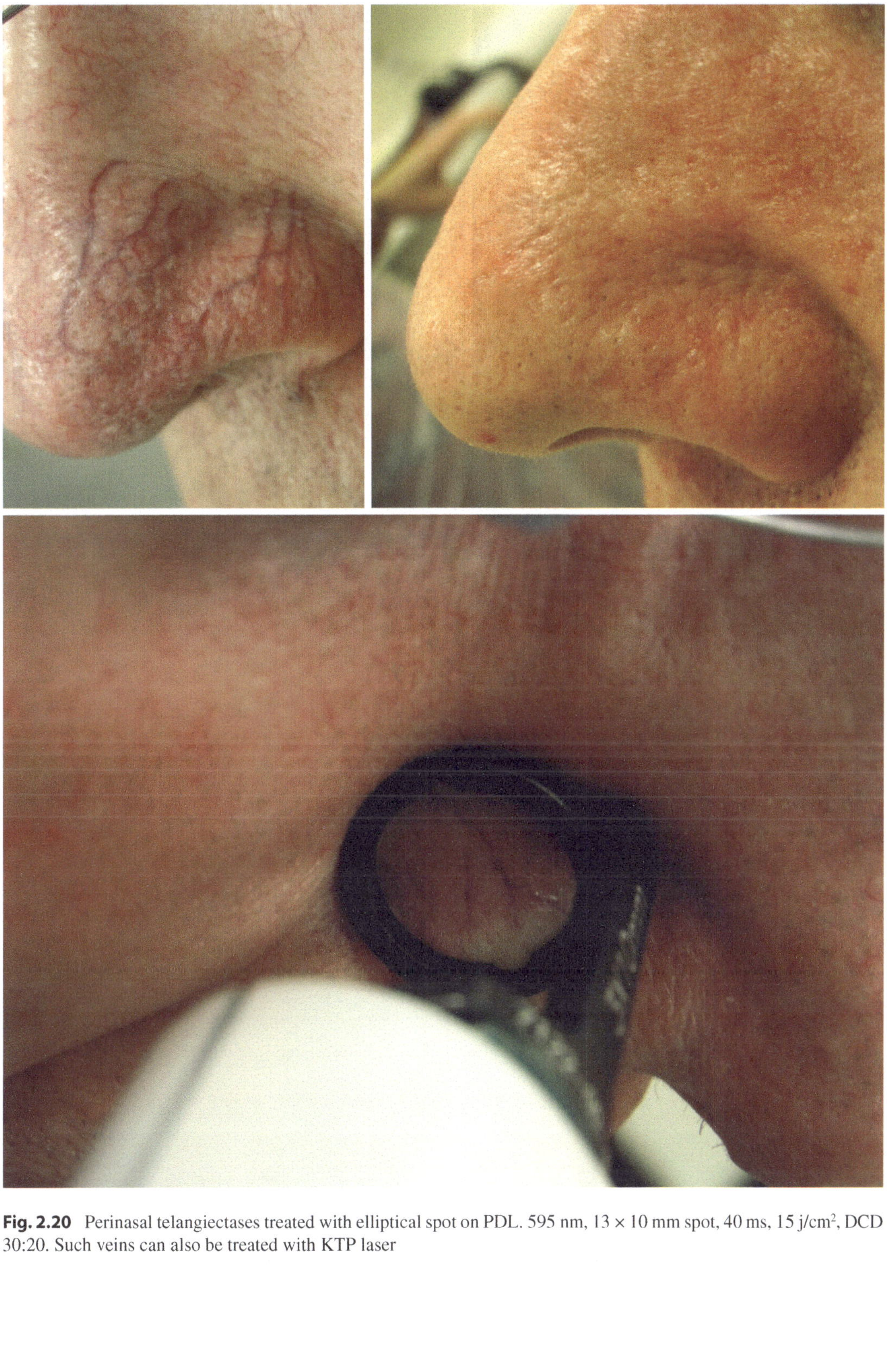

Fig. 2.20 Perinasal telangiectases treated with elliptical spot on PDL. 595 nm, 13 × 10 mm spot, 40 ms, 15 j/cm², DCD 30:20. Such veins can also be treated with KTP laser

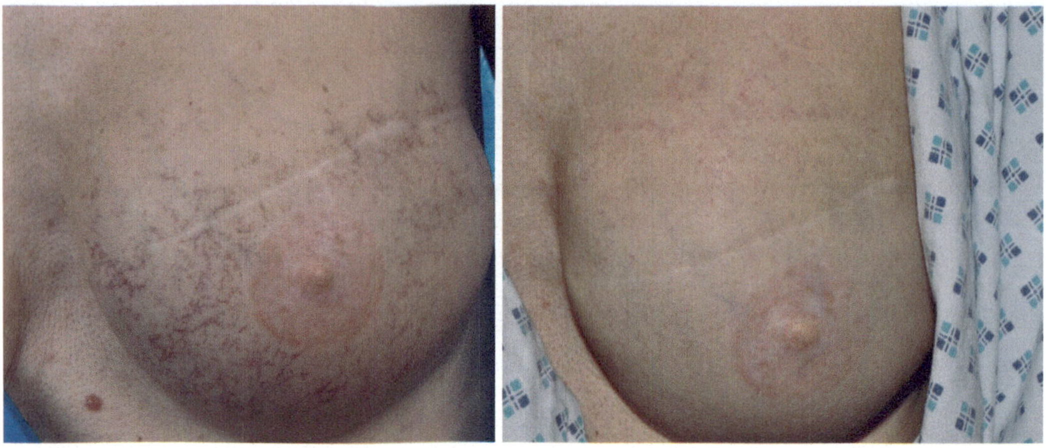

Fig. 2.21 Post radiotherapy telangiectases as seen in this case improved after 4 sessions of PDL 6 j/cm^2 10 mm spot, 1.5 ms, 30:20 DCD

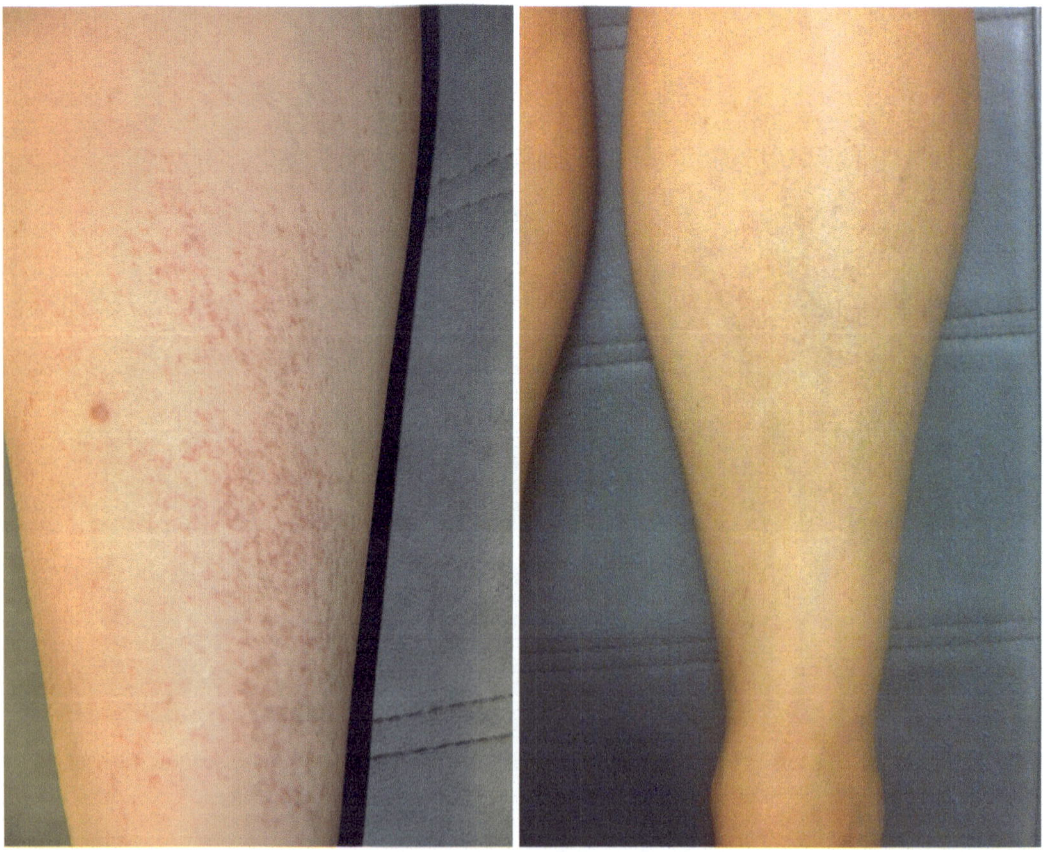

Fig. 2.22 Essential telangiectases on lower leg, before and after PDL 3 sessions. 5.5–6 j/cm^2, 10 mm, 1.5 ms, 30:20 DCD

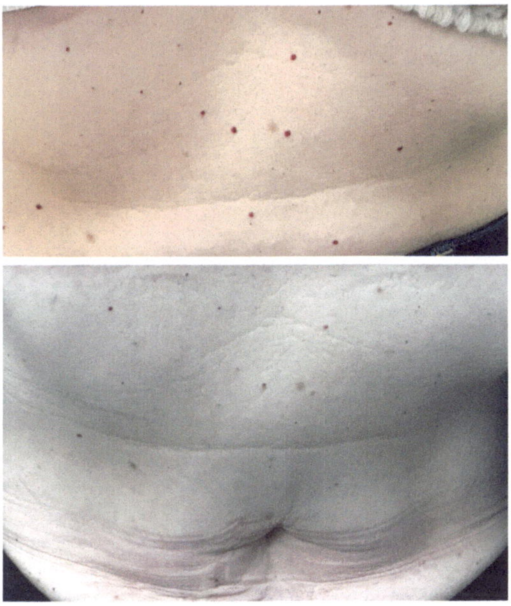

Fig. 2.23 Cherry angiomas on abdomen. Response to 1 PDL session. 595 nm, 3 mm spot, 25 j/cm^2, 3 ms; cooling 30:20 DCD

availability, liquid nitrogen cryotherapy remains the treatment of choice for warts in immunocompetent patients.

Venous Lakes

Venous lake presents as a soft compressible bluish nodules on the mucosal lip in middle aged to elderly patients. Small lesions can be treated with PDL however, larger, well established lesions do not respond to this laser. Nd:YAG and Diode lasers have been used successfully for treating venous lakes [79].

Hypertrophic Scars

PDL has a role in the treatment of post-surgical and established hypertrophic scars [80, 81]. The erythema, telangiectases and scar associated pruritus improve with PDL treatment

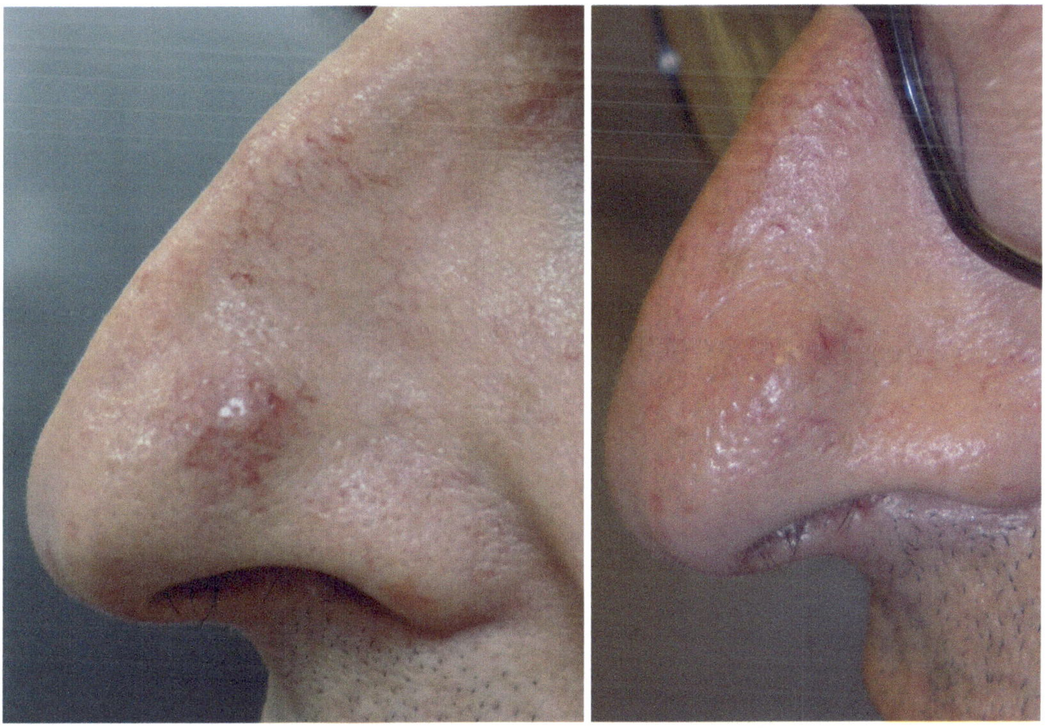

Fig. 2.24 Acquired haemangioma on nose before and after single treatment with Nd:YAG laser. Nd: YAG laser was chosen as the lesion appeared thick. 1064 nm, 3 mm spot, 220 j/cm^2, 20 ms. Air Cooling setting 7

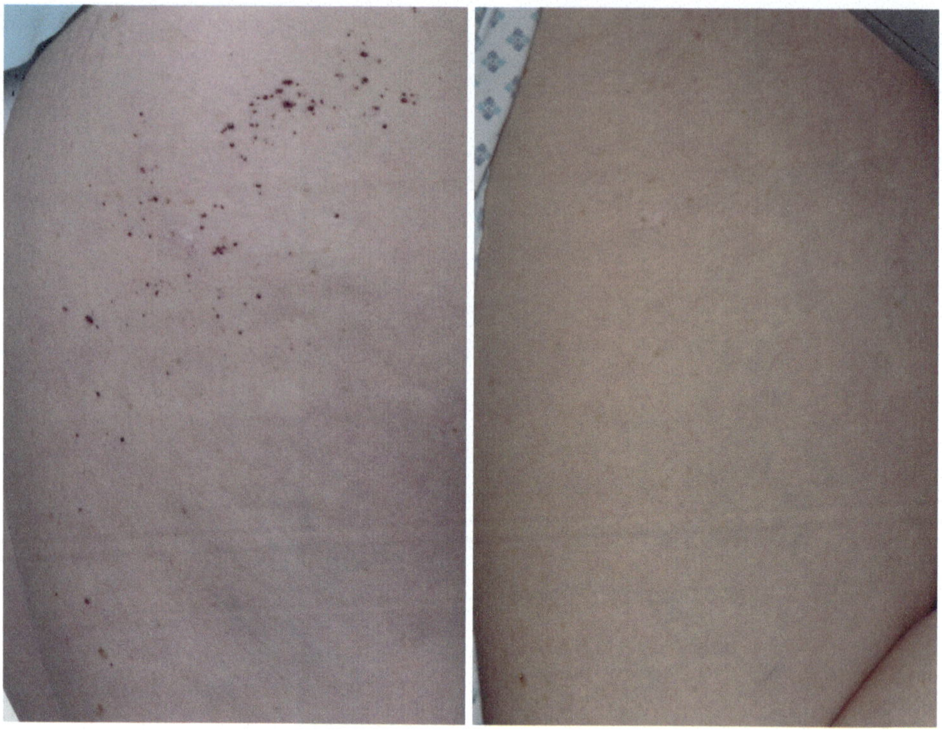

Fig. 2.25 Truncal Angiokeratomas associated with Fabry's disease. After 3 sessions of PDL. 9 j/cm^2. 7 mm spot, 1.5 ms, 30:20 DCD

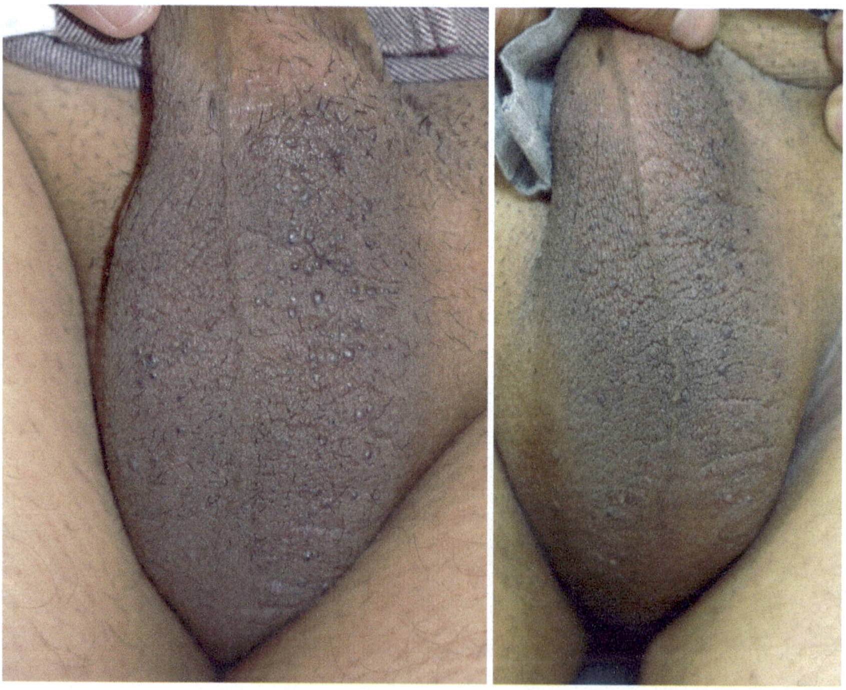

Fig. 2.26 Scrotal angiokeratomas can bleed and also become cosmetically troublesome. They respond very well to PDL as in this case. 595 nm, 20 J, 3 ms, 3 mm spot, 30:20 DCD. Results after 1 session

(Fig. 2.28). The role of lasers in the treatment of keloids is still under review. PDL is effective in reducing the keloid erythema and improves the associated pruritus. In conjunction with intralesional corticosteroids, PDL is an effective approach for fresh, hyperaemic keloids [82].

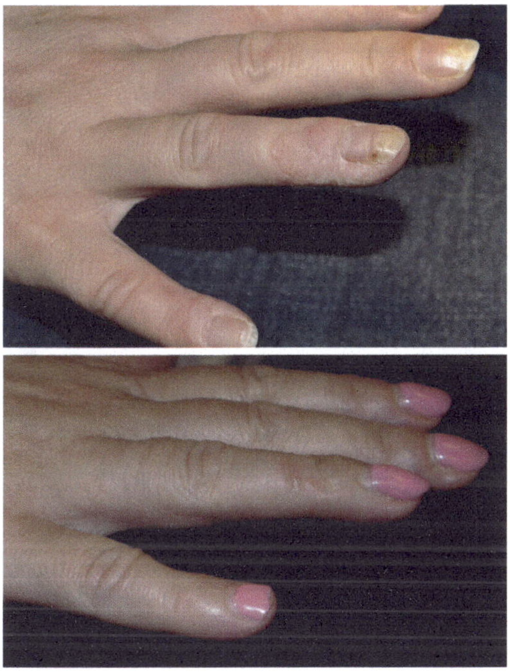

Fig. 2.27 Periungual warts before and after 4 sessions of PDL. 16–19 j/cm², 7 mm, 1.5 ms, DCD off

Role of Vascular Lasers in Inflammatory Skin Conditions

PDL is effective in the treatment of certain some inflammatory skin conditions such as psoriasis and acne [83]. The efficacy of PDL in these disorders appears to be mediated by anti-angiogenesis and photodynamic effects. Other conditions in which PDL has been found to be effective but not been established as a treatment of choice include.

Granuloma annulare
Granuloma Faciale
Lupus Erythematosus
Sarcoidosis
Jessner's lymphocytic infiltrate (Fig. 2.29)
Reticular erythematous mucinosis
Lichen sclerosus

Complications of Vascular Lasers

Laser complications arising from treatment of vascular anomalies are rare. PDL is a relatively safe laser if used judiciously. The most common complications reported after vascular laser treatments are erythema, oedema, transient pigmentation changes, blistering and scabbing [84, 85]. Rarer known complications of vascular lasers include retinal injury and scarring. Patients should have appropriate corneal shields in situ prior to periorbital laser procedures

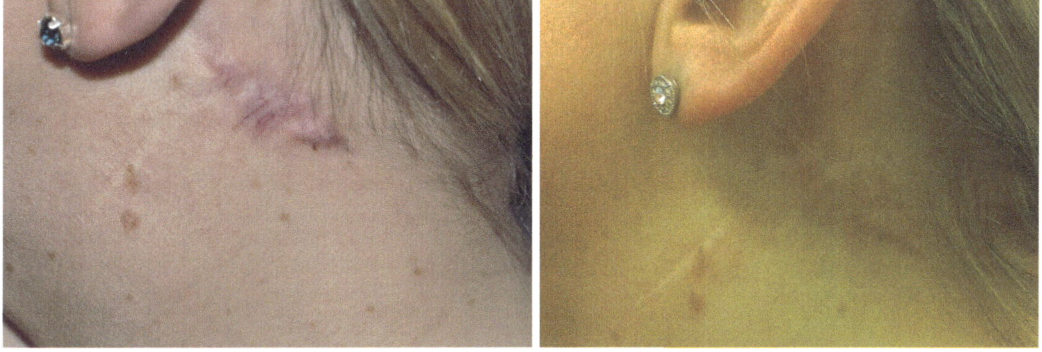

Fig. 2.28 Hypertrophic post-surgical scar treated with a combination of PDL and intralesional triamciniolone 10 mg/ml. 9 j/cm². 7 mm, 1.5 ms, 30:20DCD

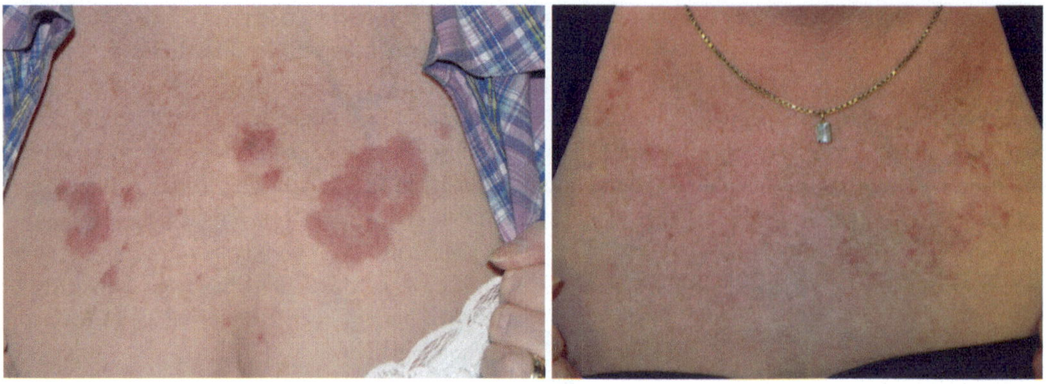

Fig. 2.29 Topical therapy resistant Jessner's lymphocytic infiltrate after 6 PDL treatments. 8–9.5 j/cm^2, 1.5 ms, 7 mm spot, 30:20 DCD

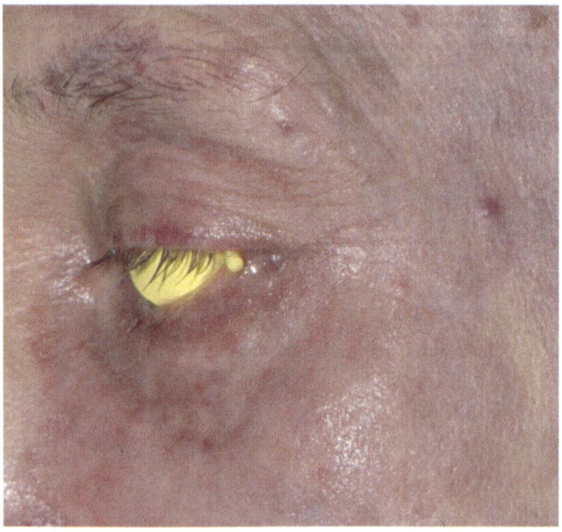

Fig. 2.30 Yellow corneal shields in situ prior to periorbital PDL treatment

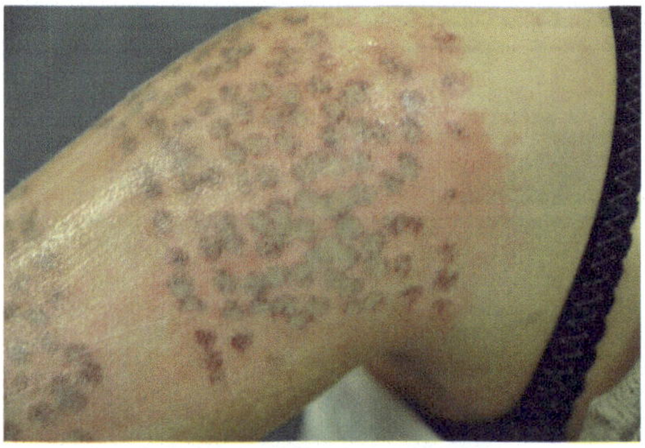

Fig. 2.31 Very high fluence PDL treatment resulting in ash grey colour of treated skin. The end point of treatment should be purpura

(Fig. 2.30). Scarring after PDL is uncommon but can be seen after KTP or Nd:YAG laser treatments.

The most common reasons for a complication arising from vascular laser treatments are inadequate cooling of the epidermis or very high fluence treatments (Fig. 2.31).

Case Studies

1. Facial Spider Naevus: A 4-year-old girl presented with a prominent spider naevus on her left cheek. This was treated with two pulses of the PDL Perfecta 595 nm laser under local anaesthetic cream at two different times. The first treatment consisted of one pulse using laser parameters of 7.5 j/cm^2, a pulse width of 0.45 ms, spot size of 10 mm and DCD 30/20 cooling system. The second treatment consisted

of one pulse of PDL Perfecta 595 nm using 9.0 j/cm^2, a pulse width of 1.5 ms, spot size of 10 mm and DCD 30/20 cooling system. The lesion completely resolved after two treatments.

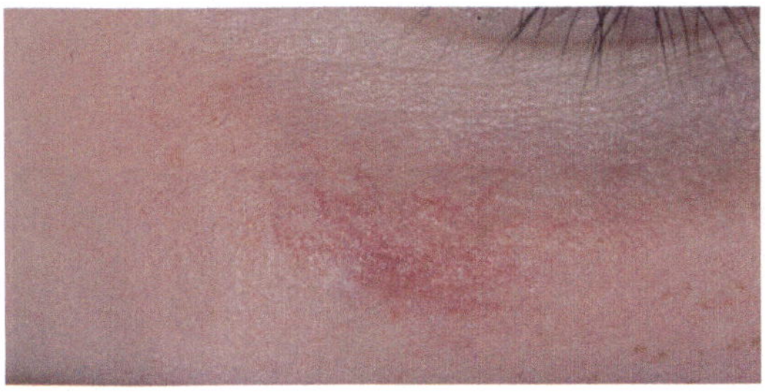

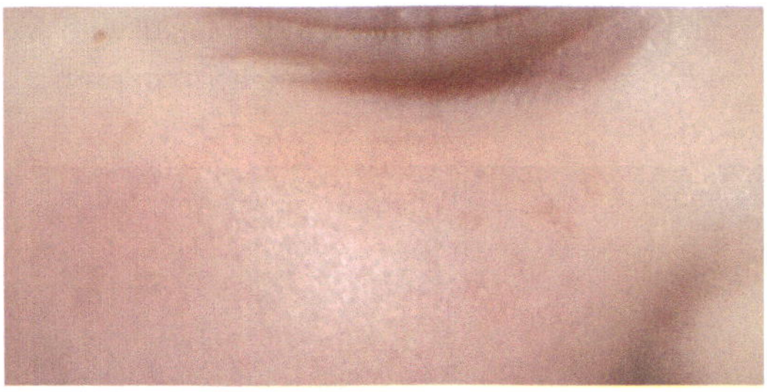

2. Lymphovenous Malformation: A seven-year-old girl presented with chronic progressive Lymphovenous malformation over her left lower thigh and knee. It was superimposed with chronic crusting and Lymphovascular blebs. She underwent the first six laser treatment sessions using Cynergy laser consisting of both PDL 585 nm and Nd:YAG 1064 nm. The laser parameters were slowly up titrated to reach parameters of PDL 585 nm 10.0 j/cm^2, Nd:YAG 60 j/cm^2, pulse group 3, spot size 10 and cryo4 cooling system was used. Her next four treatments consisted of triple pass laser therapy where Cynergy laser treatment was first performed, then after 5 min, a second pass of PDL Perfecta 595 nm was supraimposed using parameters of 595 nm 9.0 j/cm^2, 1.5 ms pulse width, spot size 10 and DCD30/20 cooling system.

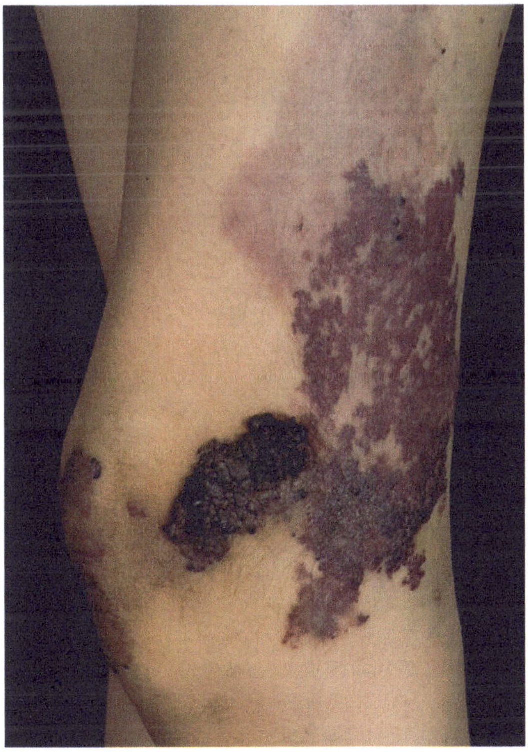

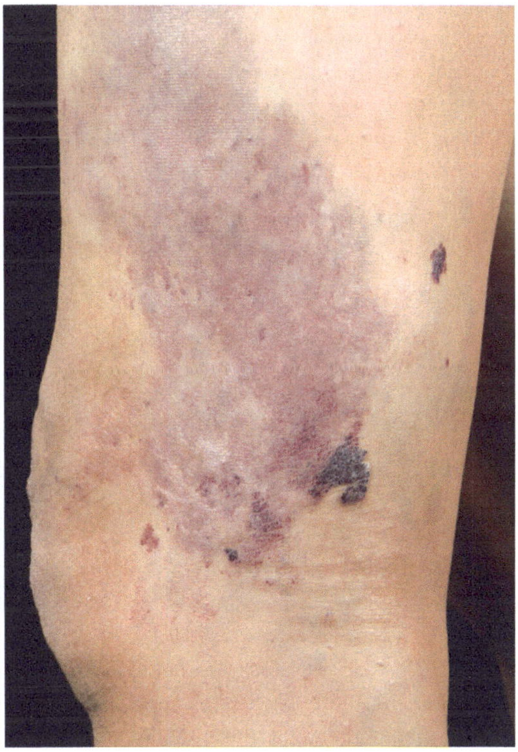

3. A 15-year-old male presented with Elastosis Perforans Serpiginosa after no response to treatment with cryotherapy, topical retinoids and 10% urea cream. He was treated with 8 sessions of PDL 585 nm using a 7 mm probe, 8–15 j/cm^2, 0.45–1.5 ms and Cryogen spray cooling system. He had a very good response and the lesions have not recurred after follow-up years later.

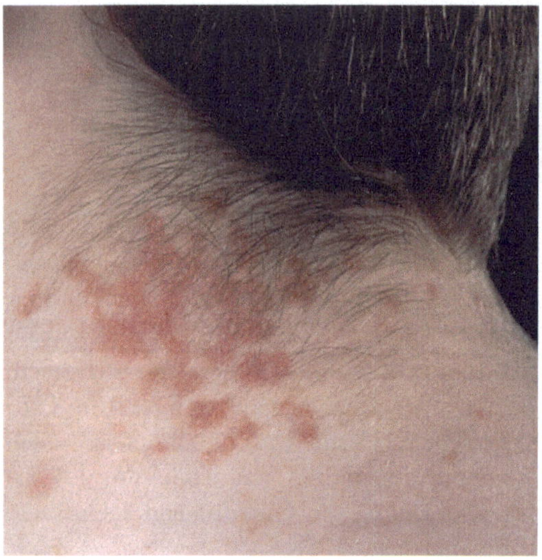

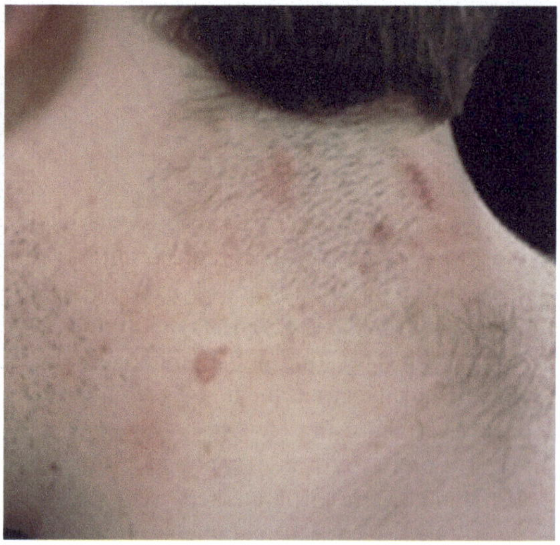

4. A 10-year-old boy presented with a remnant of a haemangioma on his right zygomatic facial area. He underwent one laser treatment with PDL 595 nm. He received 23 pulses using 10 mm probe, 8.5 j/cm^2, a pulse width of 0.45 ms and the DCD 30/20 cooling system. He also received 17 superimposed pulses to target thread veins using 10 mm probe, 12.0 j/cm^2, a pulse width of 1.5 ms and the DCD 30/20 cooling system.

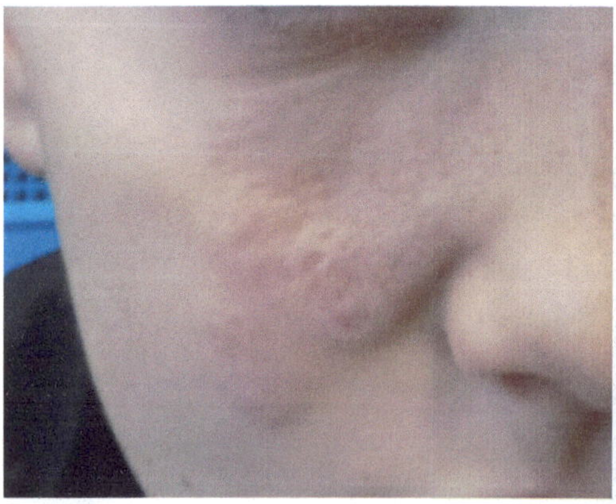

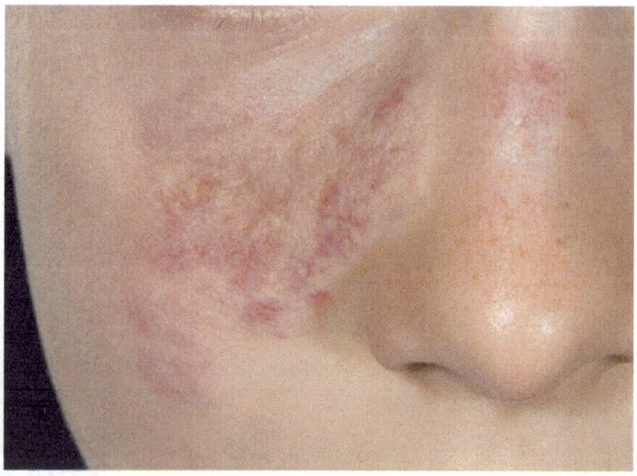

5. This 35 year old man presented with erythema on his left cheek. This appeared after a superficial chemical burn. He was treated with PDL—5 sessions spaced at 8 week intervals. 8.5–9.25 j/cm^2, 7 mm, 1.5 ms, 30:20DCD.

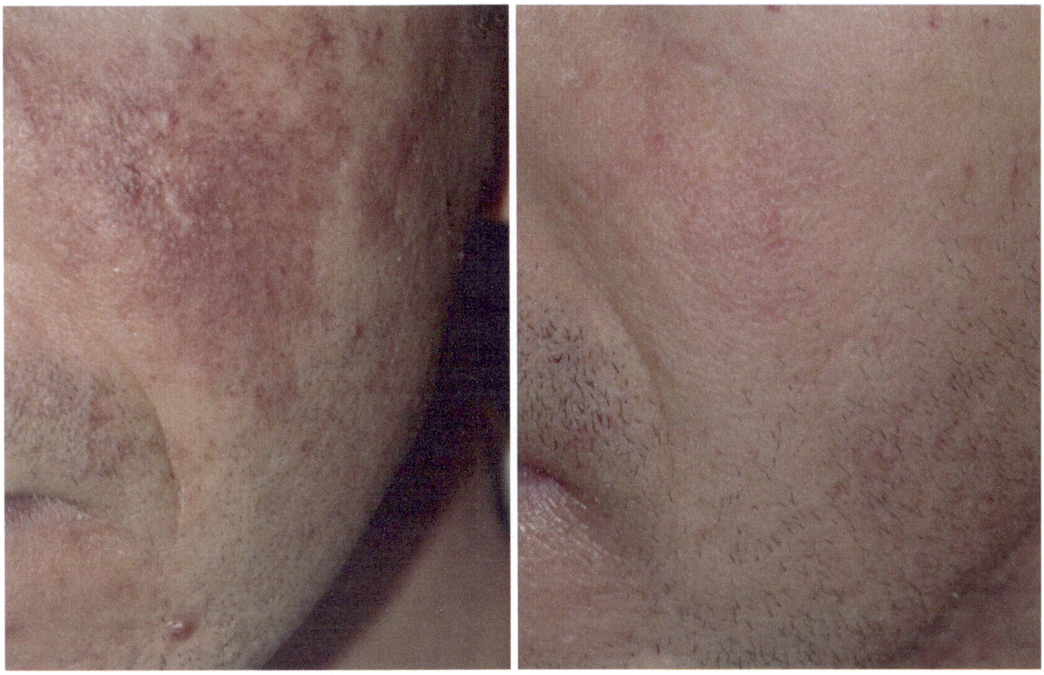

6. Certain vascular lesions readily respond to PDL. This girl had been diagnosed as having angioma serpiginosum on her thigh. Three PDL treatments were undertaken at 8 weekly intervals resulting in complete clearance of the vascular malformation.
6–6.5 j/cm^2, 10 mm spot, 1.5 ms, 30:20DCD.

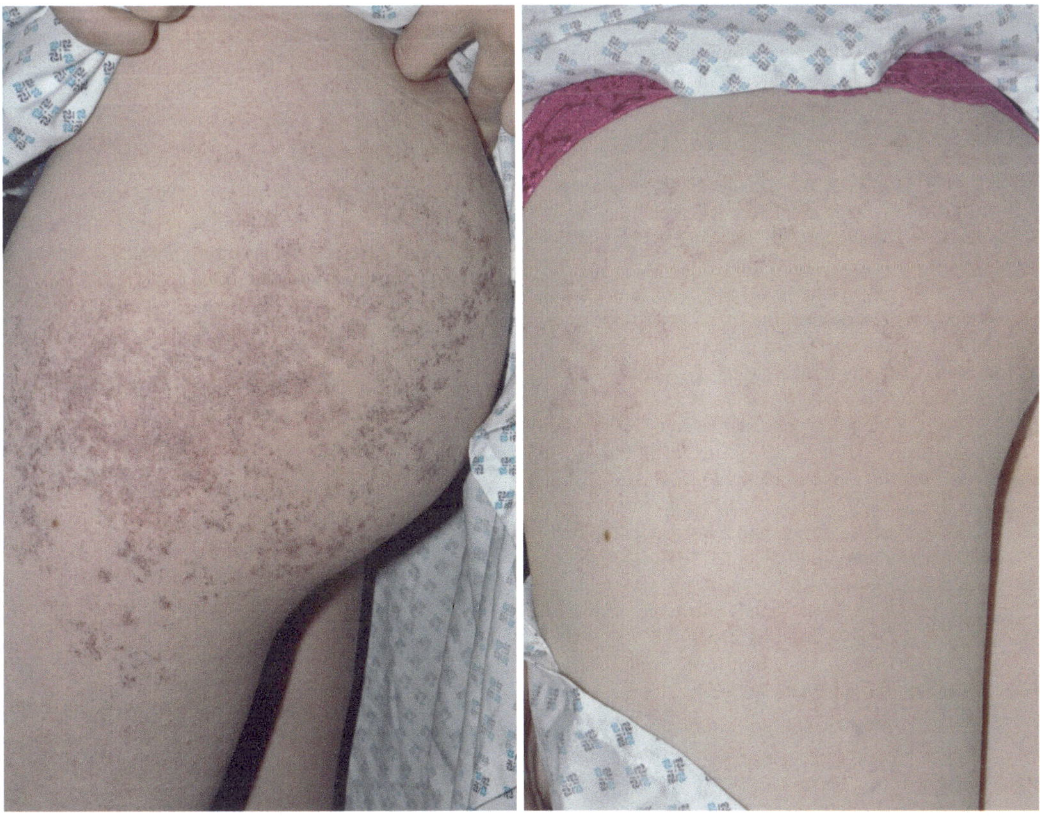

References

1. Patil UA, Dhami LD. Overview of lasers. Indian J Plast Surg [Internet]. 2008 Oct;41(Suppl):S101–13.
2. Farkas JP, Hoopman JE, Kenkel JM. Five parameters you must understand to master control of your laser/light-based devices. Aesthetic Surg J. 2013 Sep;33(7):1059–64.
3. Yadav RK. Definitions in laser technology. J Cutan Aesthet Surg [Internet]. 2009 Jan;2(1):45–6. Available from: https://www.ncbi.nlm.nih.gov/pubmed/20300375.
4. Das A, Sarda A, De A. Cooling devices in Laser therapy. J Cutan Aesthet Surg [Internet]. 2016;9(4):215–9. Available from: https://www.ncbi.nlm.nih.gov/pubmed/28163450.
5. Šulc J, Jelínková H. 5 – Solid-state lasers for medical applications. In: Jelínková HBT-L for MA, editor. Woodhead publishing series in electronic and optical materials [Internet]. Cambridge: Woodhead Publishing; 2013. pp. 127–76. Available from: http://www.sciencedirect.com/science/article/pii/B9780857092373500059
6. Goldman MP, Guex J-J, Weiss RA Chapter 13 – Treatment of leg telangiectases with laser and high-intensity pulsed light. Edinburgh: W.B. Saunders; 5 2011. p. 336–368. Available from: http://www.sciencedirect.com/science/article/pii/B9780323073677000194
7. Wall TL. Current concepts: laser treatment of adult vascular lesions. Semin Plast Surg [Internet]. 2007 Aug;21(3):147–58. Available from: https://www.ncbi.nlm.nih.gov/pubmed/20567666.
8. Chiang YZ, Al-Niaimi F, Madan V. Comparative efficacy and patient preference of topical Anaesthetics in dermatological Laser treatments and skin microneedling. J Cutan Aesthet Surg [Internet]. 2015;8(3):143–6. Available from: https://www.ncbi.nlm.nih.gov/pubmed/26644737.
9. Tollan CJ, MacLaren W, Mackay IR. Topical anaesthetic effects on skin vasculature with potential implications for laser treatment. Lasers Med Sci. 2016 May;31(4):611–7.
10. Ashinoff R, Geronemus RG. Effect of the topical anesthetic EMLA on the efficacy of pulsed dye laser treatment of port-wine stains. J Dermatol Surg Oncol [Internet]. 1990 Nov 1;16(11):1008–11. Available from: https://doi.org/10.1111/j.1524-4725.1990.tb00324.x.
11. Jacobs AH, Walton RG. The incidence of birthmarks in the neonate. Pediatrics. 1976 Aug;58(2):218–22.
12. Infantile hemangioma: epidemiology update. J Am Acad Dermatol [Internet]. 2013;68(4, Supplement 1):AB95. Available from: http://www.sciencedirect.com/science/article/pii/S019096221201674X
13. Hagen SL, Grey KR, Korta DZ, Kelly KM. Quality of life in adults with facial port-wine stains. J Am Acad Dermatol [Internet]. 2016/12/09. 2017 Apr;76(4):695–702. Available from: https://www.ncbi.nlm.nih.gov/pubmed/27955934.
14. Hein KD, Mulliken JB, Kozakewich HPW, Upton J, Burrows PE. Venous malformations of skeletal muscle. Plast Reconstr Surg. 2002 Dec;110(7):1625–35.
15. Kulungowski AM, Fishman SJ. Chapter 125 – Vascular anomalies. In: Coran AGBT-PS. 7th ed. Philadelphia: Mosby; 2012. p. 1613–30. Available from: http://www.sciencedirect.com/science/article/pii/B9780323072557001252.
16. Saxena M, Tope WD. Response of elastosis perforans serpiginosa to pulsed CO_2, Er:YAG, and Dye Lasers. Dermatologic Surg [Internet]. 2003;29(6):677–8.
17. Finley JL, Noe JM, Arndt KA, Rosen S. Port-wine stains: morphologic variations and developmental lesions. JAMA Dermatol [Internet]. 1984 Nov 1;120(11):1453–5. Available from: https://doi.org/10.1001/archderm.1984.01650470059013.
18. van der Horst CMAM, de Borgie CAJM, Knopper JL, Bossuyt PMM. Psychosocial adjustment of children and adults with port wine stains. Br J Plast Surg [Internet] 1997;50(6):463–7. Available from: http://www.sciencedirect.com/science/article/pii/S0007122697903350.
19. Troilius A, Wrangsjo B, Ljunggren B. Potential psychological benefits from early treatment of port-wine stains in children. Br J Dermatol. 1998 Jul;139(1):59–65.
20. Eubanks LE, McBurney EI. Videomicroscopy of port-wine stains: correlation of location and depth of lesion. J Am Acad Dermatol [Internet]. 2001 Jun 1;44(6):948–51. Available from: https://doi.org/10.1067/mjd.2001.113467.
21. Kwiek B, Rożalski M, Sieczych J, Paluch Ł, Kowalewski C, Ambroziak M. Predictive value of dermoscopy for the treatment of port-wine stains with large spot 532 nm laser. Lasers Surg Med [Internet]. 2019 Sep 1;51(7):569–83. Available from: https://doi.org/10.1002/lsm.23083.
22. Vázquez-López F, Coto-Segura P, Fueyo-Casado A, Pérez-Oliva N. Dermoscopy of port-wine stains. Arch Dermatol [Internet]. 2007 Jul 1;143(7):962. Available from: https://doi.org/10.1001/archderm.143.7.962.
23. Baghad B, Chiheb S, Benchikhi H. Port wine stains and pulsed dye laser: study of prognostic factors in 74 Moroccan patients. Pan Afr Med J. 2016;25:218.
24. Fu Z, Huang J, Xiang Y, Huang J, Tang Z, Chen J, Nelson JS, Tan W, Lu J. Characterization of laser-resistant port wine stain blood vessels using in vivo reflectance confocal microscopy. Lasers Surg Med [Internet]. 2019 Dec 1;51(10):841–9. Available from: https://doi.org/10.1002/lsm.23134.
25. Shi W, Wang J, Lin Y, Geng J, Wang H, Gong Y, Liu H, Zhang F. Treatment of port wine stains with pulsed dye laser: a retrospective study of 848 cases in Shandong Province, People's republic of China. Drug Des Devel Ther. 2014 Dec;8:2531–8.
26. Geronemus RG, Ashinoff R. The medical necessity of evaluation and treatment of port-wine stains. J Dermatol Surg Oncol. 1991 Jan;17(1):76–9.
27. Ho WS, Chan HH, Ying SY, Chan PC. Laser treatment of congenital facial port-wine stains: long-term

efficacy and complication in Chinese patients. Lasers Surg Med. 2002;30(1):44–7.
28. Laube S, Taibjee S, Lanigan SW. Treatment of resistant port wine stains with the V beam pulsed dye laser. Lasers Surg Med. 2003;33(5):282–7.
29. Mahendran R, Sheehan-Dare RA. Survey of the practices of laser users in the UK in the treatment of port wine stains. J Dermatolog Treat. 2004 Apr;15(2):112–7.
30. Tomson N, Lim SPR, Abdullah A, Lanigan SW. The treatment of port-wine stains with the pulsed-dye laser at 2-week and 6-week intervals: a comparative study. Br J Dermatol. 2006 Apr;154(4):676–9.
31. Yu W, Zhu J, Changc S-J, Chen H, Jin Y, Yang X, Wang T, Chang L, Chen Y, Ma G, Lin X. Shorter treatment intervals of east Asians with port-wine stain with Pulsed Dye Laser are safe and effective-A prospective side-by-side comparison. Photomed Laser Surg. 2018 Jan;36(1):37–43.
32. Beattie M, Widdowson D, Anderson W. Pulsed dye laser treatment of paediatric port wine stains—variation of practice in the UK (NHS). Lasers med Sci [Internet]. 2016;31(3):597. Available from: https://doi.org/10.1007/s10103-016-1890-2.
33. Quirke TE, Rauscher G, Heath LL. Laser treatment of leg and facial telangiectasia. Aesthetic Surg J [Internet]. 2000 Nov 1;20(6):465–70. Available from: https://doi.org/10.1067/maj.2000.112375
34. Geronemus RG. Treatment of spider telangiectases in children using the flashlamp-pumped pulsed dye laser. Pediatr Dermatol [Internet]. 1991 Mar 1;8(1):61–3. Available from: https://doi.org/10.1111/j.1525-1470.1991.tb00843.x
35. Halachmi S, Israeli H, Ben-Amitai D, Lapidoth M. Treatment of the skin manifestations of hereditary hemorrhagic telangiectasia with pulsed dye laser. Lasers Med Sci. 2014 Jan:29(1):321–4.
36. Schirra A, Schäkel K. Mat-like telangiectases. JDDG J der Dtsch Dermatologischen Gesellschaft [Internet]. 2018 Jan 1;16(1):92–4. Available from: https://doi.org/10.1111/ddg.13375.
37. Orme CM, Boyden LM, Choate KA, Antaya RJ, King BA. Capillary malformation--arteriovenous malformation syndrome: review of the literature, proposed diagnostic criteria, and recommendations for management. Pediatr Dermatol. 2013;30(4):409–15.
38. Ponnurangam VN, Paramasivam V. Cutis marmorata telangiectatica congenita. Indian Dermatol Online J [Internet]. 2014 Jan;5(1):80–2. Available from: https://www.ncbi.nlm.nih.gov/pubmed/24616866.
39. Cox JA, Bartlett E, Lee EI. Vascular malformations: a review. Semin Plast Surg [Internet]. 2014 May;28(2):58–63. Available from: https://www.ncbi.nlm.nih.gov/pubmed/25045330.
40. Karadag AS, Ozlu E, Özkanlı S, Uzuncakmak TK, Akdeniz N. Two cases of lymphangioma circumscriptum successfully treated with pulsed dye laser and cryotherapy. Indian Dermatol Online J [Internet]. 2015;6(4):291–3. Available from: https://www.ncbi.nlm.nih.gov/pubmed/26225341.
41. Lai C-H, Hanson SG, Mallory SB. Lymphangioma circumscriptum treated with pulsed dye laser. Pediatr Dermatol [Internet]. 2001 Nov 1;18(6):509–10. Available from: https://doi.org/10.1046/j.1525-1470.2001.1862001.x
42. Boccara O, Ariche-Maman S, Hadj-Rabia S, Chrétien-Marquet B, Frassati-Biaggi A, Zazurca F, Brunelle F, Soupre V, Bodemer C, Fraitag S. Verrucous hemangioma (also known as verrucous venous malformation): a vascular anomaly frequently misdiagnosed as a lymphatic malformation. Pediatr Dermatol [Internet]. 2018 Nov 1;35(6):e378–81. Available from: https://doi.org/10.1111/pde.13671
43. Laun K, Laun J, Smith D. Verrucous hemangioma. Eplasty [Internet]. 2019 Jan 7;19:ic1.
44. Madan V, August PJ, Ferguson JE. Pulsed-dye laser treatment of angioma serpiginosum. Clin Exp Dermatol. 2009 Jul;34(5):e186–8.
45. Long CC, Lanigan SW. Treatment of angioma serpiginosum using a pulsed tunable dye laser. Br J Dermatol. 1997 Apr;136(4):631–2.
46. Munden A, Butschek R, Tom WL, Marshall JS, Poeltler DM, Krohne SE, Alió AB, Ritter M, Friedlander DF, Catanzarite V, Mendoza A, Smith L, Friedlander M, Friedlander SF. Prospective study of infantile haemangiomas: incidence, clinical characteristics and association with placental anomalies. Br J Dermatol [Internet]. 2014 Apr;170(4):907–13. Available from: https://www.ncbi.nlm.nih.gov/pubmed/24641194.
47. Cordisco MR. Hemangiomas of infancy: epidemiology BT – hemangiomas and vascular malformations: an atlas of diagnosis and treatment. In: Mattassi R, loose DA, Vaghi M, editors. Milano: Springer Milan; 2009. pp. 17–21. Available from: https://doi.org/10.1007/978-88-470-0569-3_3.
48. Zheng JW, Zhang L, Zhou Q, Mai HM, Wang YA, Fan XD, Qin ZP, Wang XK, Zhao YF. A practical guide to treatment of infantile hemangiomas of the head and neck. Int J Clin Exp Med [Internet]. 2013 Oct 25;6(10):851–60.
49. Drolet BA, Frommelt PC, Chamlin SL, Haggstrom A, Bauman NM, Chiu YE, Chun RH, Garzon MC, Holland KE, Liberman L, MacLellan-Tobert S, Mancini AJ, Metry D, Puttgen KB, Seefeldt M, Sidbury R, Ward KM, Blei F, Baselga E, Cassidy L, Darrow DH, Joachim S, Kwon E-KM, Martin K, Perkins J, Siegel DH, Boucek RJ, Frieden IJ. Initiation and use of propranolol for infantile hemangioma: report of a consensus conference. Pediatrics. 2013 Jan;131(1):128–40.
50. Reddy KK, Blei F, Brauer JA, Waner M, Anolik R, Bernstein L, Brightman L, Hale E, Karen J, Weiss E, Geronemus RG. Retrospective study of the treatment of infantile hemangiomas using a combination of propranolol and pulsed dye laser. Dermatol Surg. 2013 Jun;39(6):923–33.
51. Lacour M, Syed S, Linward J, Harper JI. Role of the pulsed dye laser in the management of ulcerated capillary haemangiomas. Arch Dis Child [Internet]. 1996

Feb;74(2):161–3. Available from: https://www.ncbi.nlm.nih.gov/pubmed/8660082.
52. Morelli JG, Tan OT, Weston WL. Treatment of ulcerated hemangiomas with the pulsed tunable dye laser. Am J Dis Child. 1991 Sep;145(9):1062–4.
53. David LR, Malek MM, Argenta LC. Efficacy of pulse dye laser therapy for the treatment of ulcerated haemangiomas: a review of 78 patients. Br J Plast Surg [Internet]. 2003;56(4):317–27. Available from: http://www.sciencedirect.com/science/article/pii/S0007122603001528.
54. Wirth FA, Lowitt MH. Diagnosis and treatment of cutaneous vascular lesions. Am Fam Physician. 1998 Feb;57(4):765–73.
55. Cerrati EW, O TM, Chung H, Waner M. Diode laser for the treatment of telangiectases following hemangioma involution. Otolaryngol Head Neck Surg. 2015 Feb;152(2):239–43.
56. Rai S, Kaur M, Bhatnagar P. Laser: a powerful tool for treatment of pyogenic granuloma. J Cutan Aesthet Surg [Internet]. 2011 May;4(2):144–7. Available from: https://www.ncbi.nlm.nih.gov/pubmed/21976910.
57. Tay Y-K, Weston WL, Morelli JG. Treatment of pyogenic granuloma in children with the flashlamp-pumped pulsed dye laser. Pediatrics [Internet]. 1997 Mar 1;99(3):368LP–370. Available from: http://pediatrics.aappublications.org/content/99/3/368.abstract
58. The Birthmark Unit GOSH. Congenital haemangioma [Internet]. 2018 [Cited 2019 Oct 2].
59. de Sa KC, Martins MG, da Costa CA, Barbosa JLV, da Rosa Righi R. A mapping study on Mobile games for patients of chronic diseases. J Med Syst. 2017 Sep;41(9):138.
60. Mahendran R, White SI, Clark AH, Sheehan-Dare RA. Response of childhood tufted angioma to the pulsed-dye laser. J Am Acad Dermatol. 2002 Oct;47(4):620–2.
61. Georgesco G, Lorette G. Cutis marmorata telangiectatica congenita. Presse Med. 2010 Apr;39(4):495–8.
62. van Raath MI, Bambach CA, Dijksman LM, Wolkerstorfer A, Heger M. Prospective analysis of the port-wine stain patient population in the Netherlands in light of novel treatment modalities. J Cosmet Laser Ther [Internet]. 2018 Feb 17;20(2):77–84. https://doi.org/10.1080/14764172.2017.1368669.
63. Ortiz AE, Nelson JS. Port-wine stain laser treatments and novel approaches. Facial Plast Surg. 2012 Dec;28(6):611–20.
64. Savas JA, Ledon JA, Franca K, Chacon A, Nouri K. Pulsed dye laser-resistant port-wine stains: mechanisms of resistance and implications for treatment. Br J Dermatol. 2013 May;168(5):941–53.
65. Griffin TDJ, Foshee JP, Finney R, Saedi N. Port wine stain treated with a combination of pulsed dye laser and topical rapamycin ointment. Lasers Surg Med. 2016 Feb;48(2):193–6.
66. Lipner SR. Topical adjuncts to Pulsed Dye Laser for treatment of port wine Stains: review of the literature. Dermatol Surg. 2018;44(6):796–802.
67. Zhao Y, Tu P, Zhou G, et al. Hemoporfin photodynamic therapy for port-wine stain: a randomized controlled trial. PLoS One. 2016 26;11(5):e0156219.
68. van Drooge AM, Beek JF, van der Veen JP, et al. Hypertrophy in port-wine stains: prevalence and patient characteristics in a large patient cohort. J Am Acad Dermatol. 2012;67(6):1214–9.
69. Neuhaus IM, Zane LT, Tope WD. Comparative efficacy of nonpurpuragenic pulsed dye laser and intense pulsed light for erythematotelangiectatic rosacea. Dermatol Surg. 2009;35(6):920–8.
70. Tanghetti EA. Split-face randomized treatment of facial telangiectasia comparing pulsed dye laser and an intense pulsed light handpiece. Lasers Surg Med. 2012 Feb;44(2):97–102.
71. Schilling LM, Halvorson CR, Weiss RA, et al. Safety of combination Laser or intense Pulsed light therapies and doxycycline for the treatment of Rosacea. Dermatol Surg. 2019;45(11):1401–5.
72. Suggs AK, Macri A, Richmond H, Munavalli G, Friedman PM. Treatment of erythematotelangiectatic rosacea with pulsed-dye laser and oxymetazoline 1.0% cream: a retrospective study. Lasers Surg Med. 2019 Nov 10. https://doi.org/10.1002/lsm.23176. [Epub ahead of print].
73. Klein A, Buschmann M, Babilas P, Landthaler M, Bäumler W. Indocyanine green-augmented diode laser therapy vs. long-pulsed Nd:YAG (1064 nm) laser treatment of telangiectatic leg veins: a randomized controlled trial. Br J Dermatol. 2013;169(2):365–73.
74. Parlar B, Blazek C, Cazzaniga S, Naldi L, et al. Treatment of lower extremity telangiectasias in women by foam sclerotherapy vs. Nd:YAG laser: a prospective, comparative, randomized, open-label trial. J Eur Acad Dermatol Venereol. 2015 Mar;29(3):549–54.
75. Meesters AA, Pitassi LH, Campos V, Wolkerstorfer A, Dierickx CC. Transcutaneous laser treatment of leg veins. Lasers Med Sci. 2014 Mar;29(2):481–92.
76. Hsu VM, Aldahan AS, Tsatalis JP, et al. Efficacy of Nd:YAG laser therapy for the treatment of verrucae: a literature review. Lasers Med Sci. 2017 Jul;32(5):1207–11.
77. Veitch D, Kravvas G, Al-Niaimi F. Pulsed Dye Laser therapy in the treatment of warts: a review of the literature. Dermatol Surg. 2017 Apr;43(4):485–93.
78. Gheisari M, Iranmanesh B, Nobari NN, Amani M. Comparison of long-pulsed Nd: YAG laser with cryotherapy in treatment of acral warts. Lasers Med Sci. 2019 Mar;34(2):397–403.
79. Mlacker S, Shah VV, Aldahan AS, et al. Laser and light-based treatments of venous lakes: a literature review. Lasers Med Sci. 2016;31(7):1511–9.
80. Vazquez-Martinez O, Eichelmann K, Garcia-Melendez M, et al. Pulsed Dye Laser for early treatment of scars after dermatological surgery. J Drugs Dermatol. 2015 Nov;14(11):1209–12.
81. Manuskiatti W, Wanitphakdeedecha R, Fitzpatrick RE. Effect of pulse width of a 595-nm flashlamp-pumped pulsed dye laser on the treatment response of

keloidal and hypertrophic sternotomy scars. Dermatol Surg. 2007 Feb;33(2):152–61.
82. Stephanides S, Rai S, August P, Ferguson J, Madan V. Treatment of refractory keloids with pulsed dye laser alone and with rotational pulsed dye laser and intralesional corticosteroids: a retrospective case series. Laser Ther. 2011;20(4):279–86.
83. Erceg A, de Jong EM, van de Kerkhof PC, Seyger MM. The efficacy of pulsed dye laser treatment for inflammatory skin diseases: a systematic review. J Am Acad Dermatol. 2013 Oct;69(4):609–15.
84. Brightman LA, Geronemus RG, Reddy KK. Laser treatment of port-wine stains. Clin Cosmet Investig Dermatol. 2015 Jan;8:27–33.
85. Grunebaum LD, Bartlett K. Complications of vascular laser treatment. Aesthetic Dermatol [Internet]. 2014; 1:121–42. Available from: https://www.karger.com/DOI/10.1159/000355061

Pigment Specific Lasers and Light Devices

3

Sanjeev Aurangabadkar

Introduction

Pigmented lesions are commonly encountered in dermatology practice and pose a significant challenge to the treating dermatologist. While some hyperpigmented conditions such as post-inflammatory hyperpigmentation (PIH), melasma, etc. are best managed with topical interventions, the results are unpredictable and usually unsatisfactory; others such as naevus of Ota do not respond to topical therapy.

Skin of colour ages differently from Caucasian skin and is more prone to pigmentary alterations such as development of lentigines, pigmented seborrhoeic keratoses and dermatosis papulosa nigra (DPN). These conditions require dermatosurgical interventions as they don't respond to topical treatments.

The last decade has seen technological advancements, with new laser systems being developed that are more effective and with a favorable safety profile even in darker skin types. Q-switched (QS) lasers (Q-switched = Quality switched or Quantum switched), which produce very high peak powers in ultra-short durations of time (5–100 nanoseconds), are the mainstay lasers for treatment of pigmented lesions/conditions. Picosecond lasers (mode-locking lasers) are the new entrants in the field that show a great deal of potential in the management of pigmentary disorders.

S. Aurangabadkar (✉)
Dr. Aurangabadkar's Skin & Laser Clinic Green Lands, Begumpet, Hyderabad, Telangana, India

History

Ruby laser 694 nm was the first laser used to treat pigmented lesions and tattoos in humans by Goldman between the years 1963 and 1967. The first QS laser developed was the Ruby, followed by the neodymium: yttrium-aluminum-garnet (Nd:YAG) and alexandrite lasers. Polla et al., Dover et al. and Hruza et al. between the years 1987 and 1991 demonstrated the highly selective cellular damage occurring in melanin-containing cells following QS laser therapy [1–4].

Laser Basics and Systems

Melanin absorbs wavelength range between 290 nm up 1200 nm. At longer wavelengths, absorption is lower and the penetration is deeper (Fig. 1.34, Chap. 1). QS lasers produce ultra-short bursts of light in the nanosecond range and target melanin and ink particles in the dermis allowing removal or lightening of benign pigmented lesions and tattoos respectively [1–4].

A wavelength that penetrates 2–3 mm into the dermis is suitable for targeting deeper dermal pigmentation such as naevus of Ota. QS Nd:YAG laser with a wavelength of 1064 nm meets this

V. Madan (ed.), *Practical Introduction to Laser Dermatology*,
https://doi.org/10.1007/978-3-030-46451-6_3

requirement adequately. By passing the beam through the potassium titanyl phosphate (KTP) crystal, the frequency is doubled and the wavelength is halved (532 nm). A shorter wavelength penetrates less deeply and therefore is more useful for removal of epidermal pigment such as in ephelides. The Ruby laser (694 nm) penetrates less than 1 mm into skin and is used for treating superficial lesions such as freckles or café-au-lait macules (CALM). However, because of its high affinity for melanin and the possible risk of hypopigmentation, the QS Ruby laser should be used with extreme caution in darker skin patients. . The QS alexandrite laser (755 nm) penetrates deeper than the Ruby laser due to its longer wavelength making it suitable for removal of both epidermal and dermal pigmented lesions and some tattoos.

Besides the QS lasers, long-pulsed (millisecond) lasers such as the Diode 810 nm, long-pulsed alexandrite 755 nm, and long pulsed, pulsed dye (595 nm) lasers etc. can also be used for treating certain pigmented lesions. The intense pulsed light (IPL) systems are polychromatic light sources that use cut-off filters to block shorter wavelengths, thus producing a broad band of IPL. These systems use wavelengths from 530 nm and above, and can be used to treat superficial pigmented lesions such as freckles, lentigines, but are not recommended for dermal lesions or tattoo removal [1–4].

Fractional photothermolysis, both ablative & non-ablative have been used to treat pigmented lesions. They primarily act by eliminating pigment transepidermally through the micro ablative columns (MAC) or the micro epidermal necrotic debris (MEND). These lasers are non-selective meaning they do not specifically target melanin but work by producing vaporization or coagulation of tissue followed by remodeling in the dermis [5]. Thulium 1927 nm laser has also been used in certain pigmented lesions such as melasma.

Other lasers such as copper bromide that targets the vascular component of melasma has shown some initial promising results [6]. Picosecond lasers that use pulse duration in the range of 10^{-12} of a second are the new generation of ultra-short pulse lasers are being increasingly used for pigmented lesions and tattoos.

Mechanism of Action of QS Lasers

Definition of Q-Switch or Quality Switch

Q switching is a method for obtaining energetic pulses from lasers by modulating the intracavity losses (Page 31, Chap. 1). It is a technique for obtaining energetic short pulses from a laser by modulating the intracavity losses, the so-called the *Q* factor of the laser resonator. The technique is mainly applied for the generation of nanosecond pulses of high energy and peak power with solid-state bulk lasers. These giant pulses are responsible for the unique laser-tissue interaction that is seen with QS lasers [7].

Q-switched lasers work on the principle of selective photothermolysis and also produce an additional photoacoustic effect producing shock waves that cause explosion of target [3]. Very high energy, to the tune of 300 megawatts, is delivered in a very short period of time (5–100 ns) which leads to rapid thermal expansion. This produces shock waves that rupture the targets such as melanosomes and ink particles [4]. The ruptured fragments are cleared by tissue macrophages either to the lymphatic channels or to the regional lymph nodes. Some fragments may be eliminated transepidermally. To be selective, the pulse duration of the laser should match the thermal relaxation time (TRT) of the target. The estimated TRT of epidermis is 1–10 ms and the TRT of tattoo ink particles is 0.1–10 ns, although some newer estimates are in the range of 10–100 picoseconds. The size of the tattoo ink particles is about 10–100 nm and is generally placed at a depth of 1.1–2.9 mm. Laser tissue interaction produces intracellular steam and vacuole formation, which leads to immediate whitening. An audible popping sound is heard during the procedure due to the photoacoustic effect.

Though Q switched lasers are considered 'gold standard' for pigmented lesions, subnanosecond lasers such as picosecond lasers are now available. The picoseconds pulse width is in the range of 10^{-12} of a second. This >10 fold reduction of pulse width may allow better targeting of the tiny melanosomes and tattoo ink particles whose TRT is in subnanosecond domain [8].

Both nanosecond and subnanosecond lasers are available in various wavelengths including 1064 nm, 532 nm, 755 nm, 585 nm, 660 nm etc. All these WLs may not be available in the same system but most new QSL & picosecond lasers systems offer multiple wavelengths. In addition, some newer laser systems have both nano & subnanosecond options in the same device.

Indications

Patient selection for laser treatment of pigmented lesions is important. Pigmented lesions can be classified based on the depth of pigment deposition in the skin. Woods lamp can aid in determining the depth of pigment. Dermoscopy is invaluable in distinguishing benign from premalignant and malignant lesions and can also provide valuable information regarding the morphology of the pigmented lesion. Whenever the clinical diagnosis is in doubt, a skin biopsy should be performed. Pigmented dermatological conditions which can be treated by lasers are listed in Table 3.1 [1–3].

Some pigmented lesions amenable to laser therapy are shown in Figs. 3.1, 3.2, 3.3, 3.4, 3.5, 3.6, 3.7.

Table 3.1 Pigmented lesions amenable to treatment by lasers [9]

- **Epidermal lesions***:* CALM, lentigines, ephelides, solar lentigines, naevus spilus, pigmented seborrhoeic keratosis, DPN
- **Dermal lesions:** Naevus of Ota, blue naevus, Hori's naevus (acquired bilateral naevus of Ota-like macules), Acquired dermal melanosis eg: Lichen planus pigmentosus (LPP)
- **Epidermal-dermal lesions:** Postinflammatory hyperpigmentation, periorbital pigmentation, perioral pigmentation, benign acquired melanocytic naevi (moles), melasma and Becker's naevi, Riehl's melanosis, poikiloderma of Civatte

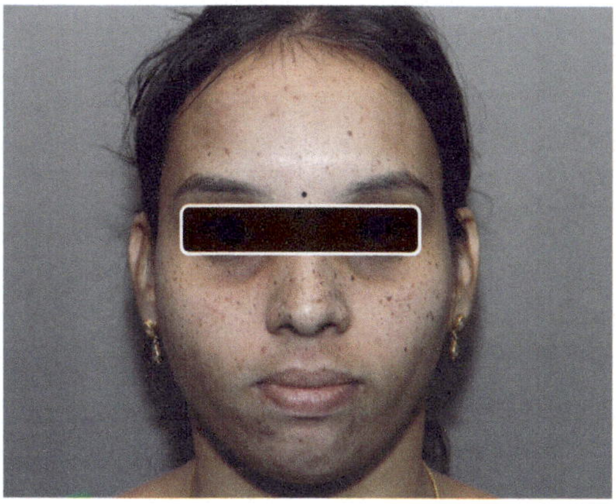

Fig. 3.1 Lentigines-centrofacial type

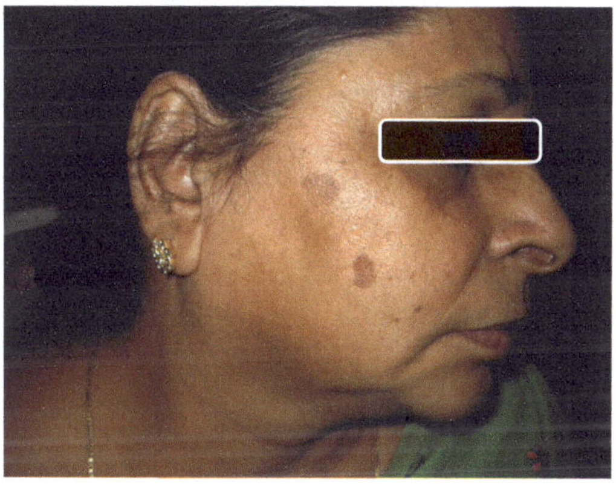

Fig. 3.2 Solar lentigos on the face

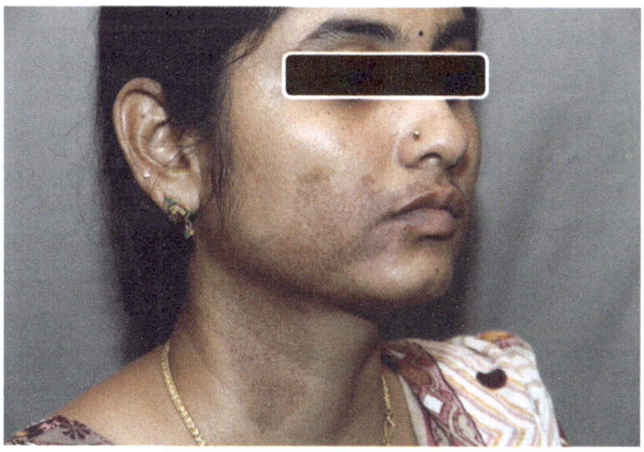

Fig. 3.3 Naevus Spilus

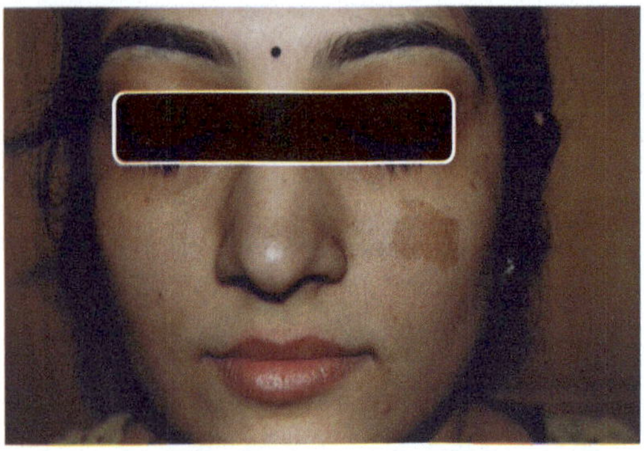

Fig. 3.4 Café au lait macule

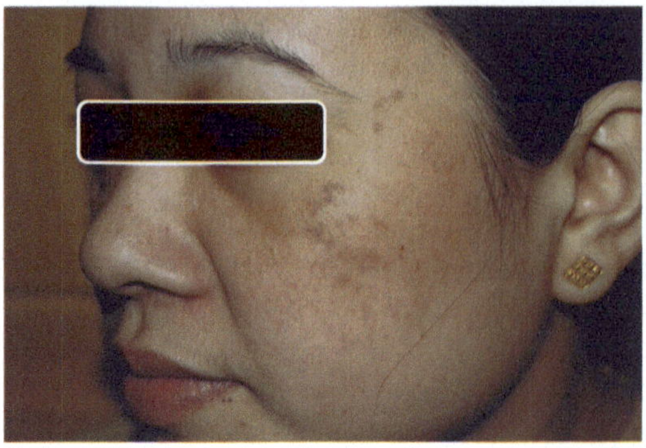

Fig. 3.7 Hori's Naevus

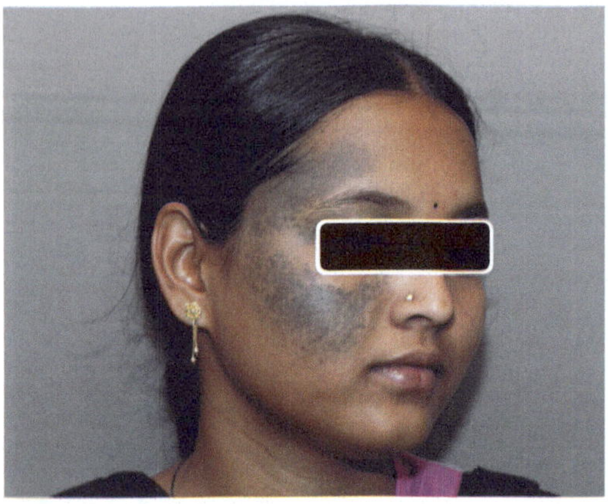

Fig. 3.5 Naevus of Ota

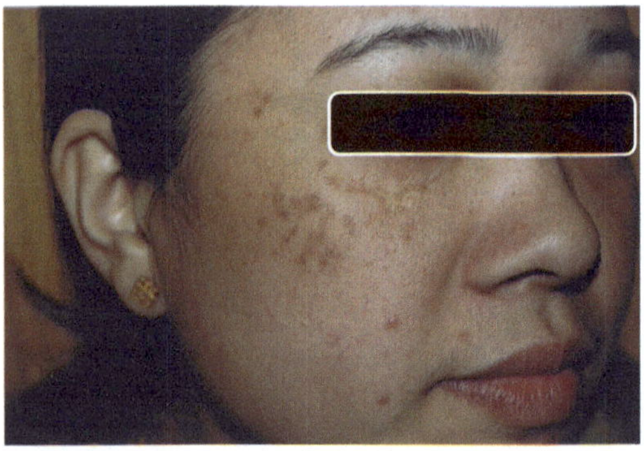

Fig. 3.6 Hori's Naevus; acquired bilateral naevus of Ota-like macules

Contraindications [10–12]

Not all pigmented lesions should be treated with lasers. The contraindications can be relative or absolute are listed hereunder.

Absolute Contraindications

- Dysplastic naevi (atypical pigmented lesions) or Melanomas
- Photoaggravated skin diseases and medical illness
- Active cutaneous infections in treatment zone, for example, herpes labialis, staphylococcal infections.
  - Unstable vitiligo and psoriasis for risk of koebnerization of treated area.
  - Pregnancy
  - Bleeding tendencies or disorders
    Medications that cause photosensitivity such as those used for photodynamic therapy (PDT), Minocycline, Doxycycline, Amiodarone, St. John's Wort. (Though minocycline and amiodarone induced pigmentation has been successfully treated with Q-switched lasers)

Relative Contraindications

In the following situations, laser has to be used with caution and should be dependent on individual patient's situation and on treating physician's experience.

- Keloidal tendency.
- Oral Isotretinoin—within 6 months (see below)
- History of herpes simplex/history of herpes for increased risk of reactivation within the treatment zone: This risk should be seriously considered prior to performing the procedure. If the treating physician decides to perform

the procedure, the risk and benefit should be explained to the patient and the procedure should be performed after proper informed consent and only after a course of acyclovir.
- Immunosuppressed patients, uncontrolled diabetes mellitus

Patient Selection and Counseling

Patient selection for laser treatment of pigmented lesions should be based on comprehensive current and past medical history, medications, allergies, previous treatments, and response to previous laser treatments [9].

Thorough counseling of the patient with informed and written consents and pretreatment and serial post treatment photographs should be considered mandatory [11–13].

Preoperative Preparation

Sun Protection

Laser treatment should be avoided on tanned skin. Epidermal melanin produced by ultraviolet (UV) light exposure may interfere with laser treatment and increase the risks for scarring, hypopigmentation or hyperpigmentation [9, 11, 13–16]. To check for tanning, it is wise to compare the color of the potential treatment site to that of an unexposed skin site, similar to the buttock or axilla. If a tan is present, treatment should be delayed until the tan has faded. Use of broad spectrum sun protection creams with UVA coverage is crucial. Protective clothing and bleaching creams can be useful in treating the tan. Patients with darker skin types and those with a tan may benefit from hydroquinone-containing compounds (2–4%) or other skin lightening agents preoperatively to minimize the risk of PIH [9].

Oral Retinoids

It has been recommended that patients on oral retinoid therapy should not undergo laser treatment of pigmented lesions and tattoos for 6–12 months following discontinuation of the medication, as they have an increased risk of keloidal scar formation [11–15]. Evidence to support such a recommendation particularly for epidermal lesions is lacking. However, caution is advised while treating patients with history of recent administration of isotretinoin.

Test Patch

A laser test patch is mandatory to determine the treatment parameters for all patients since skin type and colour do not always perfectly predict the response to treatment. It is also helpful in medico-legal situations. Always evaluate the patient 4–8 weeks after the test spots [9, 11, 13–16].

Eye Protection

Q-switched lasers produce ultra-short pulse durations that produce significant tissue splatter. QS laser beam can cause permanent retinal damage and vision loss [1, 2]. Precautions include protective clothing, goggles, masks and laser cone containment devices which should be used in each case. Eye protection in the form of optically coated glasses or goggles for the specific laser being used is necessary. All persons present in the room during laser treatment must also wear appropriate eye protection. The eye wear should block the wavelength being used and the lens should provide an optical density (OD) of at least four. Laser protective eye shields (anodized external metal eyecup) must be used when treating periorbital lesions. When treating eyelids, a metal corneal eye shield should be placed in situ to protect the globe (Table 3.2).

Anesthesia

Q-switched laser treatments usually does not require anesthesia. However, if a large area needs to be treated, topical anaesthetics such as Eutectic mixture of local anaesthetic (EMLA) or similar

Table 3.2 Checklist before laser therapy

• Right indication
• Counseling
• Rule out contraindication/s
• Sun protection and priming
Informed and written consent
Pretreatment photograph
Test patch
• Eye protection

should be applied under occlusion 1–2 h before the procedure [17, 18].

Hair Over the Treatment Area

It is best to shave the hair or trim the hair prior to laser therapy to prevent epidermal thermal injury. Q switched laser therapy tends to bleach the hair over the treated area due to the melanin present in the hair shaft but it has no impact on hair reduction as the depth of penetration is limited and fails to reach the hair bulge.

Laser Procedure

Selecting appropriate laser parameters depends upon the indication and patient's skin type. As a general rule, conservative parameters are recommended for darker skin types (longer wavelength, longer pulse width, lower fluence & larger spot size).

Fluence

It is always preferable to begin with the lowest fluence that produces a visible response. Fluence may be increased if response is suboptimal. If epidermal debris is significant, the fluence should be lowered [9, 11, 12, 16, 19–22]. **Fluence used is device specific** (not comparable across different devices) & manufacturers recommendations need to be kept in mind. This can be further tailored based on the individual situation.

Spot Size

The spot size which is just large enough to accommodate the treated lesion should be selected for epidermal lesions. While treating epidermal lesions, especially in darker individuals, it is important to avoid treating surrounding unaffected area to minimize pigmentary alterations. For dermal lesions, the spot size that elicits immediate brisk whitening on laser irradiation should be selected. Larger spot sizes allow deeper penetration and produce less tissue splatter [9–11].

Endpoint of Treatment

Appropriate endpoints are essential to ensure optimum outcome. With the QS laser, the endpoint of treatment is immediate whitening of the lesion as seen in Figs. 3.8 and 3.9. This is followed by erythema and oedema that subsides in a few hours as shown in Figs. 3.10 and 3.11. With an IPL, the endpoint is erythema. Higher fluences may produce pinpoint bleeding and blistering.

- Repetition rate: Choose higher frequency, i.e. 5–10 Hz while treating a large area. This would also depend upon the practitioner's experience. For smaller discrete lesions a frequency of 2–3 Hz gives better control [9].

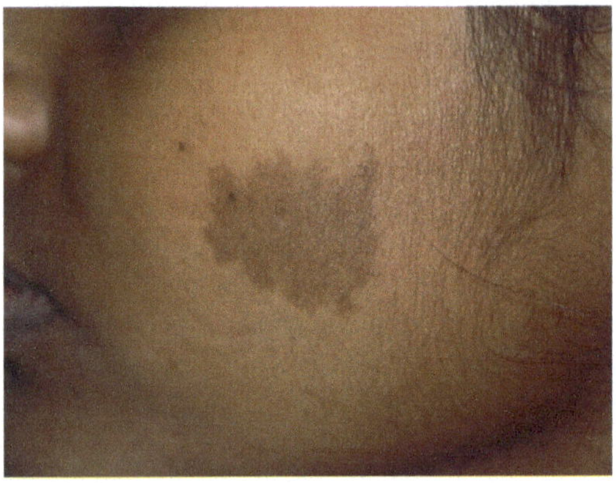

Fig. 3.8 A café au lait macule on the left cheek

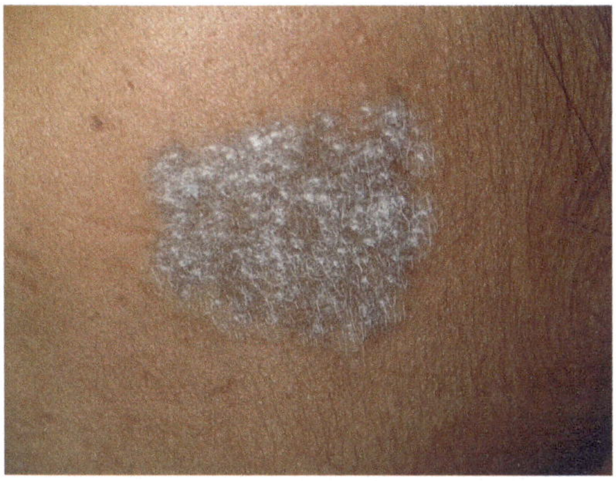

Fig. 3.9 Café au lait macule immediately following 532 nm QS ND:YAG laser showing the immediate whitening of the lesion

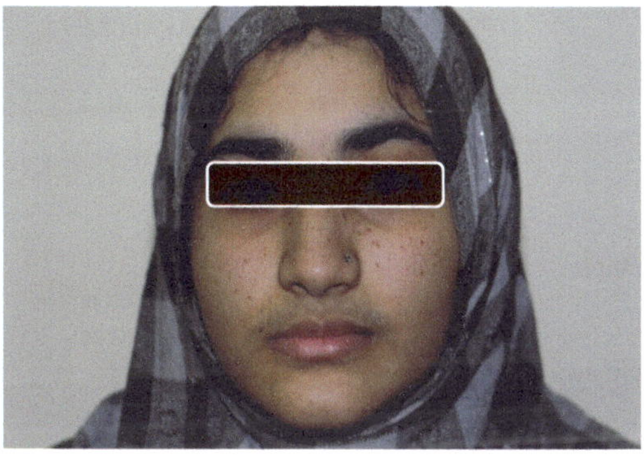

Fig. 3.10 Centro-facial lentiginosis before laser

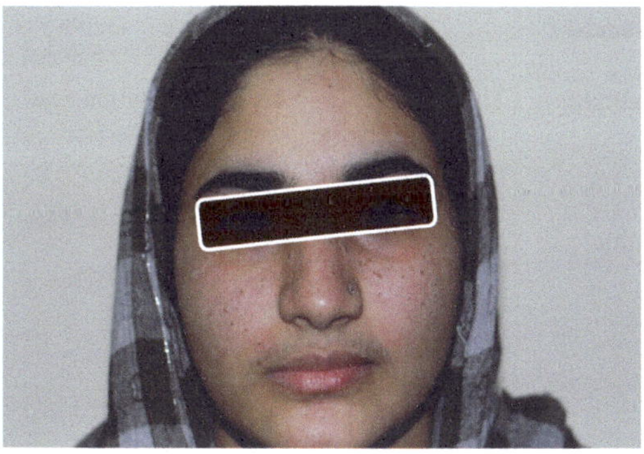

Fig. 3.11 Lentigines immediatedly after QS ND:YAG laser with 532 nm wavelength showing erythema & edema

Laser Technique

After choosing the correct spot size and fluence (J/cm^2), laser treatment is performed with the handpiece held perpendicular to the lesion and the entire area is covered with minimal overlap (up to 10%). QS laser treatment will produce an immediate whitening of the lesion. Pinpoint bleeding may occur if very high fluences and small spot sizes are used. The entire lesion is covered in one pass. A popping sound is heard with each laser shot as the cells containing melanin or ink particles explode. Laser pulses are placed close to each other with minimum overlap. The area is cooled with ice packs/air cooling (e.g. Zimmer) just before and after laser pulses to avoid a buildup of heat and to prevent collateral tissue damage.

Number of Sessions

This is dependent upon the indication however, for most epidermal lesions such as solar lentigenes one to two treatments may be sufficient; dermal lesions require 6 and 10 or even more sessions. Amateur tattoos may respond in less than 6 sessions where as multicoloured professional tattoos may require more than 20 sessions-even then complete clearance may not be possible.

Interval Between Sessions

Treatments should be undertaken at 6–8 weeks intervals. Treatment intervals of 3–6 months have been suggested for treating naevus of Ota. Continued clearance of the lesion occurs due to removal of pigment by macrophages and lymphatics between treatments. Optimal interval between treatments therefore needs to be determined on an individual basis [9, 11, 12, 16, 19–22].

Treatment of Pigmented Skin Lesions

Treatment depends on the type of lesion; epidermal lesions, dermal lesions, tattoos and mixed epidermal and dermal lesions. Table 3.3 summarizes the different indications and their treatment parameters.

Table 3.3 Summary of different indications and their treatment with lasers

Level of pigmentation	Condition	Wavelength used	Number of sessions	Remarks	Recommendations
Epidermal	Freckles and lentigines	QS 532 nm, 1064 nm, 755 nm, 660 nm QS IPL	1–3	Sun protection to avoid recurrence	QS lasers treatment of choice
	CALM	QS 532 nm (in lighter skin types)	Multiple	50% recurrence within a year	Use with caution as partial or incomplete clearance common
	Naevus spilus	532 nm	Multiple	Junctional and compound naevus components clear well, but CALM remains	Use with caution as partial or incomplete clearance common
	DPNs and seborrheic keratosis	Ablative lasers, QS lasers, long pulse lasers	1–3		
Dermal	Naevus of Ota	QS 1064 nm, 755 nm	Multiple	Recurrence uncommon though reported	QS 1064 nm is the preferred wavelength in darker skin types
	Hori's naevus	QS 1064 nm, 755 nm	Multiple		QS laser is treatment of choice
	Blue naevus	QS 1064 nm, 755 nm	Multiple		QS laser is treatment of choice
	Acquired dermal melanosis	QS 1064 nm	Multiple (average of 5–6 sessions)	Interval of 4–6 weeks	Initiate laser only after ensuring stability of the condition & withdraw any inciting factors
Mixed epidermal and dermal lesions	Becker's naevus	Long pulsed lasers and QS laser IPL, Ablative lasers	Multiple	Though many lasers have been tried, response is not satisfactory	Treat with caution, test patch recommended.
	Melasma	Fractional photothermolysis, IPL, QS lasers (low fluence QS laser), LED; 585 nm if vascular component suspected	Multiple	Response to laser unpredictable, medical management preferred	Use in selected resistant cases, test spots mandatory
	Naevocellular naevi	QS 532 nm, 755 nm, 1064 nm QS	1–3	Lesions must be dermoscopically assessed prior to treatment	QS lasers useful but treatment remains controversial
	Postinflammatory hyperpigmentation	532 nm, 1064 nm	Multiple	Response to laser unpredictable	Lasers of limited value, test spots recommended

Epidermal Lesions

Epidermal lesions respond readily to QS laser treatment. The wavelengths used include frequency doubled 532 nm QS Nd:YAG, 755 nm QS alexandrite, 1064 nm QS Nd:YAG. An average of 1–6 sessions is needed to clear most lesions. Recurrence is common after a few months to years, and patient needs to be advised regarding continued sun protection. The lesions can be retreated with QS laser without any additional risk. A spot size that is contained within the epidermal lesion should be used and the lesion treated with a single pass with minimal overlap. The QS 532 nm laser is to be used with caution in dark skin types and test spots are recommended.

Café-au-Lait Macules

Café-au-lait macules (CALM) are light to tan brown hypermelanotic flat lesions. The size varies 2–20 cm and is sharply demarcated from the surrounding normal skin. CALM are difficult to treat and usually require multiple treatments over months to years. Laser treatment may result in partial or incomplete clearance and recurrences are common, occurring in up to 50% of patients within a year of clearance. The preferred wavelength used is 532 nm particularly in light-skinned individuals. Risk of pigmentary alteration is higher in darker individuals, particularly a speckled pattern of hyperpigmentation [23–25].

Figure 3.12 shows a CALM on the right upper lip and cheek before treatment, while Fig. 3.13 shows CALM post four 1064 nm and 532 nm QS Nd:YAG laser sessions showing good lightening of the lesion.

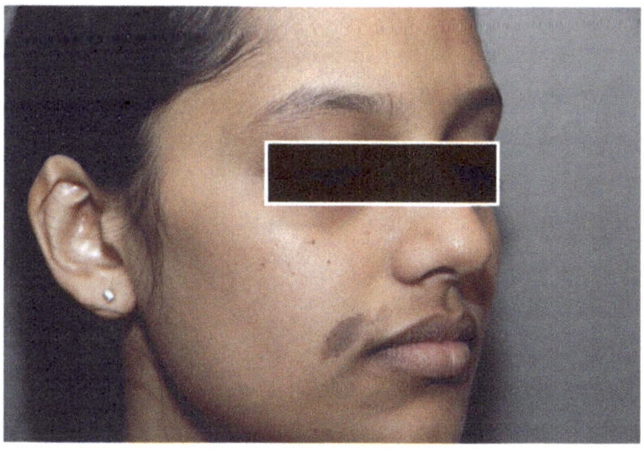

Fig. 3.12 CALM on the right cheek & upper lip before treatment with blend of 1064 nm & 532 nm QS Nd:YAG laser in same session

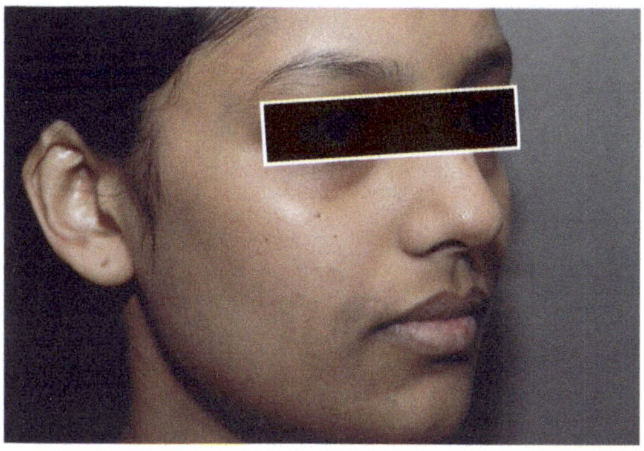

Fig. 3.13 CALM after four QS laser sessions showing significant lightening

Lentigines/Solar Lentigo

Lentigines are small, round to oval dark macules that may occur on any cutaneous surface including mucous membranes. They usually measure a few millimeters in diameter. Lentigines can usually be removed completely in 1–3 treatments with the 532 nm QS Nd:YAG laser. In darker patients, the 1064 nm QS Nd:YAG laser can also be used. The treatment of the lentigines found on the mucosal surface in Peutz-Jeghers syndrome may produce equally good results as those found on the skin surface. Treatment with Q-switched lasers is more effective than with other modalities such as liquid nitrogen, 35% trichloroacetic acid and glycolic acid peels [23, 26–32].

Figures 3.14 and 3.15 show a solar lentigo on the nose of an elderly woman, before and after a single 532 nm QS Nd:YAG laser treatment. Figures 3.16 and 3.17 show a case of segmental lentiginosis before and after 5 sessions with a 1064 nm QS Nd:YAG laser.

Freckles

Freckles are small brown macules that occur on sun-exposed skin and darken in color on exposure to sunlight. Histology shows normal epidermis without elongation or branching of rete ridges. The number of melanocytes is normal with hypermelanization confined to the basal layers. Melanosomes are larger with more active and

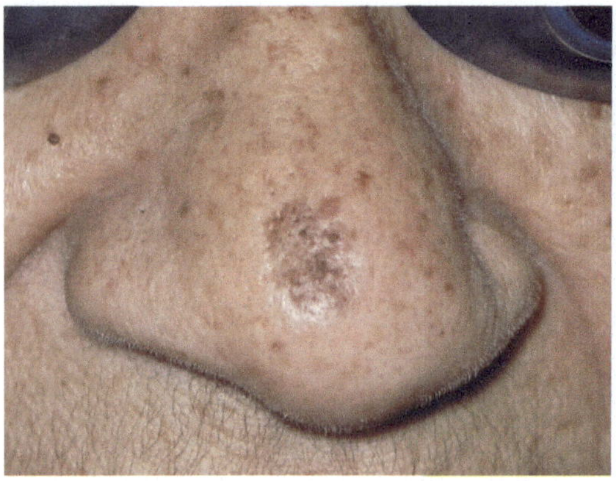

Fig. 3.14 Solar lentigo on the nose

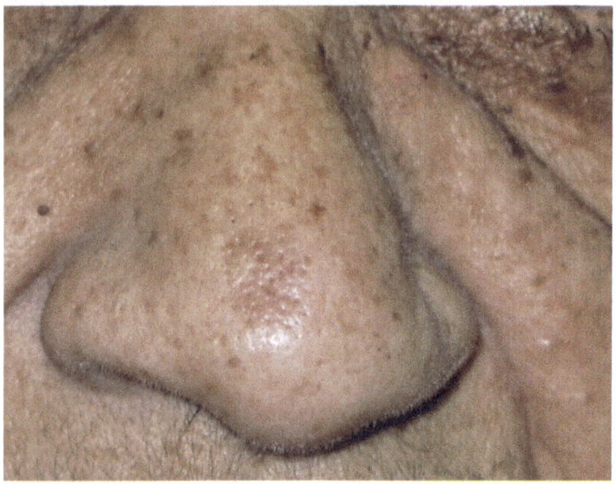

Fig. 3.15 Solar lentigo on the nose showing good clearing post one 532 nm QS Nd:YAG laser treatment

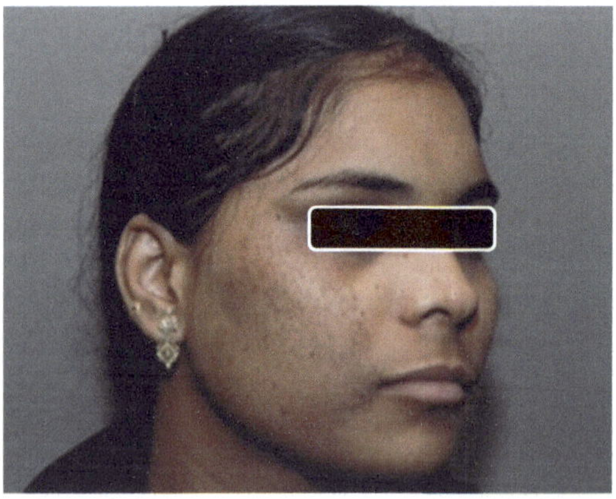

Fig. 3.16 Segmental lentiginosis

larger melanocytes. They respond very well to 532 nm QS lasers with most lesions clearing in 1–2 sessions [23, 27, 33]. Despite adequate initial clearance, freckles can recur after treatment and may require maintenance treatments . Need for adequate sun protection should be emphasized during counseling.

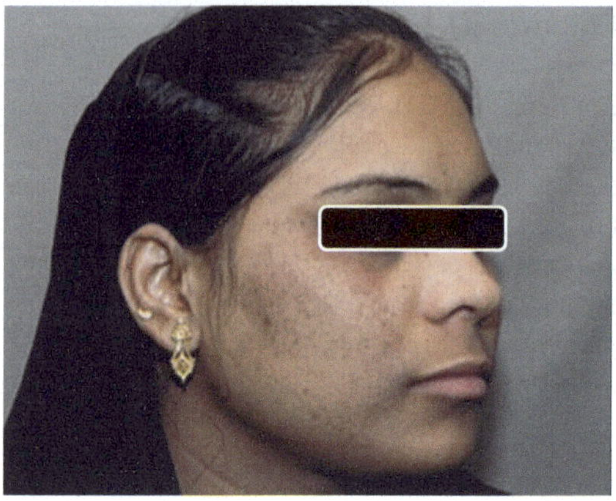

Fig. 3.17 Segmental lentiginosis post 5 sessions with QS Nd:YAG 532 nm laser

Naevus Spilus

Darker speckles of flat or raised hyperpigmentation on a background of café au lait macule are seen in naevus spilus. Histology shows lentiginous elongation and hyperpigmentation of the rete with increase in melanocytes. There may be nesting of naevus cells within the lesions. The darker speckles are either junctional or compound naevi. Since naevus spilus has a dual component of pigmentation, the entire lesion may not respond uniformly to the laser treatment. The darker macular lesions (junctional or compound melanocytic naevus component) tend to respond better than the lighter component café-au-lait macule (CALM) to the 532 nm QS Nd:YAG laser treatment. Partial or complete clearance has been reported with the use of Q-switched lasers, long-pulsed lasers and IPLs [34–37].

Figures 3.18 and 3.19 show a naevus spilus before and after 532 nm QS Nd:YAG laser treatment.

Dermatosis Papulosa Nigra and Pigmented Seborrheic Keratoses

These lesions have significant epidermal proliferation with normal to slightly increased number of melanocytes and increased melanization of

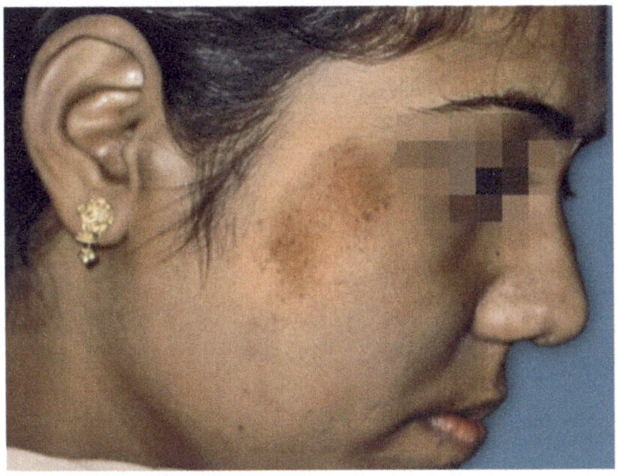

Fig. 3.18 Naevus spilus before treatment

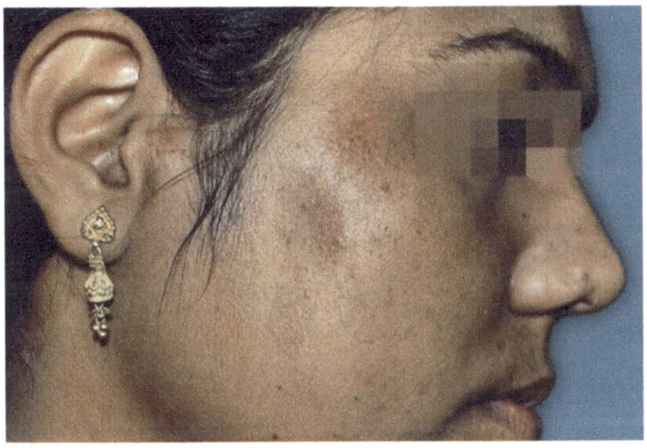

Fig. 3.19 Naevus spilus after 3 sessions with QS Nd:YAG laser at 532 nm

keratinocytes. These lesions can be readily treated by ablative devices such as ultra-pulsed carbon dioxide laser, Erbium: YAG laser, radio frequency (RF) devices and electrodessication. The QS lasers and long-pulsed lasers that target melanin can also be used to treat these lesions. Laser spot size should be limited to just below the size of the lesion. Ablative laser treatments are preferred as they produce consistently good results [38–40].

Dermal Lesions

Dermal melanosis can be broadly divided into two categories; congenital or acquired. Naevus of Ota, naevus of Ito, blue naevus, Mongolian spots etc. are congenital in nature but naevus of Ota can appear later in life. Hori's naevus (acquired bilateral naevus of Ota like macules), dermal melasma, lichen planus pigmentosus etc. are typically acquired later in life. Histologically, these lesions have melanin granules in the dermis, in melanophages or in nevoid cells. The chromophore for the laser treatment of dermal lesions includes melanin in melanosomes and ink particles, and other pigments that are located in the extracellular matrix or in melanophages. The longer wavelengths, such as 1064 nm Nd:YAG, allow deeper penetration to target these pigments with minimal damage to the overlying epidermis. Multiple sessions are required to clear the dermal lesions optimally, with an interval of at least 6–8 weeks between sessions. Recurrences are uncommon after complete clearing.

Naevus of Ota

Naevus of Ota, also known as oculodermal naevus, is an acquired bluish gray persistent macular lesion that occurs on the face in the area innervated by the first and second division of the trigeminal nerve [6, 17, 18, 38–52]. It is often associated with ipsilateral ocular pigmentation. Histological examination shows bipolar long, slender dermal melanocytes scattered largely in the upper dermis. The epidermis is usually normal, but focal basal hyperpigmentation may be seen.

Naevus of Ota readily responds to QS laser treatment. The longer wavelength 1064 nm QS Nd:YAG laser is the most widely used laser to treat, especially in darker skin types. The longer 1064 nm wavelength along with a large spot size allows deep penetration of photons and is ideally suited to treat this dermal condition. Multiple treatments are necessary (typically 6–10 sessions) with an interval of at least 2–6 months between treatments. Postinflammatory hyperpigmentation (PIH) and hypopigmentation are common problem in darker skin patients and good preoperative and postoperative care is necessary to minimize these side effects. The PIH usually clears within a few weeks, without scarring [41–55].

Figures 3.20 and 3.21 show a naevus of Ota on the left cheek before and after ten 1064 nm QS Nd:YAG laser treatments. Figures 3.22 and 3.23

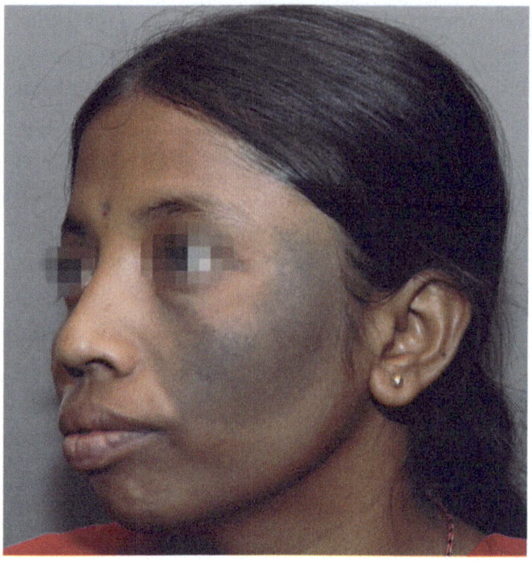

Fig. 3.20 Naevus of Ota on the left cheek

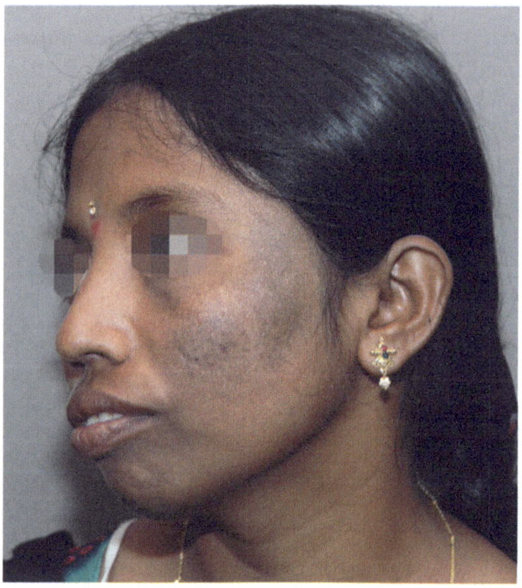

Fig. 3.21 Naevus of Ota after eight 1064 nm QS laser sessions

show another case of naevus of Ota in a patient of skin type V before and after QS Nd:YAG laser treatment.

Naevus of Ito

Naevus of Ito is a grayish blue macular hyperpigmentation seen on the shoulder or upper arm in the area innervated by the posterior supraclavicular and lateral brachial cutaneous nerves. The lesion responds well to 1064 nm QS Nd:YAG laser [9].

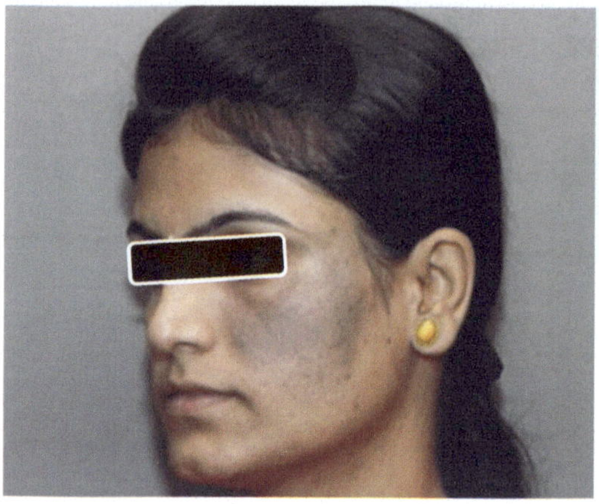

Fig. 3.22 Naevus of Ota before laser therapy

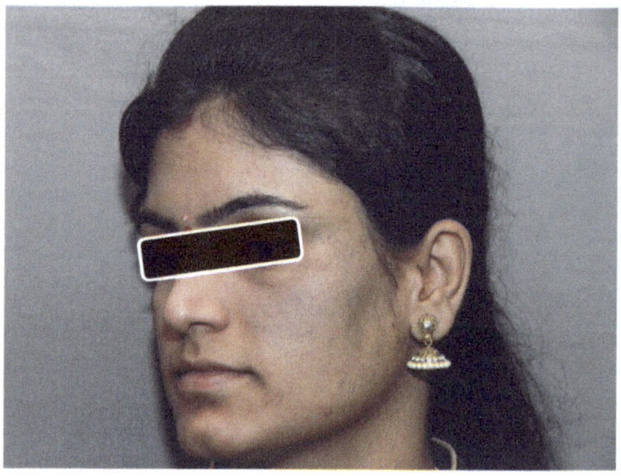

Fig. 3.23 Naevus of Ota after 61,064 nm QS ND:YAG laser sessions

Hori's Naevus (Acquired Bilateral Naevus of Ota-like Macules)

Acquired bilateral naevus of Ota-like macules or Hori's macules can mimic naevus of Ota. Late age of onset, bilateral nature of lesions, symmetry and absence of mucosal involvement are features that differentiate Hori's naevus from bilateral naevus of Ota and melasma. It is amenable to treatment by longer wavelength QS lasers [56–59]. An average of 5–6 sessions are needed for good response with an interval of 4–6 weeks.

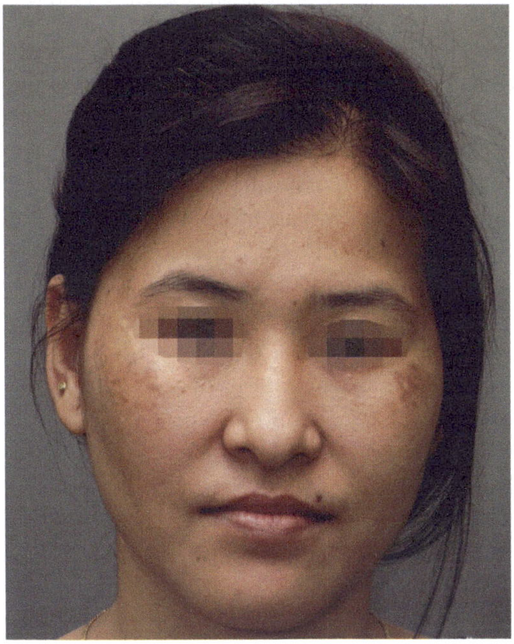

Fig. 3.24 Hori's Naevus

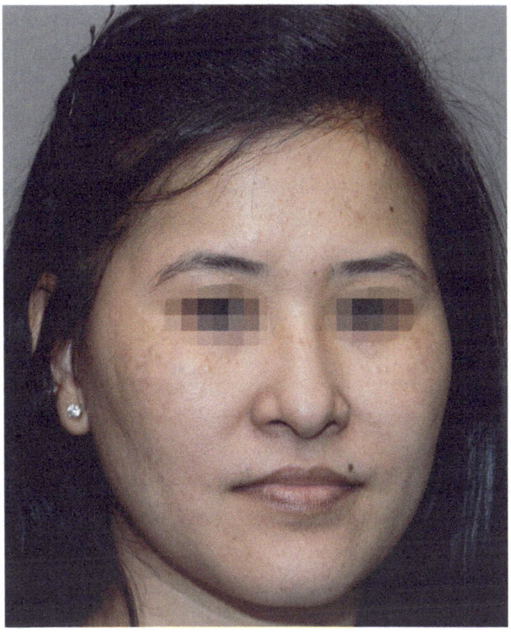

Fig. 3.25 After 5 sessions of QS ND:YAG laser at 1064 nm

Figures 3.24 and 3.25 show a case of Hori's naevus before and after QS Nd:YAG laser treatment.

Blue Naevi

Blue naevi are characterized by presence of melanocytes deep within the dermis and their blue-black color is a Tyndall effect reflected from the overlying tissues. Like naevi of Ota and Ito, blue naevi respond readily to 1064 nm QS Nd:YAG laser treatment. Lesions that extend into the subcutaneous fat are more difficult to treat [60]. Suspicious blue naevi should be excised for histology.

Mixed Epidermal and Dermal Pigmentation

Melasma

Melasma is an acquired, usually symmetrical and bilateral facial hypermelanosis. Histologically, melasma can be classified as epidermal, dermal or mixed types. Wood's light is useful in clinical assessment of the type of melasma. Epidermal melasma is enhanced on examination with Wood's light whereas dermal melasma does not show enhancement of pigmentation [61].

In epidermal melasma, the melanin deposition is seen in the basal and suprabasal layers and the melanocytes are found to contain highly melanized melanosomes. In dermal melasma, melanophages are seen in the superficial and deep dermis along with epidermal hyperpigmentation [62].

Melasma is best treated medically. Sun protection, short course fixed triple combination creams, hydroquinone (HQ) and non-HQ compounds being the mainstay of therapy. Lasers have a limited role in the treatment of melasma [6]. Lasers can be used to cause thermal destruction of melanosomes as well as elimination of epidermal pigment by resurfacing. Although successful use of QS lasers, fractional lasers, IPL and combination lasers have all been reported, response to treatment is unpredictable, and pigmentation frequently recurs. Postinflammatory hyperpigmentation is commonly seen in darker skin patients. For these reasons, lasers are not routinely recommended for treating melasma in dark skin patients. Lasers may be used in selected resistant cases, at the discretion of the treating physician, after proper counseling. A test patch should be performed prior to treating the lesion [63–68].

Recently the concept of subcellular selective photothermolysis has emerged. By using lower fluences with the QS lasers, only the organelles, such as melanosomes, are targeted thereby destroying the intracellular organelles and preventing destruction of the melanocytes. This also helps to reduce the risk of complications such as postinflammatory hyperpigmentation and hypopigmentation [69, 70]. Weekly sessions of low fluence QS Nd:YAG laser, up to 10 sessions has been used to successfully treat melasma.

The traditional QS ND:YAG laser treatment is based upon principle of selective photothermolysis which results in destruction and death of pigment containing cell [3]. As a response to this, inflammation ensues and can result in repigmentation and recurrence. The high peak power, ultrashort pulse duration [5 ns], and flat top beam results in destruction of only melanin in target cell but leaving the cell alive which could be explained by the concept of *Subcellular Selective Photothermolysis* discussed above [71].

Since low fluence is used and there is no cell death, inflammation and heating is kept to a minimum which leads to less recurrence.

A number of studies have reported the use of low-fluence QS Nd:YAG laser treatment (laser toning) at weekly intervals for 8–10 sessions with some success. Though effective, the risk of mottled hypopigmentation following multiple QS Nd:YAG laser sessions at frequent intervals has been reported in literature. Hence caution needs to be exercised while performing this procedure and the risks need to be explained to patients. Modified laser toning with low fluence and large spot size of 8–10 mm with treatments performed once in 2 weeks instead of weekly treatments for 6–8 sessions is better as it decreases the risk of hypopigmentation. Recurrence rates as high as 81% are very high after discontinuing the procedure have been reported [72].

Tranexamic acid, a lysine analogue, is a new addition in treatment of melasma and is effective in dosage of 250 mg BD for at least 4 to 8 weeks [73].

Tranexamic acid acts mainly via the plasminogen activator-plasmin system to prevent UV radiation induced pigmentation in melasma. Tranexamic acid prevents UV-induced pigmentation by interfering with the structure of plasminogen and preventing the binding of plasminogen to the lysine-binding sites of keratinocytes. The consequences of such event are less free arachidonic acid leading to a reduced ability to produce prostaglandins and thus decreased melanocyte tyrosinase activity and melanogenesis. This in turn helps reduce melasma. Tranexamic acid can be combined with lasers and light sources such as IPL or QS Nd:YAG laser.

Table 3.4 highlights the current literature evidence for lasers in melasma.

Figures 3.26 and 3.27 show melasma before and after 10 weekly low fluence 1064 nm QS Nd:YAG laser sessions demonstrating good improvement.

Table 3.4 Summary of recent studies on lasers in melasma [72, 74]

Journal	Title & authors	Conclusion	Remarks
Lasers Med Sci. 2016 Jul 23 [103]	Efficacy and safety of fractional Q-switched 1064-nm neodymium-doped yttrium aluminum garnet laser in the treatment of melasma in Chinese patients. Yue B, Yang Q, Xu J, Lu Z	The fractional mode (Pixel) QS Nd:YAG 1064-nm laser is an effective and safe treatment for melasma. The recurrence rate was relatively lower than that reported in studies treating with large-spot low-fluence QS Nd:YAG laser.	The lower recurrence could be due to lesser thermal effect due to use of fractionated beam
J Cosmet Dermatol. 2016 Jun 28 [69]	Long-term results in low-fluence 1064-nm Q-Switched Nd:YAG laser for melasma: Is it effective? Gokalp H, Akkaya AD, Oram Y	The recurrence of low-fluence 1064-nm QS-Nd:YAG laser rates in melasma was high when the long-term results were considered.	This result may be attributed to certain patient and treatment-related factors.

Table 3.4 (continued)

Journal	Title & authors	Conclusion	Remarks
Ann Dermatol. 2016 Jun;28 [70]	Treatment of Melasma with the Photoacoustic Twin Pulse Mode of Low-Fluence 1064 nm Q-Switched Nd:YAG Laser. Kim JY, Choi M, Nam CH, Kim JS, Kim MH, Park BC, Hong SP	After 5 sessions of laser therapy alone, about 60% of the subjects showed significant improvement. Few sessions of repeated laser toning treatment using the PTP mode is a safe and effective way to treat facial melasma.	PTP involves splitting of the laser pulse in to two with an interval of 100 microseconds between the two pulses. The energy is divided into half rather than a single high peak energy pulse.
Skin Therapy Lett. 2016 Jan [104]	Melasma and Post Inflammatory Hyperpigmentation: Management Update and Expert Opinion. Sofen B, Prado G, Emer J	Combining topical therapy with procedures such as chemical peels, intense pulsed light (IPL), fractional non-ablative lasers or radiofrequency, pigment lasers (microsecond, picosecond, Q-switched), and microneedling, enhances results. With proper treatment, melasma can be controlled, improved, and maintained.	Combining medical therapy with procedures enhances results in melasma
Dermatol Surg. 2016 Apr [72]	Clinical and Histopathologic Assessment of Facial Melasma After Low-Fluence Q-Switched Neodymium-Doped Yttrium Aluminium Garnet Laser. Hofbauer Parra CA, Careta MF, Valente NY, de Sanches Osório NE, Torezan LA	The results confirm the safety and effectiveness of low-fluence QS Nd:YAG laser for treating melasma; however, the high recurrence suggests poor long-term results when the laser is used as a monotherapy.	High rate of recurrence precludes use of laser toning as first line therapy
Ann Dermatol. 2015 Jun [107]	Changes in Melanin and Melanocytes in Mottled Hypopigmentation after Low-Fluence 1064-nm Q-Switched Nd:YAG Laser Treatment for Melasma Yong Hyun Jang, Ji-Youn Park, Young Joon Park, and Hee Young Kang	In conclusion, laser toning-induced hypopigmentation is characterized by almost destroyed melanosome pigments and a preserved number of melanocytes, which seem to be functionally downregulated not to produce fully matured melanosomes. Thus, early intervention aiming to restore melanocyte function would be required.	This study endorses the subcellular selective photothermolysis theory & shows that after laser toning the melanocytes are down regulated rather than destroyed.
Indian J Dermatol 2017 [105]	• Sarkar R, Aurangabadkar S, Salim T, Das A, Shah S, Majid I, *et al.* Lasers in melasma: A review with consensus recommendations by Indian pigmentary expert group. Indian J Dermatol 2017;62:477–82.	The authors suggest lasers as third line therapy for melasma	
Indian J Dermatol Venereol Leprol 2019 [106]	• Aurangabadkar SJ. Optimizing Q-switched lasers for melasma and acquired dermal melanoses. Indian J Dermatol Venereol Leprol 2019;85:10–7.	The author suggested modified laser toning with sessions performed once every fortnight for 8 to 10 sessions for melasma and use of large spot size of 10 mm at 1064 nm	The study was on skin phototypes IV to V

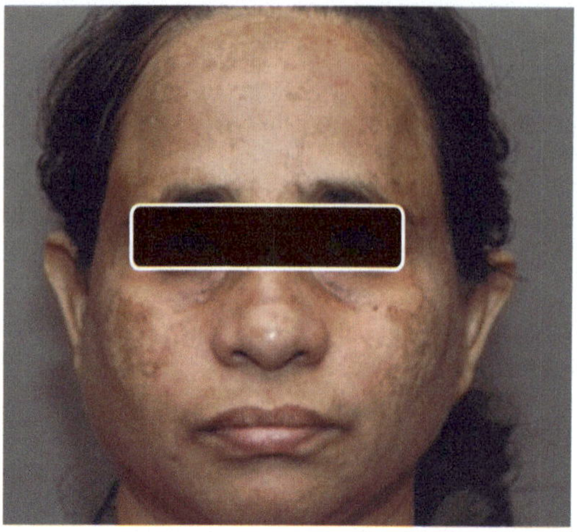

Fig. 3.26 Melasma before 1064 nm QS Nd:YAG laser treatment

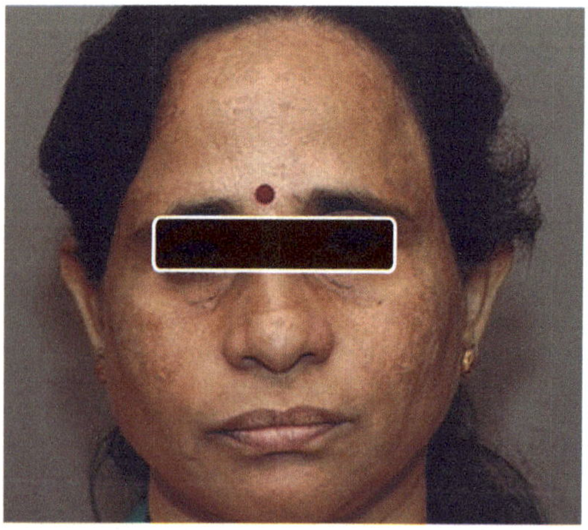

Fig. 3.27 Melasma after 10 weekly low fluence. 1064 nm QS Nd:YAG laser sessions

Becker's Naevus

Becker's naevus is a hamartomatous pigmented hairy lesion that occurs in adolescence and young adulthood. The condition is difficult to treat and uniform results are difficult to obtain. These lesions require multiple lasers for management; long-pulsed lasers for the removal of hairs, QS laser treatment for pigment reduction and fractional lasers for lesions associated with thickened skin. However, pigment reduction is variable and use of test spots with different pigment specific lasers is recommended to determine the laser (or combination of lasers) best suited to treat an individual lesion. However, it should be emphasized that the outcome of laser treatment in these conditions may be suboptimal and unpredictable [75–77].

Nevocellular Naevi

Melanocytic naevi may be congenital or acquired. Acquired naevi are further subdivided into junctional, compound and intradermal types. Such naevi should not be treated in patients with lasers if there is a personal or family history of melanoma or atypical naevus syndrome. The laser practitioner should be confident that the naevus is benign before treating it with lasers. Any of the currently available QS lasers can be used to treat naevi. Frequency-doubled Nd:YAG at 532 nm are considered suitable for superficial junctional naevi; however, longer-pulsed pigment specific lasers, with pulse duration of up to 3 ms, may also be used for the treatment of naevi. Compound and intradermal naevi are best treated by ablative lasers, radiofrequency or surgical excision. While treating junctional naevi, the response is variable. The superficial lesions may lighten or clear only partially and lesions may recur. The QS lasers at 532 nm, 694 nm and 755 nm are more effective than the 1064 nm wavelength due to better melanin absorption of these wavelengths, though the latter is safer in darker skin types. On an average, 1–3 sessions are required for clearing the pigment. The risk of dyschromia and atrophic scarring is higher in dark skin individuals. For these reasons laser treatment should be used with caution and test treatments are recommended [78–84].

Congenital melanocytic naevi (CMN), which are generally very dark and bulky, with a deep dermal component are difficult to treat and need a combination of different approaches such as excision, grafting and lasers. Combinations of QS and subsequent longer-pulsed lasers have been reported to be effective, but the lesion may clear only partially and the response is unpredictable. Three to five treatments are usually needed. Patients should be followed up regularly to check for recurrences. Non-pigmented deep nests of naevus cells may persist leading to recurrence. High powered pulsed carbon dioxide 10,600 nm laser, Er:YAG 2940 nm laser, normal mode Ruby and Q switched ruby 694 nm laser, Q switched alexandrite 755 nm lasers have all been tried for CMN [85].

CMN can be classified based on their size as small, medium and large. Small nevi are less than 1.5 cm in greatest diameter, medium are between 1.5 and 19.9 cm in their greatest diameter where as large lesions are above 20 cm in diameter. Giant nevi often have multiple smaller satellite nevi around them. A small CMN can also be defined as the one where excision and primary closure is possible. Medical management primarily revolves around sun protection and use of sunscreens. Surgical excision is recommended for either improvement of cosmesis or to prevent development of melanoma in large lesions. Serial excision, use of tissue expansion, flaps and grafts techniques are utilized for large lesions. Laser treatment of large CMN is controversial due to remnant deep nevus cells that can recur or undergo malignant transformation which can either be deep seated or masked. Curettage of CMN has been suggested in neonates and infants but again has risk of recurrence. For giant congenital melanocytic nevi, the risk of developing melanoma has been reported to be as high as 5–7% by age 60 years [86].

Figures 3.28 and 3.29 show a congenital melanocytic naevus before and after QS Nd:YAG laser treatment.

Postinflammatory Hyperpigmentation

Most commonly encountered in skin of color, PIH may have epidermal and dermal components. Although the epidermal component can

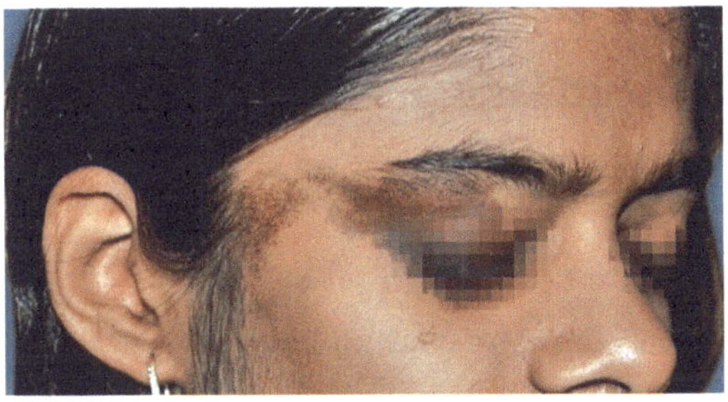

Fig. 3.28 Congenital melanocytic naevus on the upper eyelid and temple area

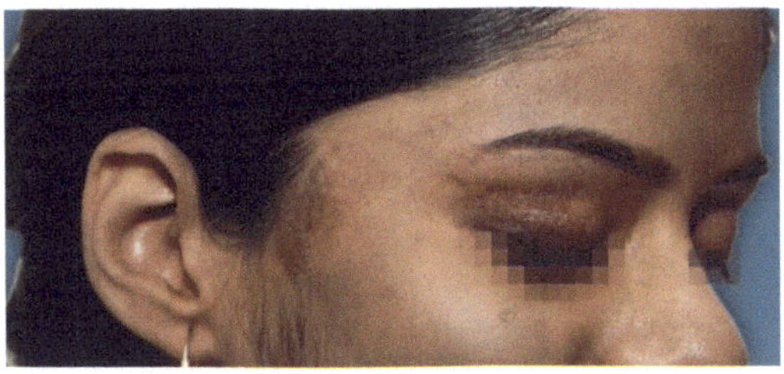

Fig. 3.29 Congenital melanocytic naevus after six QS 532 nm & 1064 nm laser treatments

be targeted with QS lasers and IPL systems, the dermal component is refractory to treatment and the pigmentation may even worsen. Hence, lasers are of limited value in the treatment of PIH [87].

Riehl's melanosis characterized by diffuse grey to black hyperpigmentation around the face is a challenge to treat. Kwon et al. in a pilot study using a triple combination approach (low fluence QS Nd:YAG, hydroquinone cream & oral tranexamic acid) for the treatment of Riehl's melanosis in 8 patients found significant improvement after 10–18 sessions [74].

Lichen planus pigmentosus (LPP) is characterized by bluish-grey macular hyperpigmentation that is often distributed on the face, neck, upper trunk & arms. It is characterized histologically by an interface dermatitis, pigment incontinence & dermal melanophages. The pigmentation can be persistent & recalcitrant to medical therapy. Once the disease activity ceases, the residual pigmentation can be tackled by QS ND:YAG laser., Multiple sessions (average 5) of QS ND:YAG at 4–6 week intervals using a large spot size & moderate fluences (which vary with the laser used) yields excellent results. In a series of 10 patients (unpublished data, author's experience SA) very good clearing was observed using this protocol as shown in Figs. 3.30, 3.31, 3.32, 3.33.

The Box 3.1 provides an algorithm for laser treatment of pigmented lesions and tattoos.

Table 3.5 summarizes the approach to pigmented lesions laser treatment.

Table 3.6 classifies the various pigmented lesions according to their response to QS laser therapy.

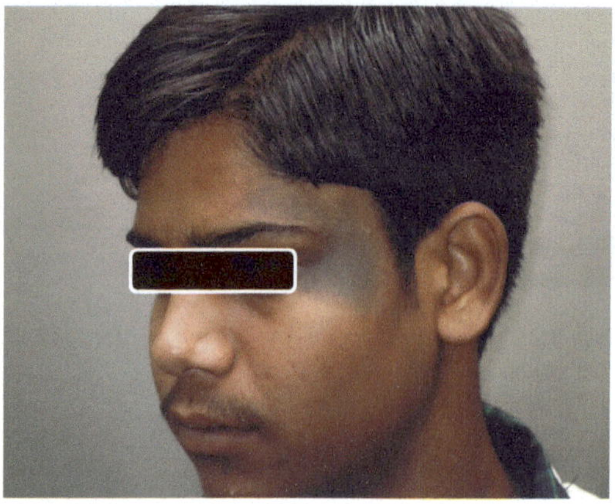

Fig. 3.30 Lichen planus pigmentosus (LPP) before laser therapy

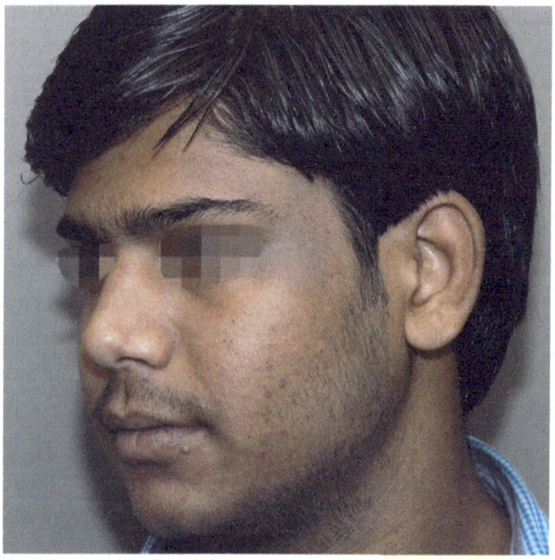

Fig. 3.31 LPP after 5 sessions of QS ND:YAG laser at 1064 nm

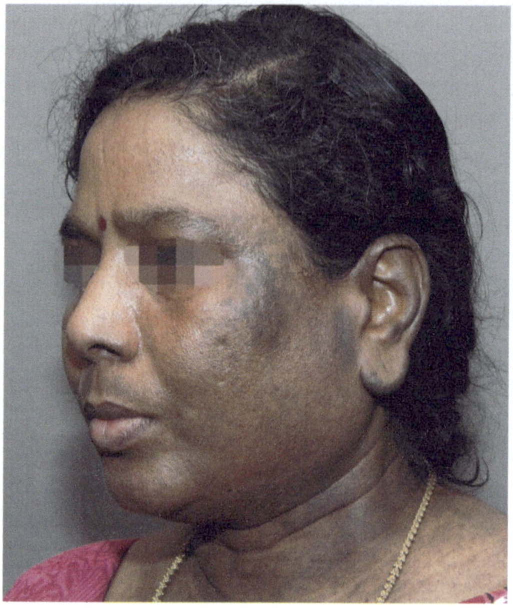

Fig. 3.32 LPP before laser

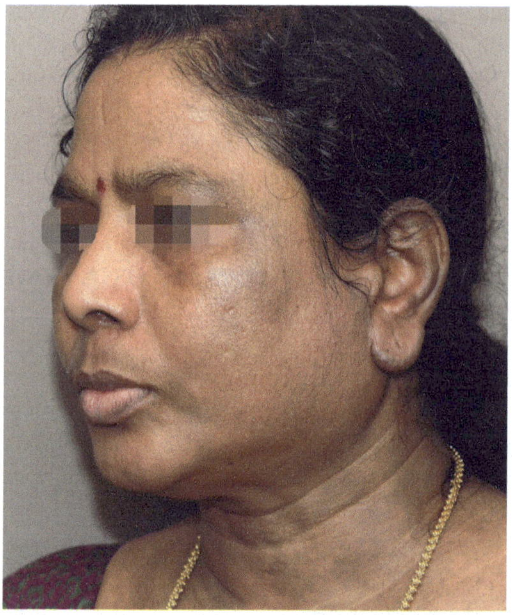

Fig. 3.33 LPP after 6 sessions of QS ND:YAG laser at 1064 nm

Postoperative Instructions

- Broad spectrum sunscreens with good UVA/UVB coverage are recommended before and throughout the treatment period.
- Immediately after laser treatment, the treated area appears abraded, and inflamed. Apply ice packs till burning sensation subsides, then apply a layer of petrolatum jelly or topical antibiotic such as mupirocin and cover with gauze. Patient is instructed to clean the area with copious amount of water and apply the ointment twice daily till lesions heal. Healing can take around 5–10 days.
- Anti-inflammatory agents may be needed while treating large lesions. Patient should be

Box 3.1 Algorithm for laser treatment of pigmented lesions and tattoos

Ephelides, lentigines and solar lentigo ↓	CALM and naevus spilus ↓	Naevus of Ota & Ito/ Hori's naevus ↓	Melasma - Medical management- sun protection, triple combination cream, chemical peels, oral tranexamic acid ↓
532 nm QS Nd:YAG/ IPL (in light skin only)	532 QS Nd:YAG (in light skin only)	1064 nm QS Nd:YAG laser (all skin types)	1064 nm QS Nd:YAG
1064 nm QS Nd:YAG (in all skin types) ↓	1064 QS Nd:YAG (in all skin types)		Low fluence-laser toning (all skin types) OR
Ablative lasers like CO_2 and Er:YAG may also be used for lentigines if QS laser not available			Fractional lasers (nonablative-1540 and 1550 nm Er:Glass)/ (ablative 2940 nm Er:YAG) OR Sequential lasers (ablative super pulsed CO_2 10,600 nm followed by QS Alexandrite 755 nm)

instructed to avoid sun exposure and cosmetics on the treated area. Treatments are scheduled at an interval of 6–8 weeks.

- Patients are instructed to apply an antibiotic ointment or petrolatum ointment for about a week after procedure. Strict sun protection is advised for darker patients.
- Post-procedure bleaching agents may be used but only after the crust subsides.

Table 3.5 Approach to laser treatment of pigmented lesions

Approach to laser treatment of pigmented lesions]
• Strict sun protection-protective clothing and use of broad spectrum sunscreens 50 SPF & UVA ++++ prior to starting laser treatment & throughout the course of therapy
• Proper priming with skin lightening agents such as hydroquinone, kojic acid etc. at least 2 to 3 weeks prior to initiation of laser therapy
• Performing test treatments/test spots to choose the right fluence
• Individualizing the treatment parameters tailored to the patient & indication
• Use of a laser with' top-hat' beam profile, large spot size, etc.
• Avoiding stacking & too much overlap while treating
• Cooling the treated area with continuous air cooling (Zimmer)- not mandatory
• Post op ice pack application for a few minutes, application of emollients, steroid-antibiotic ointment for 3 to 5 days (if blistering or crusting is anticipated)

Table 3.6 Classification of pigmented lesions according to response to QS laser therapy

Classification according to response
• **Excellent:** 532 nm/IPL—ephelides, lentigines, labial melanotic macules
• **Very good:** 1064 nm—naevus of Ota, Hori's naevus, junctional naevus
• **Variable:** CALM, naevus spilus, mongolian spots, segmental lentigines, PIH
• **Poor:** melasma, Becker's naevus

Complications and their Management

Complications may be encountered, especially in darker skin types [59, 88–94]. These may be minor and transient or major and persistent. The risk of complications increases with more aggressive treatments, poor priming, multiple treatments, choosing inappropriate laser systems and in unrealistic patients. Some of the complications which demand considerations are:

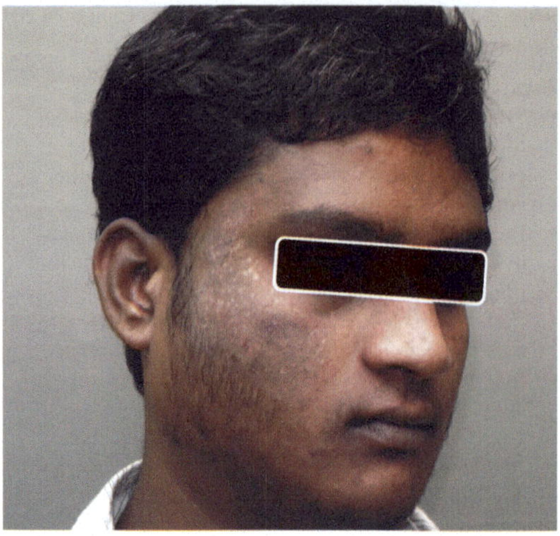

Fig. 3.34 Hypopigmentation following multiple > 10 sessions of 1064 nm QS ND:YAG using a small spot size (4 mm)

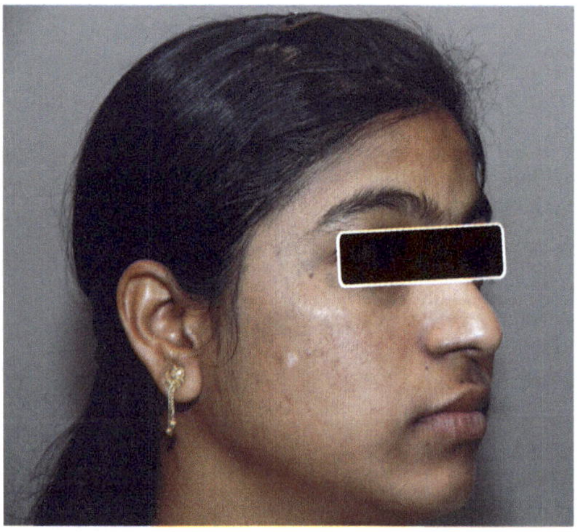

Fig. 3.35 Hypopigmentation following QS ND:YAG laser at 1064 nm in a case of naevus of Ota

- Postinflammatory hyperpigmentation resolves with time and use of bleaching agents such as hydroquinone.
- Postinflammatory hypopigmentation may persist for several weeks to months and may be difficult to treat. Figures 3.34 and 3.35 show the post inflammatory hypopigmentation following use of small spot size and excessive overlap with QS ND:YAG laser. Phototherapy (targeted or excimer laser/lamp) may be used to treat the hypopigmentation.
- Textural changes and scarring. Scarring may occur if very high fluence is used. A high fluence may result in burns which, if secondarily infected, may lead to scar formation.
- Thermal injury and burns.
- Infection, though uncommon, may occur. An antibiotic ointment and a nonadherent dressing should be applied upon completion of treatment. Patients should be instructed regarding the proper local wound care.

Tips for laser treatment of pigmented lesions

- Confirm the diagnosis (perform biopsy if diagnosis is uncertain)
- Avoid treating tanned skin
- Choose appropriate QS laser and undertake test patches.
- For epidermal lesions, for example, lentigines use 532 nm QS Nd:YAG
- For dermal lesions, for example, naevus of Ota use 1064 nm QS Nd:YAG
- Evaluate test patches after 4–8 weeks
- If needed undertake test patches again at 8 weekly intervals and only after significant improvement is seen, proceed with full treatment.

Tattoos

Lasers are the preferred modality and current gold standard for tattoo removal [95]. The nanosecond Q switched lasers (Nd:YAG at 532 and 1064 nm, Alexandrite 755 nm and Ruby 694 nm) remain the mainstay despite the availability of picosecond lasers [96].

Tattoos are classified as amateur and professional tattoos mainly by the way they are placed and the equipment used [11]. Amateur tattoos are made of carbon-based ink. They tend to be less dense than professional tattoos. These types of tattoos respond readily to Q-switched laser treatment [9]. Wavelength of 1064 nm is the preferred wavelength as it targets black ink in the dermis and also can penetrate deep. Generally, fewer sessions are needed for removal of amateur tattoos as compared to professional tattoos [9].

Professional tattoos are more complex and can be multicolored. Inks used include organic (azo dyes) or inorganic compounds (cadmium, mercury, cobalt, copper, cinnabar, ferric oxide, TiO2, carbon ink, etc.) [11]. Professional tattoos are more dense and intricate than amateur tattoos. These generally need multiple treatments (>20) and yet may not clear fully.

Tattoos can be classified as:

- Amateur (Decorative)
- Professional (Decorative)
- Cosmetic
- Traumatic, Gun-powder & Firearm tattoos
- Medical e.g. radiotherapy

Protocol for QSL tattoo removal:

- Written informed consent
- Pre treatment photo
- Test patches-followed up for 6–8 weeks
- No anesthesia-EMLA for large lesions
- Sunscreens & Bleaching agents pre-op
- Average of 6 sessions (Range 2–20)
- 6–8 weeks interval between each session
- Amateur tattoos require fewer sessions than professional tattoos
- Serial photographs taken to access improvement
- Sunscreens & topical antibiotics post-op

Factors affecting number of treatments needed for tattoo removal:

Characteristics	Easy sessions	Difficult sessions
Tattoo type	Amateur, traumatic	Professional, cosmetic
Colour	Black	Multi-coloured
Age	Old	New
Intensity	Faded	Dark
Layering	No	Yes
Skin Type	Lighter	Darker
Scarring	No	Yes
Location	Proximal	Distal

Tips for approach to laser treatment of tattoos in skin of colour

- Avoid treating a tanned patient
- Use of sunscreens and skin lightening agents prior to laser therapy
- Choose appropriate QS laser and wavelength and do a test area
- Red tattoo: use: 532 nm QS Nd:YAG
- Dark blue and black tattoo: use 1064 nm QS Nd:YAG
- Green tattoo: use 694 nm QS Ruby or 755 QS Alexandrite laser
- Evaluate test spots after 4–8 weeks
- If the test patch lesion clears well, treat the remaining area
- If any worsening or scarring occurs, stop further treatments.

Q-Switched lasers are very effective for dark-blue, black and green tattoos, whereas red and yellow tattoos are more difficult to treat as the absorption spectrum for these colors lies in the 500–600 nm spectrum (green light) The QS ND:YAG 532 nm laser can be used to treat red ink but use of high fluence is difficult in patients with darker skin types due to higher risk of adverse effects [15]. The QS 660 nm can also be used for yellow/red colors. The risk of dyschromias is high with these lasers. Pigments containing iron oxide tend to darken on exposure to laser; hence a test patch is desirable [97]. Some professional tattoos may not clear completely, in spite of repeated treatments, and a ghost image of the design may be left behind.

The Kirby-Desai Scale has been proposed to be used to estimate the approximate number of sessions needed for a given tattoo based on the following factors [98]:

- Fitzpatrick skin type.
- Location.
- Color.
- Amount of ink used.
- Scarring and tissue damage.
- Ink layering.

Each of these six factors are given numerical score and the total of these will give an estimate of the approximate number of sessions required for tattoo removal.

Figures 3.36, 3.37, 3.38, 3.39 show before and after tattoo removal with QS Nd:YAG laser at 1064 nm.

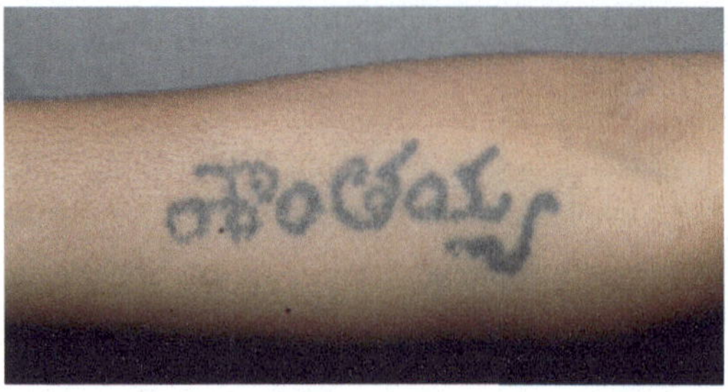

Fig. 3.36 Tattoo on forearm

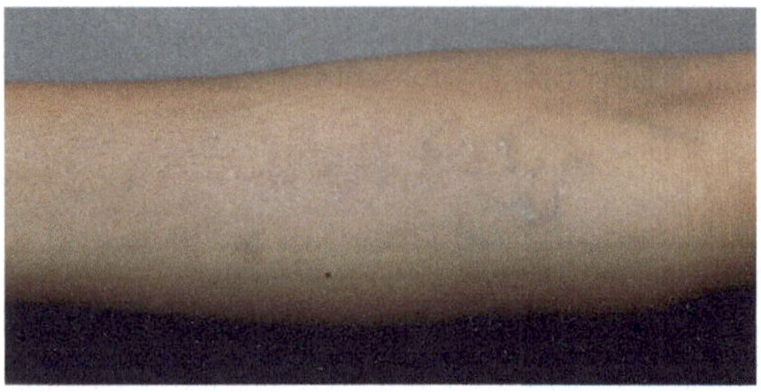

Fig. 3.37 Tattoo clearance after QS ND:YAG laser

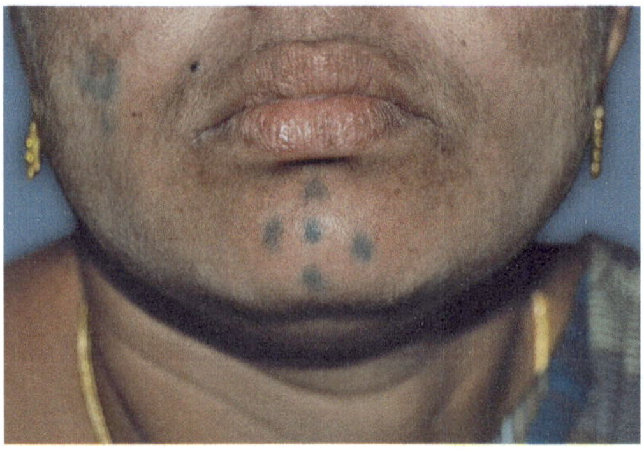

Fig. 3.38 Amateur tattoo on chin and cheek

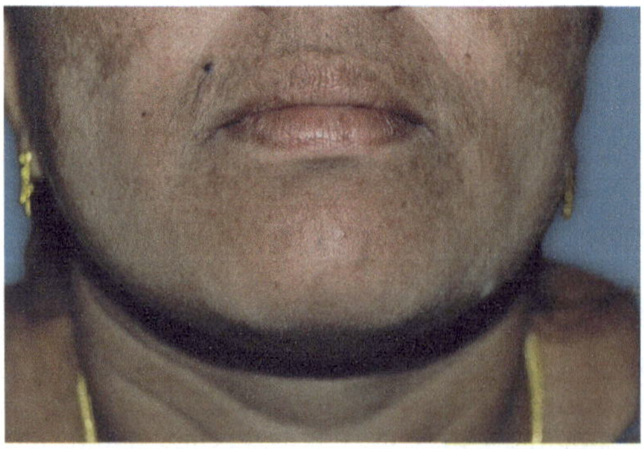

Fig. 3.39 Tattoo clearance after a single QS ND:YAG laser

Picosecond Lasers

Current QSL laser has pulse duration in nanosecond [10^{-9} of a second]. If the pulse duration is narrowed further, the peak energy of the laser beam becomes very high. The picosecond lasers have a pulse duration of 10^{-12} of a second. This results in more rapid heating of the tattoos and finer fragmentation [99]. The lymphatic elimination of these finer particles is easier resulting in faster clearing of the tattoos. The picosecond lasers with pulse durations in the range of 450–750 picosecond were introduced commercially in the early part of 2013. At present, there are 3 or more systems with a wavelength of 755 nm and 1064 nm and pulse duration of 450–750 picoseconds.

Au et al. analyzed the incidence of bulla formation after tattoo treatment using the combination of the picoseconds alexandrite laser and a fractionated carbon dioxide (CO_2) laser ablation [100]. In their study, 32% of patients treated with the picosecond laser alone experienced blistering, whereas none of the patients treated with the combination developed blistering. The study showed a statistically significant decrease in bulla formation associated with tattoo treatment when fractionated CO_2 ablation was added to the picosecond alexandrite laser.

Recent studies by Brauer et al. demonstrated the efficacy of 755 nm picosecond laser in treating blue and green tattoos [101]. They demonstrated 75% clearance in just 1 or 2 treatment. Saedi et al. also reported similar efficacy. However, they also reported complications such as hypo and hyperpigmentation at 3 months follow-up in few of their patients [102]. Although effective and safe in white skin, their safety remains to be evaluated in pigmented skin.

Case Studies

1. Café au lait macules: are challenging to treat with lasers. Histologically, they are characterized by presence of giant melanosomes. Though these lesions lighten up with QS ND:YAG laser treatment, they often recur with chances of relapse as high as 50%. In skin types I to III, shorter WL of 532 nm is used whereas in darker skin types the risk of

dyschromias is very high and caution needs to be exercised to avoid PIH. In skin types IV to VI, it is preferable to use 1064 nm. In the author's experience, a blend of 1064 nm and 532 nm in the same session often yields good results. Multiple sessions are generally needed for improvement. Parameters used were 1064 nm, 6 mm spot, 3.4 J & 532 nm,4 mm spot, 0.8 J.

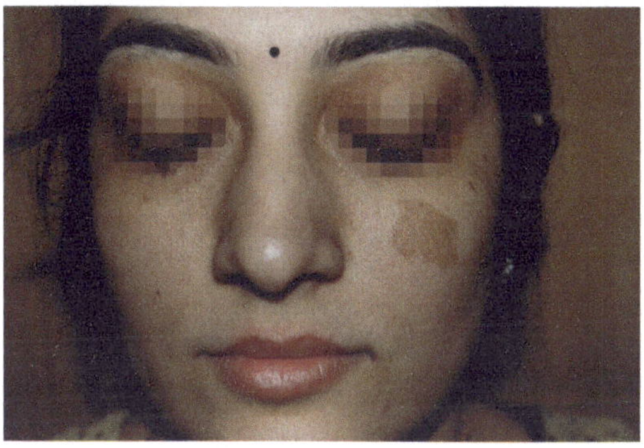

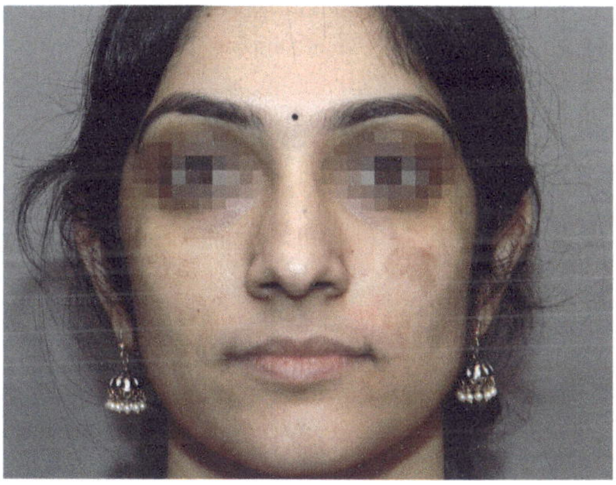

2. Naevus of Ota with scar: This young female patient had a naevus of Ota on the right cheek and underwent a surgery to remove the naevus but ended up with a linear post-surgical scar due to partial excision. This case was treated with combination of fractional CO_2 (FCO_2) laser and QS ND:YAG laser at 1064 nm in order to improve the scarring and to clear the pigment. FCO_2 parameters were 120 micron tip, 100 density and 30 W power and a fluence of 30mj per micro beam, followed by 1064 nm QS ND:YAG at 5 mm spot size, 5 joules and 2–5 ns pulse duration.

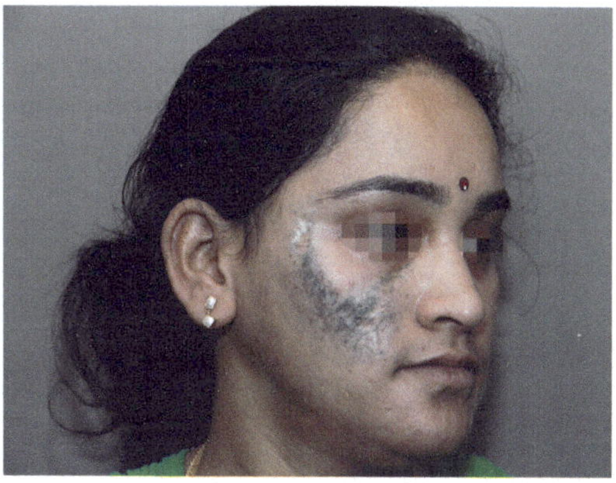

Case no 3: Tattoo with hypertrophic scar:

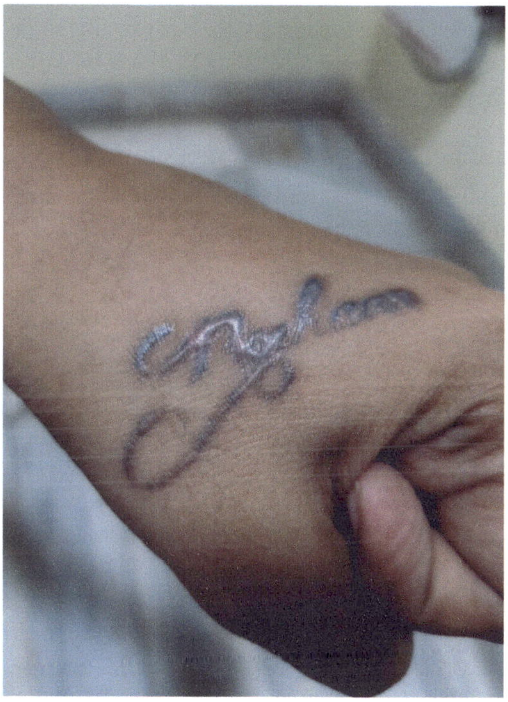

A 25 year old female patient presented with a tattoo on the dorsum of her left hand. The patient had developed a hypertrophic scar following blistering after a previous QS Nd:YAG laser session (in a different centre). Due to the partial clearance, scarring and dyschromia, the best option in such a case is to use a fractional CO_2 laser immediately followed by a QS ND:YAG laser in same session. In effect, a combination can be used to reduce the scarring and clear the residual pigment. Trans-dermal drug delivery with topical triamcinolone immediately following fractional laser can also be used to reduce the hypertrophic scar.

Conclusion

The current gold standard for pigmented lesion removal remains the QS ND:YAG laser, the versatility of the system with the availability of multiple wavelengths, quasi-long pulse mode and large spot size makes this the laser of choice for treating pigmented lesions. Though the picosecond laser are available in various wavelengths and spot sizes, the early results show they may not yet replace the QS ND:YAG laser. They are very expensive when compared to the QSLs hence are not yet widely available. The newer techniques of laser toning and its modifications hold some promise and fine tuning of the protocols will ensure better outcomes.

Acknowledgements Dr. Venkat Mysore, editor of the ACS(I) Textbook of cutaneous and aesthetic surgery & Jaypee Brothers, India.

References

1. Barlow RJ, Hruza GJ. Lasers and light tissue interactions. In: Goldberg DJ, Dover JS, Alam M, editors. Procedures in cosmetic dermatology: laser and lights. 1st ed. Philadelphia: Elsevier; 2005. p. 1–11.
2. OíShea DC, Callen WR, Rhodes WT. Introduction to lasers and their applications. Indian J Dermatol Venereol Leprol. Menlo Park, CA: Addison-Wesley, 1978.
3. Anderson RR, Parrish JA. Selective photothermolysis: precise microsurgery by selective absorption of pulsed radiation. Science. 1983;220:524–7.
4. Polla LL, Margolis RJ, Dover JS, et al. Melanosomes are a primary target of Q-switches ruby laser irradiation in guinea pig skin. J Invest Dermatol. 1987;89:281–6.
5. Goel A, Krupashankar DS, Aurangabadkar S, Nischal KC, Omprakash HM, Mysore V. Fractional lasers in dermatology – current status and recommendations. Indian J Dermatol Venereol Leprol. 2011;77:369–79.
6. Lee HI, Lim YY, Kim BJ, Kim MN, Min HJ, Hwang JH, et al. Clinicopathologic efficacy of copper bromide plus/yellow laser (578 nm with 511 nm) for treatment of melasma in Asian patients. Dermatol Surg. 2010;36:885–93.
7. McClung FJ, Hellwarth RW. Giant optical pulsations from ruby. J Appl Phys. 1962;33:828.
8. Ross V, Naseef G, Lin G, Kelly M, Michaud N, Flotte TJ, et al. Comparison of responses of tattoos to picosecond and nanosecond Q-switched neodymium: YAG lasers. Arch Dermatol. 1998;134(2):167–71.
9. Aurangabadkar S, Mysore V. Standard guidelines of care: lasers for tattoos and pigmented lesions. Indian J Dermatol Venereol Leprol. 2009;75:111–26.
10. Kilmer SL. Laser eradication of pigmented lesions and tattoos. Dermatol Clin. 2002;20:37–53.
11. Goldberg DJ. Pigmented lesions, tattoos, and disorders of hypopigmentation. In: Goldberg DJ, editor. Laser dermatology pearls and problems. 1st ed. Massachusetts: Blackwell; 2008. p. 71–114.
12. Kilmer SL, Garden JM. Laser treatment of pigmented lesions and tattoos. Semin Cutan Med Surg. 2000;19:232–44.
13. Schmults CD, Wheeland RG. Pigmented lesions and tattoos. In: Goldberg DJ, Dover JS, Alam M, editors. Procedures in cosmetic dermatology: laser and lights. 1st ed. Philadelphia: Elsevier; 2005. p. 41–66.
14. Kilmer SL. Laser treatment of tattoos. Dermatol Clin. 1997;15:409–17.
15. Grevelink JM, Duke D, van Leeuwen RL, et al. Laser treatment of tattoos in darkly pigmented patients: efficacy and side effects. J Am Acad Dermatol. 1996;34:653–6.
16. Adrian RM, Griffin L. Laser tattoo removal. Clin Plast Surg. 2000;27:181–92.
17. Koay J, Orengo I. Application of local anesthetics in dermatologic surgery. Dermatol Surg. 2002;28:143–8.
18. Drake LA, Dinehart SM, Goltz RW. Guidelines of care for local and regional anesthesia in cutaneous surgery. Guidelines/Outcomes Committee: American Academy of Dermatology. J Am Acad Dermatol. 1995;33:504–9.
19. Kilmer SL, Farinelli WF, Tearney G, et al. Use of a larger spot size for the treatment of tattoos increases clinical efficacy and decreases potential side effects. Lasers Surg Med. 1994;6:S51.
20. Chan HH, Lam LK, Wong DS, et al. Naevus of Ota: new classification based on the response to laser treatment. Lasers Surg Med. 2001;28: 267–72.
21. Ueda S, Isoda M, Imayama S. Response of naevus of Ota to Q-switched ruby laser reatment according to lesion color. Br J Dermatol. 2000;142:77–83.
22. Kilmer SL, Lee MS, Grevelink JM, et al. The Q-switched Nd:YAG laser (1064 nm) effectively treats tattoos. A controlled, dose-response study. Arch Dermatol. 1993;129:971–8.
23. Kilmer SL, Wheeland RJ, Goldberg DJ, et al. Treatment of epidermal pigmented lesions with

the frequency-doubled Q-switched Nd:YAG laser. A controlled, single-impact, dose-response, multi-center trial. Arch Dermatol. 1994;130:1515–9.
24. Levy JL, Mordon S, Pizzi-Anselme M. Treatment of individual cafe au lait macules with the Q-switched Nd:YAG: a clinicopathologic correlation. J Cutan Laser Ther. 1999;1:217–23.
25. Grossman MC, Anderson RR, Farinelli W, et al. Treatment of cafe au lait macules with lasers. A clinicopathologic correlation. Arch Dermatol. 1995;131:1416–20.
26. Jiang SB, Levine V, Ashinoff R. The treatment of solar lentigines with the Diode (Diolite 532 nm) and the Q-switched ruby laser: a comparative study. Laser Surg Med Suppl. 2000;12:55.
27. Wang CC, Sue YM, Yang CH, et al. A comparison of Q-switched alexandrite laser and intense pulse light for the treatment of freckles and lentigines in Asian persons: a randomized, physician-blinded, split-face comparative trial. J Am Acad Dermatol. 2006;54:804–10.
28. Todd MM, Rallis TM, Gerwels JW, et al. A comparison of 3 lasers and liquid nitrogen in the treatment of solar lentigines: a randomized, controlled, comparative trial. Arch Dermatol. 2000;136:841–6.
29. Li YT, Yang KC. Comparison of frequency-doubled Q-switched Nd:YAG laser and 35% trichloroacetic acid for the treatment of face lentigines. Dermatol Surg. 1999;25:202–4.
30. Bjerring P, Christiansen K. Intense pulsed light source for treatment of small melanocytic naevi and solar lentigines. J Cutan Laser Ther. 2000;2:177–81.
31. Kono T, Manstein D, Chan HH, et al. Q-switched ruby versus long-pulsed dye laser delivered with compression for treatment of facial lentigines in Asians. Lasers Surg Med. 2006;38:94–7.
32. Chan HH, Fung WK, Ying SY, et al. An in vivo trial comparing the use of different types of 532 nm Nd:YAG lasers in the treatment of facial lentigines in oriental patients. Dermatol Surg. 2000;26:743–9.
33. Jang KA, Chung EC, Choi JH. Successful removal of freckles in Asian skin with a Q-switched alexandrite laser. Dermatol Surg. 2000;26:231–4.
34. Grevelink JM, Gonzalez S, Bonoan R, et al. Treatment of naevus spilus with the Q-switched Ruby laser. Dermatol Surg. 1997;23:365–9.
35. Gold MH, Foster TD, Bell MW. Naevus spilus successfully treated with an intense pulsed light source. Dermatol Surg. 1999;25:254–5.
36. Moreno-Arias GA, Bulla F, Vilata-Corell JJ, et al. Treatment of widespread segmental naevus spilus by Q-switched alexandrite laser (755 nm, 100 nsec). Dermatol Surg. 2001;27:841–3.
37. Abecassis S, Spatz A, Cazeneuve C, et al. Melanoma within naevus spilus: 5 cases. Ann Dermatol Venereol. 2006;133:323–8.
38. Fitzpatrick RE, Goldman MP, Ruiz-Esparza, et al. Clinical advantage of the CO2 laser superpulsed mode. Treatment of verucca vulgaris, seborrheic keratoses, lentigines, and actinic chelitis. J Dermatol Surg Oncol. 1994;20:449–56.
39. Khatri KA. Ablation of cutaneous lesions using erbium:YAG laser. J Cosmet Laser Ther. 2003;5:150–3.
40. Mehrabi D, Brodell RT. Use of the alexandrite laser for the treatment of seborrheic keratoses. Dermatol Surg. 2002;28:437–9.
41. Chan HH, Leung RS, Ying SY, et al. A retrospective analysis of complications in the treatment of naevus of Ota with the Q-switched Alexandrite and Q-switched Nd:YAG lasers. Dermatol Surg. 2000;26:1000–6.
42. Chan HH, King WW, Chan ES, et al. *In vivo* trial comparing patients' tolerance of Q-switched Alexandrite (QS Alex) and Q-switched neodymium:yttrium-aluminum-garnet (QS Nd:YAG) lasers in the treatment of naevus of Ota. Lasers Surg Med. 1999;24:24–8.
43. Chan HH, Ying SY, Ho WS, et al. An *in vivo* trial comparing the clinical efficacy and complications of Q-switched 755 nm alexandrite and Q-switched 1064 nm Nd:YAG lasers in the treatment of naevus of Ota. Dermatol Surg. 2000;26:919–22.
44. Kono T, Nozaki M, Chan HH, et al. A retrospective study looking at the long-term complications of Q-switched ruby laser in the treatment of naevus of Ota. Lasers Surg Med. 2001;29:156–9.
45. Kilmer SL, Anderson RR. Clinical uses of Q-switched ruby and Q-switched Nd:YAG (1064 nm and 532 nm) lasers for treatment of tattoos. J Dermatol Surg Oncol. 1993;19:330–8.
46. Goldberg DJ, Nychay SG. Q-switched ruby laser treatment of naevus of Ota. J Dermatol Surg Oncol. 1992;18:817–21.
47. Watanabe S, Takahashi H. Treatment of naevus of Ota with the Q-switched ruby laser. N Engl J Med. 1994;331:1745–50.
48. Geronemus RG. Q-switched ruby laser therapy of naevus of Ota. Arch Dermatol. 1992;128:1618–22.
49. Alster TS, Williams CM. Treatment of naevus of Ota by the Q-switched Alexandrite laser. Dermatol Surg. 1995;21:592–6.
50. Turnbull JR, Assaf C, Zouboulis C, et al. Bilateral naevus of Ota: a rare manifestation in a Caucasian. J Eur Acad Dermatol Venereol. 2004;18:353–5.
51. Kopf AW, Bart RS. Malignant blue (Ota's?) naevus. J Dermatol Surg Oncol. 1982;8:442–5.
52. Patel BC, Egan CA, Lucius RW, et al. Cutaneous malignant melanoma and oculodermal melanocytosis (naevus of Ota): report of a case and review of the literature. J Am Acad Dermatol. 1998;38:862–5.
53. Lowe NJ, Wieder JM, Sawcer D, et al. Naevus of Ota: treatment with high energy fluences of the Q-switched ruby laser. J Am Acad Dermatol. 1993;29:997–1001.
54. Chan HH, Lam LK, Wong DS, et al. Role of skin cooling in improving patient tolerability of

Q-switched alexandrite (QS Alex) laser in naevus of Ota treatment. Lasers Surg Med. 2003;32:148–51.
55. Aurangabadkar S. QYAG5 Q-switched Nd:YAG laser treatment of naevus of Ota: an Indian study of 50 patients. J Cutan Aesthet Surg. 2008;1:80–4.
56. Kunachak S, Leelaudomlipi P. Q-switched Nd:YAG laser treatment for acquired bilateral naevus of ota-like maculae: a long-term follow-up. Lasers Surg Med. 2000;26:376–9.
57. Polnikorn N, Tanrattanakorn S, Goldberg DJ. Treatment of Hori's naevus with the Q-switched Nd:YAG laser. Dermatol Surg. 2000;26:477–80.
58. Lee B, Kim YC, Kang WH, et al. Comparison of characteristics of acquired bilateral naevus of Ota-like macules and naevus of Ota according to therapeutic outcome. J Korean Med Sci. 2004;19:554–9.
59. Lam AY, Wong DS, Lam LK, et al. A retrospective study on the efficacy and complications of Q-switched alexandrite laser in the treatment of acquired bilateral naevus of Ota-like macules. Dermatol Surg. 2001;27:937–41.
60. Milgraum SS, Cohen ME, Auletta MJ. Treatment of blue naevi with the Q-switched ruby laser. J Am Acad Dermatol. 1995;32:307–10.
61. Katsambas A, Antoniou C. Melasma. Classification and treatment. J Eur Acad Dermatol Venereol. 1995;4:217–23.
62. Kang WH, Yoon KH, Lee ES, Kim J, Lee KB, Yim H, et al. Melasma: Histopathological characteristics in 56 Korean patients. Br J Dermatol. 2002;146:228–37.
63. Nouri K, Bowes L, Chartier T, et al. Combination treatment of melasma with pulsed CO2 laser followed by Q-switched alexandrite laser: a pilot study. Dermatol Surg. 1999;25:494–7.
64. Wang CC, Hui CY, Sue YM, et al. Intense pulse light for the treatment of refractory melasma in Asian persons. Dermatol Surg. 2004;30:1196–200.
65. Manaloto RM, Alster T. Erbium:YAG laser resurfacing for refractory melasma. Dermatol Surg. 1999;25:121–3.
66. Rokhsar CK, Fitzpatrick RE. The treatment of melasma with fractional photothermolysis: a pilot study. Dermatol Surg. 2005;31:1645–50.
67. Polnikorn N. Treatment of refractory dermal melasma with the MedLite C6 Q-switched Nd:YAG laser: two case reports. J Cosmet Laser Ther. 2008;10:167–73.
68. Jeong SY, Chang SE, Bak H, et al. New melasma treatment by collimated low fluence Q-switched Nd:YAG laser. Korean J Dermatol. 2008;46:1163–70.
69. Gokalp H, Akkaya AD, Oram Y. Long-term results in low-fluence 1064-nm Q-Switched Nd:YAG laser for melasma: Is it effective? J Cosmet Dermatol. 2016;15(4):420–6. https://doi.org/10.1111/jocd.12253. Epub ahead of print.
70. Kim JY, Choi M, Nam CH, Kim JS, Kim MH, Park BC, et al. Treatment of melasma with the photoacoustic twin pulse mode of low-fluence 1,064 nm Q-switched Nd:YAG laser. Ann Dermatol. 2016;28(3):290–6.
71. Mun JY, Jeong SY, Kim JH, Han SS, Kim IH. A low fluence Q-switched Nd:YAG laser modifies the 3D structure of melanocyte and ultrastructure of melanosome by subcellular-selective photothermolysis. J Electron Microsc. 2011;60(1):11–8.
72. Hofbauer Parra CA, Careta MF, Valente NY, de Sanches Osório NE, Torezan LA. Clinical and histopathologic assessment of facial melasma after low-fluence Q-switched neodymium-doped yttrium aluminium garnet laser. Dermatol Surg. 2016;42(4):507–12.
73. Dashore S, Mishra K. Tranexamic acid in melasma: why and how? Indian J Drugs Dermatol. 2017;3:61–3.
74. Kwon HH, Ohn J, Suh DH, Park HY, Choi SC, Jung JY, et al. A pilot study for triple combination therapy with a low-fluence 1064 nm Q-switched Nd:YAG laser, hydroquinone cream and oral tranexamic acid for recalcitrant Riehl's Melanosis. J Dermatolog Treat. 2016;27:1–5.
75. Nanni CA, Alster T. Treatment of a Becker's naevus using 694-nm long-pulsed ruby laser. Dermatol Surg. 1998;24:1032–4.
76. Trelles MA, Allones I, Moreno-Arias GA, et al. Becker's naevus: a comparative study between erbium: YAG and Q-switched neodimiyum: YAG; clinical and histopathological findings. Br J Dermatol. 2005;152:308–13.
77. Kopera D, Hohenleutner U, Landthaler M. Quality-switched ruby laser treatment of solar lentigines and Becker's naevus: a histopathological and immunohistochemical study. Dermatology. 1997;194:338–43.
78. Goldberg DJ, Stampien T. Q-switched ruby laser treatment of congenital naevi. Arch Dermatol. 1995;131:621–3.
79. Grevelink JM, van Leeuwen RL, Anderson RR, et al. Clinical and histological responses of congenital melanocytic naevi after single treatment with Q-switched lasers. Arch Dermatol. 1997;133:349–53.
80. Rosenbach A, Williams CM, Alster TS. Comparison of the Q-switched alexandrite (755 nm) and Q-switched Nd:YAG (1064 nm) lasers in the treatment of benign melanocytic naevi. Dermatol Surg. 1997;23:239–44.
81. Waldorf HA, Kauvar AN, Geronemus RG. Treatment of small and medium congenital naevi with Q-switched ruby laser. Arch Dermatol. 1996;132:301–4.
82. Ueda S, Imayama S. Normal-mode ruby laser for treating congenital naevi. Arch Dermatol. 1997;133:355–9.
83. Kono T, Ercocen AR, Chan HH, et al. Effectiveness of the normal-mode ruby laser and the combined (normal-mode plus Q-switched) ruby laser

in the treatment of congenital melanocytic naevi: a comparative study. Ann Plast Surg. 2002;49:476–85.
84. Kono T, Ercocen AR, Nozaki M. Treatment of congenital melanocytic naevi using the combined (normal-mode plus Q-switched) ruby laser in Asians: clinical response in relation to histological type. Ann Plast Surg. 2005;54:494–501.
85. Michel JL. Laser therapy of giant congenital melanocytic nevi. Eur J Dermatol. 2003;13(1):57–64.
86. Bett BJ. Large or multiple congenital melanocytic nevi: occurrence of cutaneous melanoma in 1008 persons. J Am Acad Dermatol. 2005;52(5):793–7.
87. Taylor CR, Anderson RR. Ineffective treatment of refractory melasma and postinflammatory hyperpigmentation by Q-switched ruby laser. J Dermatol Surg Oncol. 1994;20:592–7.
88. Rheingold LM, Fater MC, Courtiss EH. Compartment syndrome of the upper extremity following cutaneous laser surgery. Plast Recontr Surg. 1997;99:1418–20.
89. Bhardwaj SS, Brodell RT, Taylor JS. Red tattoo reactions. Contact Dermatitis. 2003;48:236–7.
90. Ashinoff R, Levine VJ, Soter NA. Allergic reactions to tattoo pigment after laser treatment. Dermatol Surg. 1995;21:291–4.
91. England RW, Vogel P, Hagan L. Immediate cutaneous hypersensitivity after treatment of tattoo with Nd:YAG laser: a case report and review of the literature. Ann Allergy Asthma Immunol. 2002;89:215–7.
92. Kyanko ME, Pontasch MJ, Brodell RT. Red tattoo reactions: treatment with the carbon dioxide laser. J Dermatol Surg Oncol. 1989;15:652–6.
93. De Argila D, Chaves A, Moreno JC. Erbium:Yag laser therapy of lichenoid red tattoo reactions. J Eur Acad Dermatol Venereol. 2004;18:332–3.
94. Jimenez G, Weiss E, Spencer JM. Multiple color changes following laser therapy of cosmetic tattoos. Dermatol Surg. 2002;28:177–9.
95. Shah SD, Aurangabadkar SJ. Newer trends in laser tattoo removal. J Cutan Aesthet Surg. 2015;8:25–9.
96. Aurangabadkar SJ. Shifting paradigm in laser tattoo removal. J Cutan Aesthet Surg. 2015;8:3–4.
97. Anderson RR, Geronemus R, Kilmer SL, et al. Cosmetic tattoo ink darkening. A complication of Q-switched and pulsed-laser treatment. Arch Dermatol. 1993;129:1010–4.
98. Kirby W, Desai A, Desai T, et al. The Kirby-Desai scale: a proposed scale to assess tattoo-removal treatments. J Clin Aesthet Dermatol. 2009;2:32–7.
99. Ross V, Naseef G, Lin G, et al. Comparison of responses of tattoos to picosecond and nanosecond Q-switched neodymium: YAG lasers. Arch Dermatol. 1998;134(2):167–71.
100. Au S, Liolios AM, Goldman MP. Analysis of incidence of bulla formation after tattoo treatment using the combination of the picosecond Alexandrite laser and fractionated CO2 ablation. Dermatol Surg. 2015;41(2):242–5.
101. Brauer JA, Reddy KK, Anolik R, et al. Successful and rapid treatment of blue and green tattoo pigment with a novel picosecond laser. Arch Dermatol. 2012;148(7):820–3.
102. Saedi N, Metelitsa A, Petrell K, et al. Treatment of tattoos with a picosecond alexandrite laser: a prospective trial. Arch Dermatol. 2012;148:1360–3.
103. Yue B, Yang Q, Xu J, Lu Z. Efficacy and safety of fractional Q-switched 1064-nm neodymium-doped yttrium aluminum garnet laser in the treatment of melasma in Chinese patients. Lasers Med Sci. 2016;31(8):1657–63.
104. Sofen B, Prado G, Emer J. Melasma and post inflammatory hyperpigmentation: management update and expert opinion. Skin Therapy Lett. 2016;21(1):1–7.
105. Sarkar R, Aurangabadkar S, Salim T, Das A, Shah S, Majid I, et al. Lasers in melasma: a review with consensus recommendations by Indian pigmentary expert group. Indian J Dermatol. 2017;62:477–82.
106. Aurangabadkar SJ. Optimizing Q-switched lasers for melasma and acquired dermal melanoses. Indian J Dermatol Venereol Leprol. 2019;85:10–7.
107. Jang YH, Park J-Y, Park YJ, Kang HY. Changes in melanin and melanocytes in mottled hypopigmentation after low-fluence 1,064-nm Q-switched Nd:YAG laser treatment for melasma. Ann Dermatol. 2015;27(3):340–2.

Epilation Lasers

4

Samantha Hills and Daron Seukeran

Introduction

Cultural norms in many countries dictate that excessive or visible hair on certain areas of the body is problematic at worst and unattractive at best. With a global hair removal market predicted to grow to $1.5 billion by 2025 [1], the drive to rid ourselves of facial and body hair shows no signs of abating.

Laser and light-assisted hair removal is increasingly considered the treatment of choice for long term reduction of unwanted hair. In 1997, the FDA approved the use of the first laser for cosmetic hair reduction, and since then, it has been widely used in clinical practice and is considered to be a safe and effective alternative to other methods of hair removal. Despite this, a 2009 Cochrane Review concluded that the lack of high-quality studies meant that data were insufficient to support long-term hair clearance from laser and IPL [2].

Although initially promoted as a means of achieving permanent hair removal for all skin types, many clinicians have revised this claim and now hold more realistic expectations. Depending on factors such as the colour, texture and location of the hair, as well as a patient's skin type and hormonal status, it is now generally accepted that complete hair *removal* may not be achieved. Rather, the absence of hair growth in a 12-month period is classed as "permanent hair *reduction*" with any regrowth generally being lighter in colour, finer in texture and reduced in number.

The Ruby laser was the first laser to be demonstrated in 1960. Although some early studies looked at using lasers on the skin to remove tattoos, it wasn't until 1996 that Grossman et al. showed that the Ruby laser could be used for successful long-term hair reduction for cosmetic applications. Since then, long-pulsed Alexandrite, Diode, and Nd:YAG lasers have all been cultivated for use in hair removal. In the late 1990s, the first Intense Pulsed Light (IPL) system was introduced, and since then countless other IPL systems have come to market, and these Intense Light Sources (ILS) are also commonly used for hair removal.

Mode of Action

Most lasers and light sources use the principle of Selective Photothermolysis, which describes how light can be delivered to the skin, such that it can selectively destroy certain biological targets, whilst avoiding damage to the surrounding areas. In order for long-term hair loss to occur, the cells that make up the hair follicle must be irreversibly

S. Hills (✉)
Lynton Lasers Ltd, Cheshire, UK
e-mail: shills@lynton.co.uk

D. Seukeran
James Cook University Hospital, Middlesbrough, UK

SK:N Laser Clinics, London, UK

V. Madan (ed.), *Practical Introduction to Laser Dermatology*,
https://doi.org/10.1007/978-3-030-46451-6_4

damaged. Following this damage to the follicle, the cells responsible for hair growth are destroyed and long-term hair reduction is achieved. This damage to the hair follicle can be achieved using laser or light systems due to the absorption of light by the chromophore melanin, which is present in the hair shaft and skin.

In order to achieve this damage, the light must be delivered over a time period matching the approximate Thermal Relaxation Time (TRT), or Cooling Time, of the target. In the case of the hair, the TRT is of the order of 10–100 ms, so for laser hair removal, long-pulsed lasers (rather than Q-Switched lasers) are used.

Light of the correct pulse duration (approximately tens of milliseconds), is directed at the skin and absorbed by the melanin in the hair shaft producing heat (photothermal reaction). This heat is conducted down the shaft and outwards into the surrounding follicle—the hair is in fact acting as an 'intermediary' for the transmission of heat into the follicle. The hair must therefore always be present in the follicle for laser hair removal to work—hair that has been plucked or waxed or otherwise removed from the follicle is not suitable for treatment.

If the heating effect is sufficient, *the follicular cells within the matrix and hair bulge that are responsible for re-growth are damaged* to the extent that re-growth is inhibited and long term hair reduction is achieved.

This can be summarized as follows:

1. The light is selectively absorbed by the melanin within the hair shaft.
2. This light causes the hair to heat rapidly and conducts heat to the follicle and the neighbouring cells.
3. The cells responsible for re-growth of the hair are heated and damaged, resulting in either the complete destruction of the hair or a transition to a finer, fairer hair.
4. New hair growth appears as surrounding hairs enter the anagen (growing) phase.
5. New hair growth is treated and the percentage of re-growth decreases with each subsequent treatment.

When considering the mechanisms involved using light sources for hair removal, it is crucial to consider the effect of wavelength selection. In order to effectively remove hair with lasers or light it is necessary to target the melanin contained within the hair shaft. Hair lacking in melanin (i.e. grey or white hair) will show limited light absorption and heat production, so it is therefore difficult to treat this type of hair with any laser or light system. According to the principle of Selective Photothermolysis, to target the pigment in hair it is necessary to use a wavelength that will be selectively absorbed by melanin. The ideal wavelength should be readily absorbed in melanin but not well absorbed in other chromophores such as water or blood.

The commonly used hair removal lasers all use wavelengths within the 'Optical Window for Melanin' which stretches from approximately 650–1200 nm. This region contains wavelengths which are readily absorbed by melanin, but avoids the main absorption peaks of blood, minimizing the possibility of vascular damage, and avoiding the longer infrared wavelengths that will cause heating of water present in the tissue.

In order for hair to be treated without damaging the surrounding tissue, Laser and IPL hair removal relies on the absorption of light by the melanin contained in the hair shaft in preference to absorption by melanin in the skin. As it is usual for melanin to exist in the epidermis, at the junction between the epidermis and the dermis, within the dermis, as well as within the hair, the process can become quite complex. It is essential however, that the hair is darker than the skin for preferential absorption to occur. *The best results will normally be seen for people with dark hair and fair skin.* The treatment is effective when the hair follicle reaches a temperature high enough to destroy the follicle whilst the epidermis remains below the damage threshold temperature.

Cooling the skin before, during and after treatment can reduce damage to the epidermis. Thermal damage can occur if skin temperatures reach more than 45 °C [3], so cooling the epidermis allows the use of higher fluences without increasing the risk of complications. Common cooling methods include ice packs, cold gel, forced air cooling, contact cooling or cryogen sprays.

Hair Structure

The hair follicles (bulb, papilla and surrounding connective tissue) develop before birth and cannot be replaced if they die. The total number of hair follicles for an adult human is estimated to be at least five million (with one million of these on the head).

Hair is made of keratin and nourished by blood supply from dermal papilla, with the hair epithelium being continuous with epidermis. The hair shaft grows from matrix cells within the hair bulb, but epithelial stem cells are also contained with the hair bulge, at the junction of the erector pili muscle.

A cross-section of a terminal hair consists of:

1. Cuticle: the outermost layer, which is thin and colourless
2. Cortex: the middle layer which accounts for greatest proportion of hair shaft
3. Medulla: the central portion of the hair shaft which contains the hair pigment

Hair can be classified into two major types:

- Terminal hairs are thick, long and pigmented with melanin
- Vellus hairs are small in diameter, short and often non-pigmented

It is generally terminal hair that causes the greatest cosmetic concern, as fine vellus hair is often not immediately visible. Vellus hairs can be converted to terminal hairs by hormones (as happens during the onset of puberty) or by mechanical stimulation of the hair, such as that which arises from plucking the hair. Plucking, threading and waxing of unwanted hair should therefore be discouraged.

Hair Growth Cycle

Every hair has a cycle of growth—in fact it has a cycle of growing, resting and shedding. Not all of the hairs on our body are in the same stage at the same time. The three phases of growth are Anagen, Catagen and Telogen.

1. Anagen—the stage at which hairs are in active growth and when melanin synthesis occurs. At this stage, melanocyte stem cells located in the bulge start to produce melanosomes which give the hair shaft its colour [4]. In addition, anagen hairs are attached to the papilla and at maximum depth within the dermis.
2. Catagen—the stage at which hair growth is arrested but the hair continues to be nourished from the papilla
3. Telogen—the stage at which hair growth ceases altogether, the hair detaches from the papilla and contracts to almost one-third its original depth. The hair then falls out and the process begins once more with the early anagen phase.

Probably the most important phase for laser or light assisted hair removal is anagen, as the hair is connected to, and nourished by the papilla, which is still relatively close to the surface. The hair follicle is also comparatively richer in melanin at this phase of growth. It therefore makes it easier to deposit sufficient energy into the hair shaft, the papilla and the hair bulb to cause permanent damage which will delay or prevent future hair re-growth. It is because of the need to treat hair in this early anagen phase that several treatments are always required to successfully target an entire anatomical area.

The duration of the anagen phase varies greatly depending upon age, season, anatomic region, sex and genetic disposition, and can be as long as 6 years on the scalp, with 80–90% of hair in the anagen phase. The catagen phase is relatively constant for most body sites, at around 3 weeks, whereas the telogen phase usually lasts approximately 3 months. Hair in the catagen or telogen phase is thought to be less susceptible to the effects of the light. This explains why legs or backs, which have only about 20% of hair in the anagen phase at any time, may take some time to show long term results as the majority of the hair is not actively growing at any one time.

In addition, the hair cycle is under the influence of a number of hormones: oestrogens, testosterone, adrenal glucocorticoids, prolactin and growth hormone. Testosterone and its active metabolite, dihydrotestosterone (present in conditions such as Polycystic Ovaries) exerts the strongest effect. Most people seeking hair removal generally are in good health but excess hair growth can also result from many inherited syndromes and it is useful to be aware of such cases.

Lasers and Light Sources Used for Photoepilation

The key properties of the light required for successful photo-epilation are:

- Wavelength
- Pulse duration
- Fluence

Wavelength

The method utilized to heat the hair follicle relies on the absorption of light by the chromophore melanin. There are five different laser/light sources that are commonly used for hair removal. They all deliver 'long-pulses' in the millisecond range for a photothermal effect. They are:

1. Ruby laser (694 nm)
2. Alexandrite laser (755 nm)
3. Diode laser (various wavelengths, usually 810 nm or 920 nm)
4. Nd:YAG laser (1064 nm)
5. IPL or ILS sources (filtered broadband light, typically 620–1200 nm)

Lasers at the shorter end of the wavelength spectrum show enhanced melanin absorption, making them particularly effective for the treatment of finer, lighter hairs. However, the high melanin affinity means that these shorter wavelengths are more likely to interact with pigment within the skin, and they are therefore not suitable for the treatment of skin of colour.

Fluence

The fluence, also known as Energy Density, is a measure of the amount of energy delivered in a given area, and is measured in Joules per centimeter square (J/cm^2). In order to achieve destruction of the hair follicle, the fluence must be sufficient to obtain temperatures high enough to damage the follicular stem cells. For a fixed energy, fluence can be increased by using smaller spot sizes, but this will impact on treatment times and effective penetration depths.

The fluence required to achieve follicular damage is largely determined from experiment and will often vary significantly depending upon various factors. The skin type and the colour of hair are major factors in determining a suitable (safe but effective) fluence. However, there are also variations due to the parameters of a particular system, in general, systems with longer wavelengths (and reduced melanin affinity) require much higher fluences to achieve the same clinical results as those with shorter wavelengths.

Pulse Duration

The pulse duration (sometimes known as pulse width) represents the on-time of the light pulse. According to the Theory of Selective Photothermolysis, the pulse duration of the laser should match the Thermal Relaxation Time (TRT) of the target. The Thermal Relaxation Time is defined as the time taken for an object to lose 50% of its induced thermal energy to surrounding tissues through thermal diffusion. For a hair, the TRT is approximately 40–100 milliseconds [5], so lasers/light sources using pulse durations of this order can efficiently heat the hair follicle whilst the epidermis conducts heat to surrounding tissue.

Thicker hairs have longer TRT and can therefore be treated effectively with longer pulse durations, however, very fine hairs will need shorter pulses in order to achieve high peak temperatures within the follicle. Keeping all else equal, reducing pulse durations will make treatments more effective (and more aggressive), whilst increasing pulse durations will reduce peak powers delivered, therefore making treatments safer for skin of colour.

Hair Removal Lasers and Light Sources

Ruby Lasers

The ruby laser at 694 nm was the first selective laser to be used for hair removal. At the shorter end of the wavelength range, melanin absorption is high, resulting in effective heating of the hair follicle, but also resulting in undesirable heating of the melanin within the skin. Multiple studies have shown an increased incidence of side effects with this wavelength, such as superficial burns or pigment disruption [6, 7]. For this reason, the Ruby laser is only suitable for Fitzpatrick skin types 1 and 2.

Technological difficulties with long-pulsed Ruby lasers (the inefficient lasing process results in high operating temperatures within the laser cavity) mean that high repetition rates and high energies are difficult to reliably achieve, which has limited their use as hair removal systems in recent years.

Alexandrite Lasers

At 755 nm, the Alexandrite is often the preferred choice for the treatment of lighter skin types. The high melanin absorption means that it can effectively treat even fine and fair hairs (although some melanin is always required within the hair shaft, so blonde or white hair will not respond to any laser or light treatment). Short pulse durations are achievable with Alex lasers, increasing efficacy, however, they are not suitable for the treatment of skin types 5 and 6, and should be used with extreme caution in skin type 4.

Diode Lasers

Diode lasers are increasingly popular due to their ability to treat a wide range of skin types (1 to 5). They were also the first lasers to be used for in-motion or 'pain-free' treatments, and are delivered to the skin directly, via a laser handpiece. Some diode systems struggle to deliver sufficient energy in short pulse durations, which may affect the efficacy of the treatment of finer hairs.

Neodymium YAG Lasers

The long pulsed Nd:YAG laser has the longest wavelength (1064 nm) of all the lasers commonly used for hair removal and as such shows a decreased affinity for absorption in the epidermal melanin. This reduced absorption results in less skin heating in comparison to other hair removal laser systems. Therefore there is a lower associated risk of epidermal damage and the Nd:YAG is considered to be the safest laser for skin of colour, especially for the treatment of skin type VI. The reduced melanin absorption also means that skin penetration depths are relatively high. This enables the laser energy to easily reach the hair bulb and bulge region and cause lethal follicular damage, resulting in long-lasting hair reduction, however this increased penetration can make treatment more painful than with other laser systems, and results can be limited on fine and fair hair.

Intense Light Sources

Intense Light Sources (ILS), often known as Intense Pulsed Light (IPL) are now perhaps the most common method of light-assisted hair removal on the high-street. Their relative simplicity means that they are generally lower priced than lasers, and the ability to use filters to target additional skin chromophores mean that these can be very versatile systems, also being used for the treatment of superficial vascular lesions and rosacea, lentigines and photo-damaged skin (see Chap. 9 for further details).

ILS are generally comprised of a Xenon flashlamp which produces a wide spectrum of wavelengths ranging from ultra violet to near infrared. The output therefore requires some form of filtration, and for hair removal treatments, a cut-off filter is usually employed to remove all wavelengths below approximately 650 nm. This results in an emitted wavelength range from about 650 nm to 1200 nm. These wavelengths are readily absorbed in melanin but avoid the main absorption peaks of blood, therefore avoiding the possibility of vascular damage.

The treatment outcomes are very dependent on pulse duration and peak powers achievable, and there is a wide range of pulsing profiles available from different systems, which are not always easy to decipher from the manufacturers' specifications. This means there tends to be much more variation in technical specification and price with IPL systems than is commonly seen with lasers, with a resultant variation in treatment outcomes.

A comparison of different devices for LHR is shown in Table 4.1.

Table 4.1 A brief comparison of different laser/light sources suitable for Hair Removal

Light source	Advantages	Disadvantages
Ruby nm (694 nm)	Greatest melanin absorption of all commonly used hair removal lasers, making it effective for the treatment of fine hair, and hair with lower levels of pigment	Not suitable for darker skin types due to high risk of epidermal blistering or pigment disruption. Slow treatment times due to inherent limitations of laser repetition rates and available spot sizes
Alexandrite laser (755 nm)	Considered by most to be the 'gold standard' for laser hair removal due to the high levels of melanin absorption. Effective results on skin-types 1–3 Short pulse durations can be obtained meaning high peak powers can be achieved. Available in low fluence, high-repetition versions, for 'pain-free treatment'	Not suitable for treatment of skin types 5 and 6 (extreme caution required for the treatment of skin type 4)
Diode laser (Variable, usually 810 or 920 nm)	Generally compact, table-top devices. Can effectively treat a wide range of skin types. Diode arrays usually result in large spot sizes for fast treatments. Available in low fluence, high-repetition versions, for 'pain-free treatment'	Difficult to achieve very short pulse durations, which can limit max power. Reduced melanin absorption at this wavelength can reduce efficacy when treating fine or fair hairs.
Nd:YAG laser (1064 nm)	Limited melanin absorption means it's the safest laser to use for the treatment of the skin types 4–6 and tanned skin.	Will generally require more treatments than other hair removal devices. Deep penetration can make treatment particularly uncomfortable. Reduced melanin absorption at this wavelength can reduce efficacy when treating fine or fair hairs.

Table 4.1 (continued)

Light source	Advantages	Disadvantages
Intense Light Source/ILS (variable, usually from approx. 600–1200 nm)	Large treatment area and machine versatility (by use of filters to offer Skin Rejuvenation/ vascular treatments) make these attractive options Lower cost than most lasers	Lots of variation between systems. Low quality systems may have reduced efficacy when compared to laser systems

Pre-Treatment Preparation and Precautions

Prior to treatment, each patient should undergo a thorough consultation, informed consent should be obtained, and a test patch should be carried out. During the consultation a full medical history will be taken and the treatment will be fully explained. Generally, the following circumstances would contraindicate treatment:

Contraindications

- Recently UV-exposed or tanned skin (real or fake, including tanning injections)
- Skin pigmentation problems such as melasma (in or near the treatment area)
- A history of keloid scarring
- Pregnancy/Breastfeeding
- Severely photosensitive skin or photosensitising conditions such as porphyria
- Epilepsy within the last 12 months
- Skin Cancer or other malignant disease
- Any active inflammatory skin condition e.g. eczema, psoriasis, Herpes Simplex in the treatment area
- Healing disorders such as those caused by Diabetes Mellitus, connective tissue disease (e.g. lupus), radiation therapy or chemotherapy
- Patients with unrealistic expectations, or those who are unlikely to follow post treatment guidelines
- Do not treat over any tattoos, semi-permanent make-up or moles.
- Use of St John's Wort, minocycline or amiodarone in the past month
- Use of Isotretinoin (Roaccutane) or any drugs for Photodynamic Therapy (PDT) in the previous 6 months
- Use of topical retinoids such as Tretinoin, (Retin-A, Aknemycin Plus,) Isotretinoin (Isotrexin), Adapalene (Differin) in the last 2 weeks on the area to be treated
- Use of high dose systemic (oral or injectable) steroids in the past month
- Use of topical steroids in the past week (in or near the treatment area)

After a medical history is obtained it is important to also:

- Assess the condition to be treated. For example, hair thickness and colour. If there is a possibility of an underlying endocrine disorder, then explain that the cause of the hair growth is not being treated, so maintenance treatments may be necessary.
- Show examples to the patient of the likely results of treatment. Answer any questions the patient has regarding treatment and make sure the patient has realistic expectations of the outcome of the treatment. The patient should be informed that 100% clearance can not be guaranteed and results may not be permanent, and the effectiveness of treatment is related to skin/hair type.
- Explain that treatment efficacy is related to patient skin and hair colour so results may vary. Dark hair with light skin responds best, whilst white, blonde and red hair rarely responds.
- Ensure the patient knows that multiple treatments will be required because hair grows in cycles and can only be treated effectively in the growing phase. Explain that alternative methods of hair removal exist, include waxing, shaving, threading and depilatory creams, but prior to laser/IPL hair removal, the hair must be shaven.

- Explain the treatment process to the patient. Discuss pain control and aftercare. Possible side effects of treatment should be discussed in detail.
- Explain the hazards of Intense Pulsed Light/ laser radiation and the need for appropriate goggles to be worn at all times.
- Carefully record the patient's reaction to sun exposure and assign skin type using the Fitzpatrick Scale.
- Provide estimates of the total cost of treatment and methods of payment.
- Photograph the treatment site for the patient's records.
- Answer any questions that the patient might have and record patient comments. Each patient should be provided with written information about the treatment
- Ask the patient to read, sign and date the consent form if he/she has understood its contents. Countersign the consent form and give the patient a copy if requested.

Informed Consent

Prior to any examination, skin test patch or treatment, every patient is required to provide informed consent to LASER or ILS treatment. Patients need sufficient information concerning the benefits, risks, alternative treatments, expected outcomes and fees before they can decide whether to give their consent. If the patient is not offered as much information as they reasonably need to make their decision, and in language they can understand, their consent may not be valid. If the patient is suitable for treatment, continue with patch-testing. A patch test must be performed on or as near as possible to the area prior to any course of treatment.

Test-Patching

Once eligibility has been established, it is recommended that a test patch is completed for all patients before treatment commences. The aim of the test patch is to determine the most effective treatment parameters for the patient's skin and hair type and lesion type, and to judge how the skin will respond to treatment. The test patch should always be carried out in a small area, in or near the area for treatment, and if other body sites are to be treated subsequently, then a test patch must be carried out in the new treatment area.

Select the lowest recommended settings, taking into account skin type, body site and density and thickness of hair in the area. Observe the skin response and patient's tolerance to treatment, settings can be increased if an appropriate skin reaction is not observed, but keep in mind that reactions may not always be obvious on test patch. The presence of follicular erythema and oedema, and a smell of burning hair are good indicators that the treatment settings are suitable. Very pronounced erythema is not expected following most hair removal treatments and may be a sign of over-treatment. Typically, a test patch consists of a few shots only. Complete patient records, noting observed skin and patient reaction, sign, date and schedule an appointment for treatment.

An appropriate amount of time should pass before proceeding with treatment—this might be as short as 24 h, but more often will be approximately 7 days, especially for darker skin types. Subsequent treatment intervals will typically be around 4–8 weeks.

Typical Skin Reactions and End Points of Treatment

Patients should be made aware of likely effects following treatment including:

- Redness and/or tenderness of the treatment area.
- Itchiness, mild irritation or swelling of the follicles which normally subsides within 48 h (see Fig. 4.1)
- Hair should fall out within approximately 2 weeks
- Some hair may regrow thinner and lighter than before

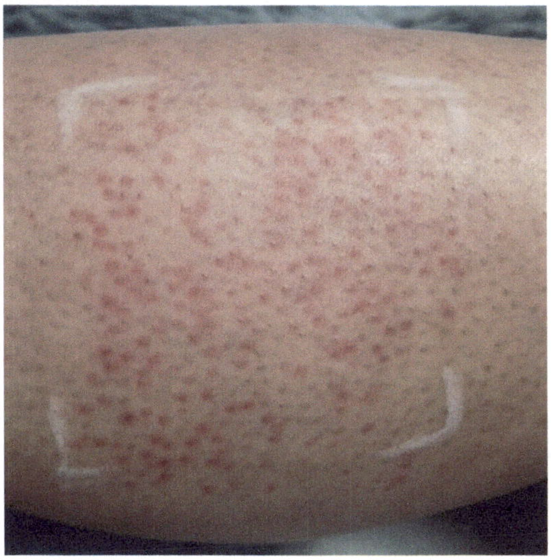

Fig. 4.1 Pronounced follicular erythema following treatment with a low-fluence, high rep-rate Alexandrite laser (Motus AY, DEKA lasers). Although not always seen, when present, it's a good indicator of a successful treatment

- Shaving of the area may be restarted as soon as hair growth becomes apparent.
- Folliculitis and/or histamine reactions can occur on occasion, and can be reduced by increased personal hygiene (new razor, fresh towels and face cloths) and by using anti-inflammatory/antibacterial and skin-calming lotions

Epilation Laser Medical Indications

- Hirsutism
- Polycystic Ovarian Syndrome
- Limb Prosthesis in Amputees
- Reduction of Body Odour
- Pilonidal Sinus
- Hidradenitis Suppurativa
- Dissecting Folliculitis of the Scalp
- Trichostasis Spinulosa
- Pseudofolliculitis Barbae
- Hairy Intraoral flaps
- Transgender laser hair removal and Genital Gender reaffirming surgery
- Peristomal hair growth
- Hair restoration surgery to redesign frontal hairline in women

Hirsuitism

Hirsutism is often defined as excessive hair in an androgen dependent distribution e.g. beard area, lower abdomen in females. The prevalence of hirsutism varies from 5% to 32% in different population groups. It is recognized that hirsutism is a distressing symptom with a negative impact on psychosocial aspects and quality of life [8].

It is important to recognize patient's perceptions of the severity of their hirsutism can differ greatly from doctors, nurses and the wider population. One study showed a significant reduction in the hirsutism related Disability Life Quality Index score (DLQI) after treatment with an Alexandrite laser. The same study also showed that LHR led to an increase in social and interpersonal activities [8].

Many women choose LHR over alternative methods of hair removal for axillary, legs, bikini line hair. Alternative methods such as depilatory creams and electrolysis are becoming less popular. Depilatory creams can often cause an irritant reaction and plucking can result in folliculitis and post inflammatory pigmentation. Waxing can cause similar problems. Electrolysis is an effective method, and can lead to permanent hair reduction, but the process is slow and painful, and results and side effect profile are very operator dependent.

On the basis of this, LHR has become a popular option, despite the fact that original reports of permanent hair removal have now been revised to longer periods of remission and delayed hair growth (Fig. 4.2). However, many people, especially women with facial hirsutism, find that having several months of remission is more acceptable than daily treatments such as shaving or plucking.

Non androgen dependent hair growth in areas such as the forearms or back is termed hypertrichosis. Patients with hirsutism require a full evaluation to exclude treatable causes of androgen excess, including some tumours. Other causes of hypertrichosis include drug induced hair growth, congenital hair and hair growth from grafted donor sites [9].

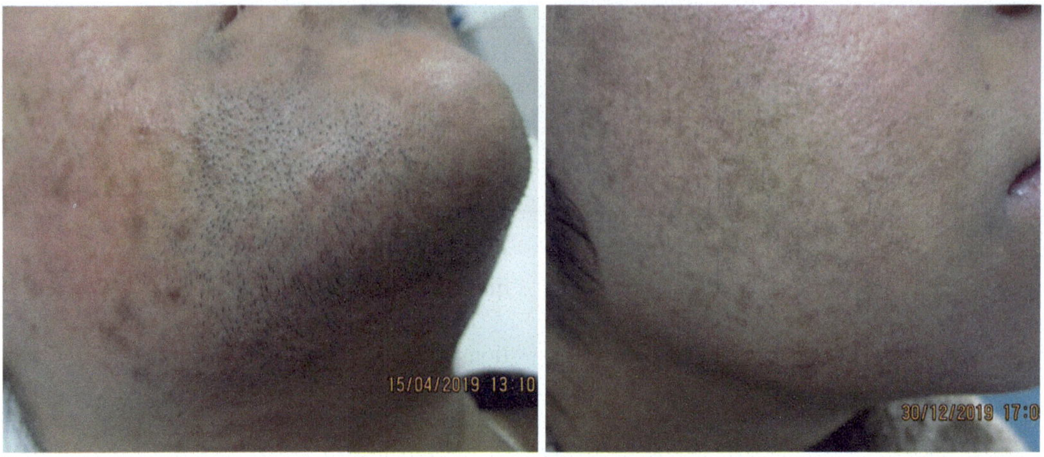

Fig. 4.2 Female patient before and after nine treatments with Long pulsed ND Yag 20–30 J/cm^2 12 mm spot size 3 ms pulse duration for Laser Hair reduction

There are also an increasing number of men who are having laser hair removal in areas such as the chest and back. It is becoming increasingly commonplace for men, particularly under 30s to remove hair from their body. 19% of men claim they feel expected to remove hair from their torso [10].

Poly Cystic Ovarian Syndrome

Polycystic ovarian syndrome (PCOS) is a condition affecting 4–8% of women of reproductive age. Characteristic features include polycystic ovaries, menstrual disturbances and hyperandrogenism. Up to 70% of women with hyperandrogenism present with hirsutism. Suppression of ovarian androgen production using oral contraceptives, androgen receptor blockers are often tried to reduce hirsutism but results are variable [11].

Laser hair removal has been a significant advance of treatment for these individuals as medical treatment has provided limited results. Compared with idiopathic hirsutism, PCOS patients require more treatment sessions and 'top up' sessions to achieve hair reduction.

Limb Prosthetics in Amputees

Hair growth at the residual limb-prosthetic interface in individuals with traumatic lower limb amputation can lead to a folliculitis. This can cause significant irritation and limit the time the prosthesis can be worn. Laser hair removal in this area can lead to reduction in the folliculitis and improve symptoms which can lead to a significant improvement in quality of life due to the improved comfort in wearing a prosthesis (Fig. 4.3) [12]. Studies have shown a marked decrease in hair density and disease exacerbations at follow-up were noted after Alexandrite LHR for below knee amputation stump [13].

Use of Laser Hair Removal in the Axillae to Reduce Body Odour

Body odour, in particular axillary odour, is perceived as unpleasant by many cultures worldwide. Reducing or eliminating body odour is an important part of the daily personal care routine for many individuals. Over the last decade, removal of underarm hair has become more commonplace for hygiene as well as aesthetic reasons [14].

Hair Follicle Pathology

A number of dermatological conditions associated with hair follicular pathology as the primary dysfunction have been treated with LHR. These include chronic inflammatory disorders such as pilonidal sinus disease (PSD), hidradenitis suppurativa (HS), dissecting folliculitis, and pseudofolliculitis barbae (PFB). These diseases are thought to result from occlusion, rupture, and inflammation of the follicular unit [15]. Laser-

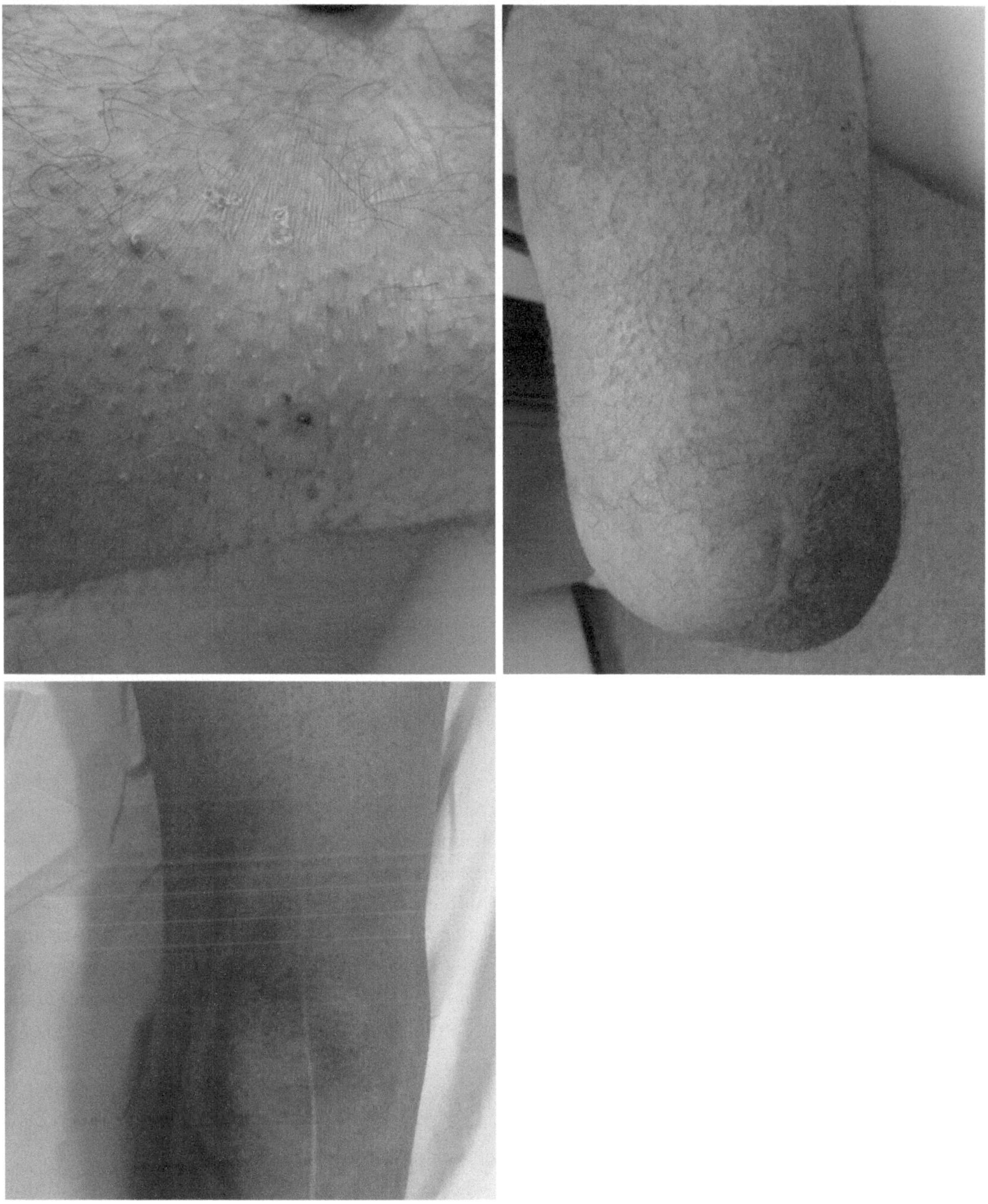

Fig. 4.3 Lower leg amputee presenting with folliculitis which showed marked improvement after 4 Alexandrite laser treatments 755 nm 18 mm 3 ms 16–20 J/cm^2

induced damage and epilation of hair follicles has led to a significant improvement in these disorders, which is helpful where current medical treatment options often have limited results with frequent relapses.

Pilonidal Sinus

A pilonidal sinus (PNS) or sacrococcygeal fistula is a cyst or abscess on the natal cleft of the buttocks that often contains hair and skin debris (Fig. 4.4).

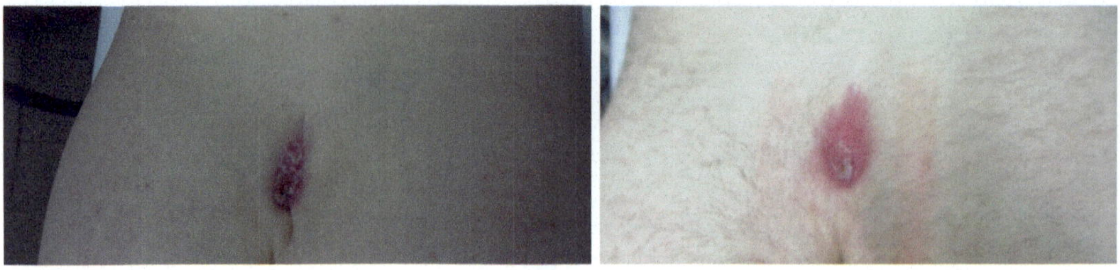

Fig. 4.4 Pilonidal sinus in male before and after 7 treatments with Alexandrite laser 755 nm 18 mm spot size, 3 ms pulse duration 16–20 J/cm^2

PNS of the natal cleft is painful and causes significant disability. Complete surgical excision of the sinus tract is the standard treatment but there is significant risk of recurrence. Due to the association with excessive hair in sacrococcygeal region, laser epilation has been reported to be beneficial as an additional treatment to surgery [16–24].

The conventional treatment of PNS involve use of depilatory creams, but with this recurrence is a common due to recurring hair growth at the site. However, with five to six sessions of LHR, chances of recurrence reduce [25, 26]. Diode, Nd:YAG and Alexandrite lasers as well as IPL systems have been used in different studies in this indication and all of these devices have shown promising results [27].

Jain et al. [28] treated three patients of PNS but the disease recurred. The patients were then treated with a combination of CO_2 laser with 1064 nm Nd:YAG laser with the aim of deroofing with CO_2 laser and use of long pulse Nd:YAG laser to destroy hair follicles in five patients with PNS with follow up of up to 3 years. Long Pulse Nd:YAG was repeated in all patients at a 2–3 month gap for four to five times. During this time, no recurrence was observed.

Relapse rates are high if fewer than four sessions are used; one study with mean of 2.7 sessions reported a recurrence rate of 13.3% over a follow-up period of 4.4 years [23]. LHR in PSD is usually well tolerated and without any major complications. A long-term follow-up study reported no recurrence in 86.6% of patients following LHR over a period of 5–7 years [13].

Hidradenitis Suppurativa (HS)

HS is a chronic disabling disorder, often affecting the axillae, inframammary areas and groin, characterized by exacerbations, recurrence, and progression despite medical and surgical treatment. There has been increasing evidence for a primary follicular pathogenesis, which has led to LHR being used in the treatment of HS.

Significant improvement of HS has been reported in this condition after LHR with diode and Nd:YAG lasers, and IPL devices [29–31].

Long pulse Nd:YAG laser has deeper tissue penetration than other lasers and due to this, has been considered to be the preferred laser for this indication. Histopathological changes in 20 patients of HS were followed using biopsy specimens obtained at specified intervals before and after treatment and this correlated with the degree of clinical improvement in them after treatment with a long-pulsed 1064-nm Nd:YAG laser. Patients received two treatments to an affected area; Laser parameters ranged from 25 to 50 J/cm^2 with a 10-mm spot size and a 20- to 35-ms pulse duration. Double pulse stacking was used at the first treatment, and triple at the second treatment on all inflammatory lesions. By 1 month, inflammation had decreased and broken hair shafts were noted. At 2 months, the investigators found scarring, fibrosis, and minimal inflammation. As measured by a Lesion Area and Severity Index score modified for HS, a significant improvement of 32% in treated areas was noted 2 months after the second treatment [32].

Pseudofolliculitis Barbae

PFB is a common chronic disorder predominantly in those of African descent with tightly curled hairs curving back into the skin. Shaving is a predisposing factor because it results in sharp and short hairs, which re-enter the skin. LHR has been shown to be helpful by reducing the number and/or thickness of hair shafts. Greater than 50% improvement has been observed in long-standing PFB after LHR [33–35]. In PFB, LHR with Nd:YAG laser has been reported as a safe and effective option for reducing hair and subsequent papule formation. Papule counts performed 90 days after treatment in dark skins (type IV–VI) were significantly reduced in the laser-irradiated area as compared to the control [36]. Another study reported 56% mean reduction in PFB lesions after using three passes of Nd:YAG laser [37]. A low-fluence (12 J/cm^2) laser treatment at 1064 nm at 5-week intervals also achieved significant temporary reduction in PFB on the neck which had been unresponsive to other treatments [38].

Dissecting Cellulitis

Dissecting cellulitis is an inflammatory condition of the scalp characterized by nodules, sinus tract formation, and scarring alopecia. A severe case of recalcitrant dissecting cellulitis of the scalp had no recurrence at 6-month follow-up after four treatment sessions of diode laser as monotherapy [39]. In addition, some patients have reported regrowth of terminal hairs in treatment sites, 1 year after initiating laser treatment [40].

Folliculitis Decalvans

Folliculitis decalvans (FD) is another inflammatory condition of the scalp characterized by follicular papules and pustules. It often leads to a scarring alopecia. The long pulse Nd:YAG laser was used in in several cases of FD with good results in a few studies [41–43].

Trichostasis Spinulosa

Trichostasis spinulosa is a disorder consisting of asymptomatic comedo-like lesions that contain keratin and multiple vellus hairs primarily on the face associated with dilated hair follicles. LHR therapy has been reported to be helpful, removing the hair responsible for the plugged appearance. The alexandrite laser has been reported as being effective [44, 45], with one study reporting no recurrence in 90% of the treated cases [46].

Hair-Bearing Skin Flaps and Grafts

Following surgical reconstruction hair-bearing skin flaps and grafts result in hair growth at sites where it is inappropriate. LHR has been used on the nose following basal cell carcinoma excision, after reconstruction in breast cancer, and other traumatic injuries requiring skin grafts [47, 48].

Hairy Intraoral Flaps

A variety of flaps used to reconstruct defects of the head and neck region following surgery for malignant disease contain hair follicles that may result in unwanted hair growth. This can lead to with irritation, pooling of saliva and trapping of food. Several lasers have been used to deal with this but the most common has been the long pulsed alexandrite laser [49]. The long pulsed Nd:YAG laser has also been used.

Shields et al. demonstrated that these lasers provided safe and effective treatment and improved patient quality of life following intraoral flap repair following excision of malignancy [50].

LHR is very difficult in such cases due to poor visibility and the bulky hand piece of laser in the confined oropharyngeal space. Marked symptom improvement was noted in a patient with reconstructed hypopharynx post laryngopharyngectomy using Alexandrite laser, with a 7-mm hand piece with 90° side-firing fiber-optic attachment passed through the lumen of a suspension laryngoscope [51].

Transgender Laser Hair Removal and Genital Gender Affirming Surgery

The trans gender community often desire hair removal and lasers provide an effective method of achieving this (Fig. 4.5).

Genital gender affirming surgery (GAS) involves reconstruction of the genitals to match the patients identified sex. The use of hair-bearing flaps can result in postoperative intravaginal and

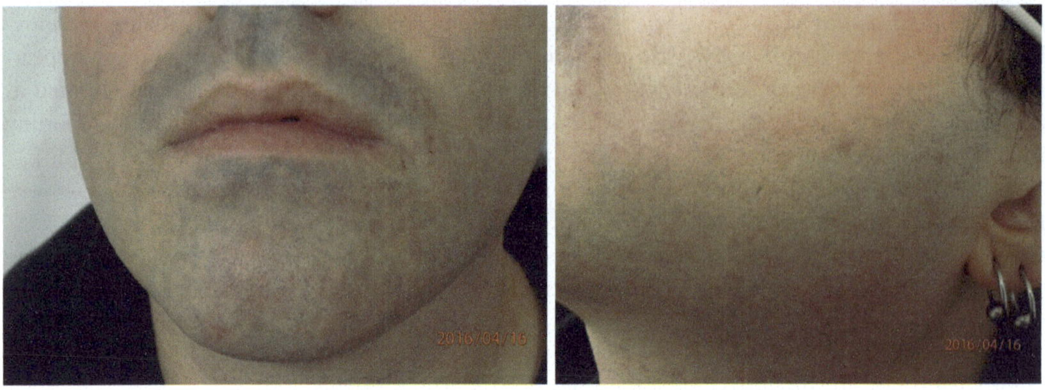

Fig. 4.5 Male to female gender reassignment patient. Alexandrite laser 755 nm. over 30 treatments 20 J/cm^2–30 J/cm^2 12 mm. In addition to eight electrolysis sessions

intraurethral growth hair growth and associated complications [52, 53]. Electrolysis has been used for hair removal prior to GAS but LHR has been shown to be superior [54, 55]. It is best to wait 3 months after the last planned hair removal treatment before proceeding with surgery, in order to confirm that no further hair regrowth will occur [56].

Peristomal Hair Growth

Peristomal hair growth following an ileostomy can cause difficulty for adhesion of the stomal appliance to the skin. LHR has resulted in effective epilation, resulting in improved stoma appliance adhesion and reduced risk of trauma and infection [57, 58].

Redesign Frontal Hairline in Women in Hair Restoration Surgery

Hair transplantation in women for hairline correction can be associated with an unnatural appearance due to thicker donor hair from occipital region. LHR has been used as a nonsurgical method for revising hairline following hair transplantation in women. Study carried out by Park et al. [59], resulted in subjective improvement in 87.5% of the cases as well as significant reduction in hair diameter.

Complications of Hair Removal Laser Treatments and How to Treat and Avoid Them

Typical end points following hair removal treatment are usually restricted to mild erythema, peri-follicular swelling and smell of burning hair. Laser and light-assisted hair removal is generally a low-risk procedure and when complications do arise they are generally transient, with permanent sequalae being very uncommon. Good clinical practice and sensible precautionary measures can minimize this risk, and most importantly, it's essential that patients are treated with the laser most appropriate for their skin type.

During the consultation procedures, it is important to be clear on possible risks of treatment. These are outlined below:

Burning, Blistering and Scarring

If inappropriate settings are used (fluence too high, incorrect wavelength for skin type etc.), cooling is not adequate or tanned skin is treated, then thermal damage can occur to the skin, presenting as pronounced erythema, grazing or even blistering (Figs. 4.6 and 4.7).

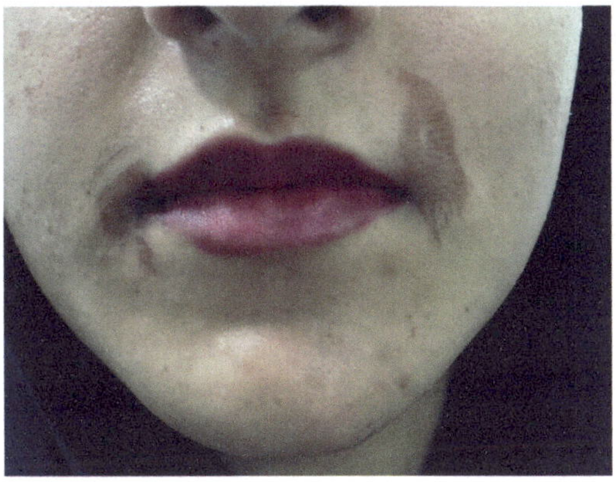

Fig. 4.6 Adverse skin reactions due to excessive overlapping and incomplete removal of make-up. Figure courtesy Dr. Vishal Madan

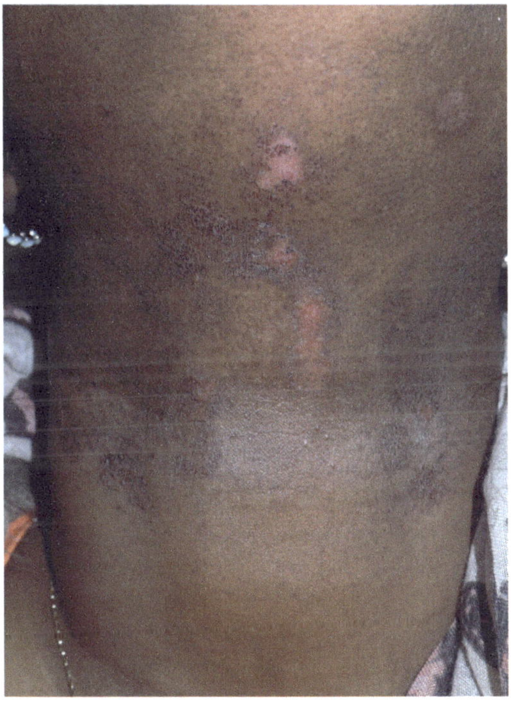

Fig. 4.7 Adverse skin reactions due to excessive overlapping and incomplete removal of make-up. Figure courtesy Dr. Vishal Madan

It is essential that any blisters or grazes which form following the treatment are not popped, picked, or scratched and the area kept clean and dry. Once the blister subsides, the skin may be dry and flaky, do not exfoliate and let the skin flake at its own speed. Sun avoidance is essential, and once the area has healed, a high-factor sunscreen should be applied daily for up to 12 months to reduce the risk of pigmentation changes occurring.

Generally IPL/Laser burns are superficial and will heal without issue, but if infection is suspected, immediate treatment is required to minimize the risk of scarring or permanent pigmentation change.

Pigmentation Changes

Hyper and hypo pigmentation may arise either following the presence of a burn or just occur spontaneously after treatment (Figs. 4.8, 4.9, and 4.10). Avoidance of sun exposure before and after treatment can lessen the risk of pigmentary changes occurring. Permanent pigmentary alteration is rare, but is more common in darker skins.

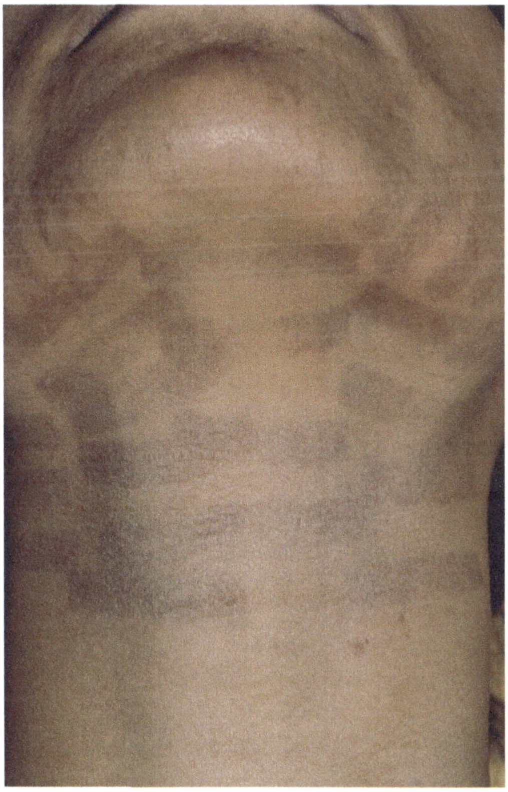

Fig. 4.8 Transient hyperpigmentation following IPL treatment, due to presence of tan or inappropriate settings for skin type. Figure courtesy Dr. Vishal Madan

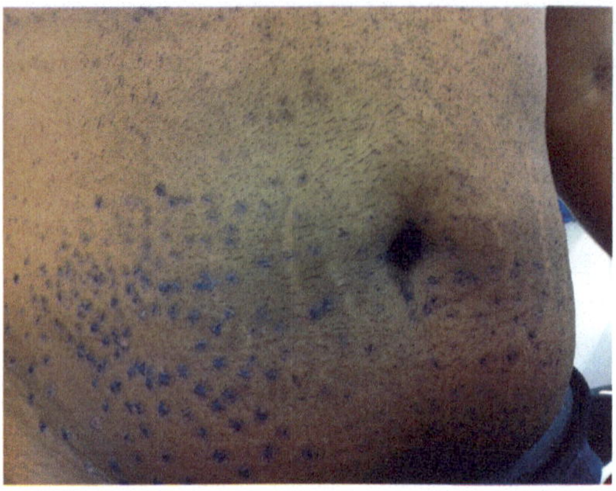

Fig. 4.9 Pronounced skin reaction following treatment due to excessive fluence. Figure Courtesy Dr. Vishal Madan

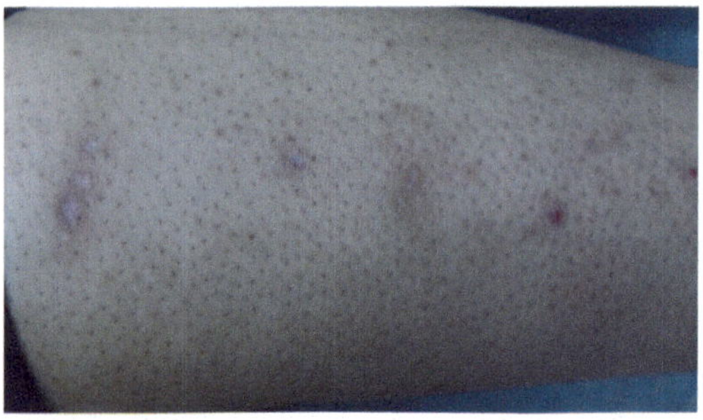

Fig. 4.10 Hypopigmentation on a skin type 2 following LHR. Figure courtesy Dr. Vishal Madan

The presence of melasma appears to increase the risk of post-inflammatory hyperpigmentation occurring, so facial hair removal should proceed with caution in patients with this condition, and pigment suppressants are recommended prior to treatment.

Hyperpigmentation should be treated with daily use of sunscreen in the first instance. Topical products containing hydroquinone and retinoids can be used to expedite improvement.

Paradoxical Hypertrichosis

A rare but distressing adverse effect of laser hair removal is an increase in hair growth on, or adjacent to, the LASER or IPL treatment site (Fig. 4.11). This is called 'paradoxical hair growth' and is thought to affect 0.6–10% of all patients having treatment [60]. Paradoxical growth has been reported with all types of laser and IPL [61], and the aetiology is unclear. Many mechanisms have been proposed, including sub-therapeutic thermal injury affecting the follicular cycling so that terminal hair growth is induced whilst other studies indicate that it is the thermally-induced inflammatory response which induces activation of dormant hair follicles in untreated areas close to hirsute-treated areas [62]. Another hypothesis is that hair removal simply synchronizes the cycling of hairs growing within the laser treatment, thereby causing the overall hair density to appear to be greater [63].

It is certainly the case that this affect appears to be more prevalent in patients of Mediterranean, Middle-Eastern and Asian descent (skin types 3 to 5 [64]), and one study reported that it was more common in patients suffering from underlying hormonal conditions such as Poly Cystic Ovarian Syndrome and associated ovarian hyperandrogenism [65]. It generally occurs when treating fine, vellus hair on the neck and jawline in women, but it has also been reported in men, usually on the back and shoulders, although it is unclear whether this predominance is simply due to those areas being treated more commonly in men than other body sites.

The increased hair growth can be treated with further laser/IPL treatments, with the use of higher laser fluences widely recommended. Wiley et al. [66] suggest actively cooling the neighbouring (non-treated) areas to prevent stimulation of the follicles by sub-therapeutic light. They also recommend double passing over the treatment area, although caution is advised with this method, especially when treating darker skin types.

Other Unusual Side Effects

Leukotrichia has been reported following treatment with IPL [67] and other lasers [68]. This seems to occur when fluences are used that are insufficient to damage the germinative hair follicle, but sufficient to damage the melanocytes either permanently or temporarily. It appears to

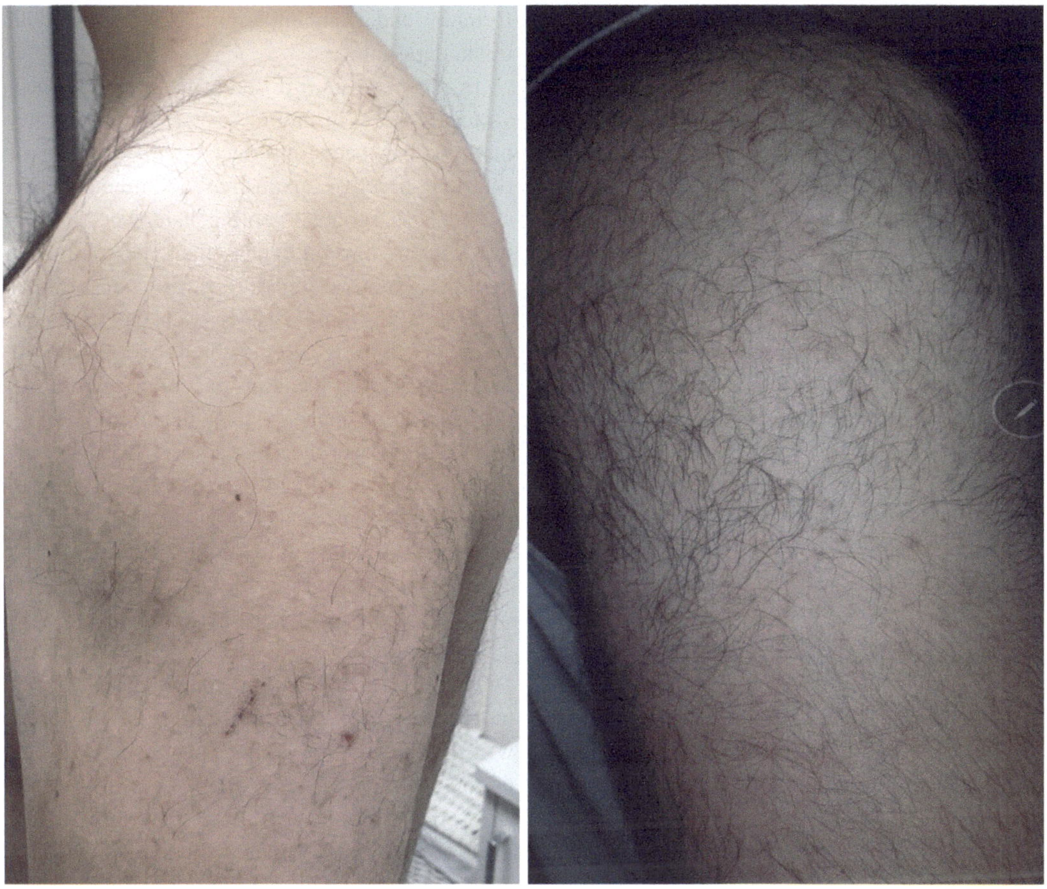

Fig. 4.11 Reactive hair growth on shoulder before and after five treatments with an Alexandrite laser

be more common in patients who already have some white or grey hair.

Folliculitis can arise following treatment—this may be as a result of shaving the area prior to treatment, or may be due to the hair shaft burning and causing orificial oedema which may occlude the follicular canal.

Common Causes of Adverse Reactions

1. *Treating tanned or recently UV exposed skin*—Perhaps the most common cause of unwanted skin reactions is treatment of tanned skin. Skin that has been recently exposed to UV, or self-tanning products, should not be treated, and exposure to UV should also be avoided for 4 weeks after treatment. Some lasers, such as the Nd:YAG or pain-free lasers, are less likely to cause problems when treating tanned skin. Nonetheless, lower fluences will have to be used, so general advice is to avoid tanning where possible, even with systems suitable for tanned skins.

In recent years, a number of tanning supplements have become available such as tanning injections, melonotan, tanning oral supplements and tanning nasal sprays. Many of these are unlicensed and untested, so although it's probable that they will also increase the risk of epidermal damage, we do not know how long they will have an effect—some anecdotal evidence suggests tanning injections in particular can be very long-lasting. Their use is therefore a contraindication for LHR.

2. *Inappropriate wavelength selection*—unwanted reaction incidence is higher when using shorter wavelengths, especially on darker skins. The Ruby and Alexandrite lasers are particularly inappropriate for use in darker skin types.
3. *Treating unshaven hair*—reactions can occur when hair has not been shaved sufficiently. Although it can be useful for visualization for the hair to protrude from the follicle by a millimeter or so, if it is any longer than this, absorption by the hair shaft can cause frazzling of the hair and subsequent epidermal damage.
4. *Treating over thin skin*—Settings should be reduced when treating over bony prominences or thin skin, for example, when treating the neck and décolleté, over shins or elderly patients.
5. *Treating thick, coarse hair*—when treating over very concentrated target (for example pubic hair or facial hair in men) more absorption will occur, and settings will therefore need to be adjusted to account for this.
6. *Inadequate cooling*—most hair removal systems will require some form of cooling. Some are built into the system, such as contact cooling handpieces or cryogen cooling, others recommend the use of separate devices such as forced air cooling or even just ice-packs. Too much cooling can limit efficacy but some cooling is generally recommended, especially when treating darker skin types.

Latest Advances

Pain-Free Hair Removal

A factor in many people's decision not to continue with LHR is the discomfort associated with treatment, especially for those with thick, dense hair, or darker skin. Although different cooling methods are employed to protect the epidermis and lessen discomfort, the traditional single-shot method of treatment, delivers high fluences in one pulse, resulting in high-peak temperatures within the skin. This can make treatment uncomfortable, and even intolerable, for people with thick, dark hair.

In recent years a different technique, known variously as 'in-motion' or 'high rep-rate' method, has been introduced with the aim of offering effective, 'pain-free' treatment. These systems use a contact-cooling handpiece, delivering light at lower fluences than the traditional methods, but at very high repetition rates. Rather than stamping single shots over the treatment area, the light is administered by sliding the handpiece across the skin in a series of continuous circular or linear movements, aiming to pass several times over the same area. Delivering multiple passes over a given area (usually 100 cm^2) in this fashion, causes cause gradual heating of the vital parts of the hair follicle, leading to its destruction with significantly less discomfort and with a very low incidence of side effects [69, 70]. These treatments are typically delivered with a Diode laser at a 800–810 nm wavelength, but more recently Alexandrite and Nd:YAG lasers with similar technology have also been launched on the market [69].

In general, more treatments may be required in pain-free modes, and many manufacturers suggest moving to standard emission for the final treatments for residual finer hair. Nonetheless, studies show that results are comparable to traditional lasers, with fewer side effects and high patient satisfaction [71].

Home-Use Devices

A number of laser/light sources are now available for home-use. These generally use diode or IPL technology and operate at fluences lower than those of professional devices. They usually have an in-built contact sensor to stop the system firing unless it is in contact with the skin, thereby making them eye safe and avoiding the requirement for safety eyewear [72]. However, it is more difficult to ensure that these systems are only used by people of appropriate skin type, or those without an active tan. The lack of training of the users means that there is also a real risk of people misjudging skin type and therefore using inappropriate settings that may result either in reduced efficacy or unwanted skin reactions.

Several studies report hair reduction with light-based home use devices [73, 74], however, there is some evidence that the low fluences used are only damaging the hair follicles to the extent that the hair is moved into catagen or telogen phase, thus delaying regrowth rather than causing permanent hair reduction [75].

Case Studies

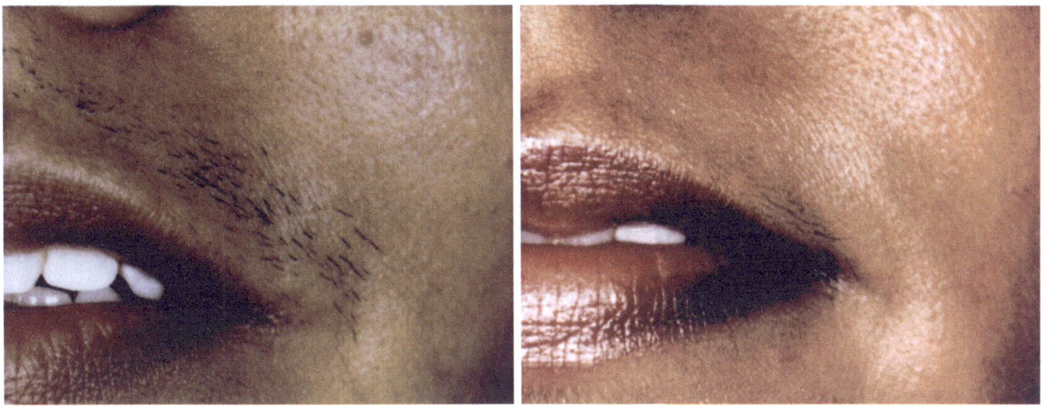

Case Study 1: A 29 year old lady, Fitzpatrick skin type 5 presented with coarse hair on her top lip, previously managed by threading. Before and after four treatments with Lumina IPL system (Lynton Lasers). Fluence 14–18 J/cm^2. Note remaining hair is much finer.

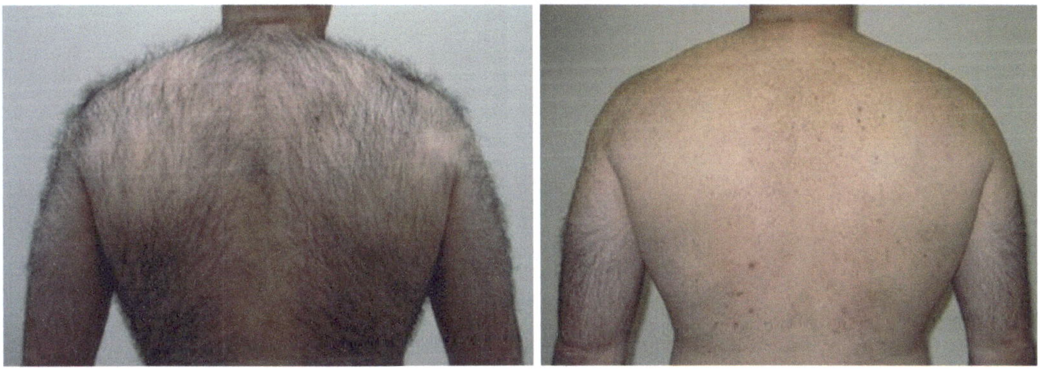

Case Study 2: A 36 year old man requested hair removal for dense hair growth on his back. Before and after four treatments with Lumina IPL system (Lynton Lasers). Skin Type 2, Fluence 20–26 J/cm^2. Note that in cases such as this, consideration is required to determine whereabouts on the arms to terminate treatment. In this case, the upper arms were treated every other treatment to avoid an abrupt change in growth. Due to the long hair growth cycle on the back, treatments should be spaced no less than 8 weeks apart.

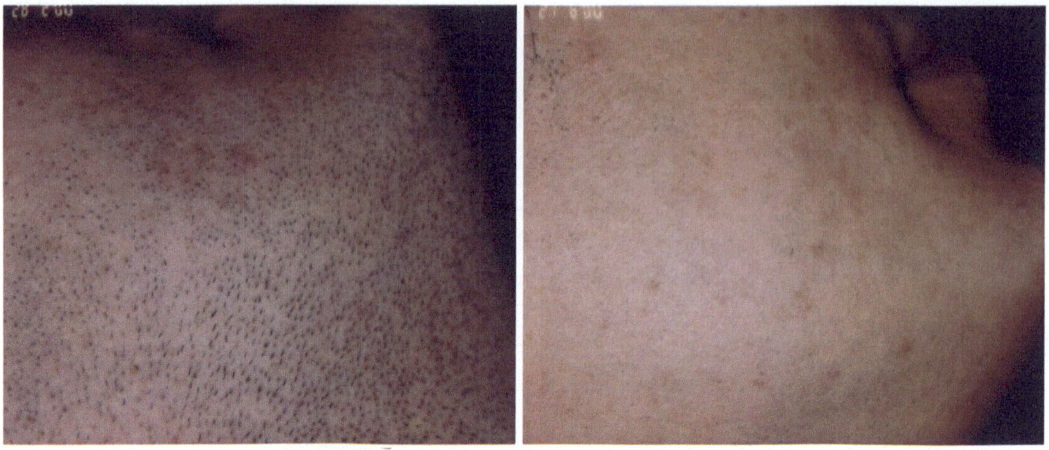

Case Study 3: Facial hair removal in a 32 year old man, before and after six treatments with Lumina IPL system (Lynton Lasers). Skin Type 2, Fluence 20–26 J/cm^2.

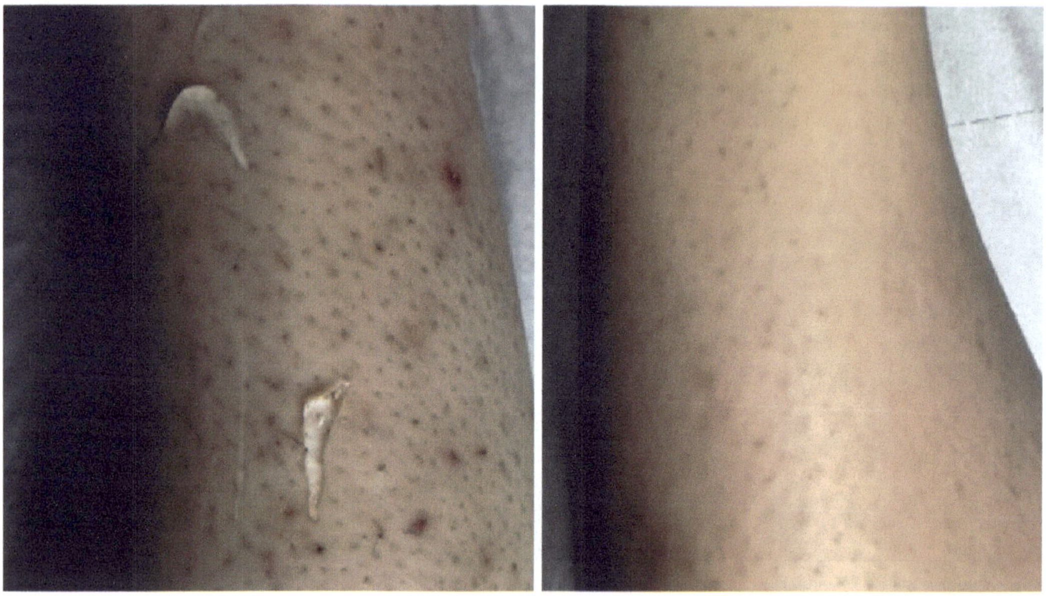

Case Study 4: A 27 year old woman presented for hair removal on her lower legs. This had preciously been managed with waxing, but had resulted in unsightly ingrowing hairs. Before and after nine treatments with Lumina IPL system (Lynton Lasers). Skin Type 4, Fluence 16–20 J/cm^2, 4–5 pulses with a 40–50 ms delay. Note the improvement in in-grown hairs and skin tone.

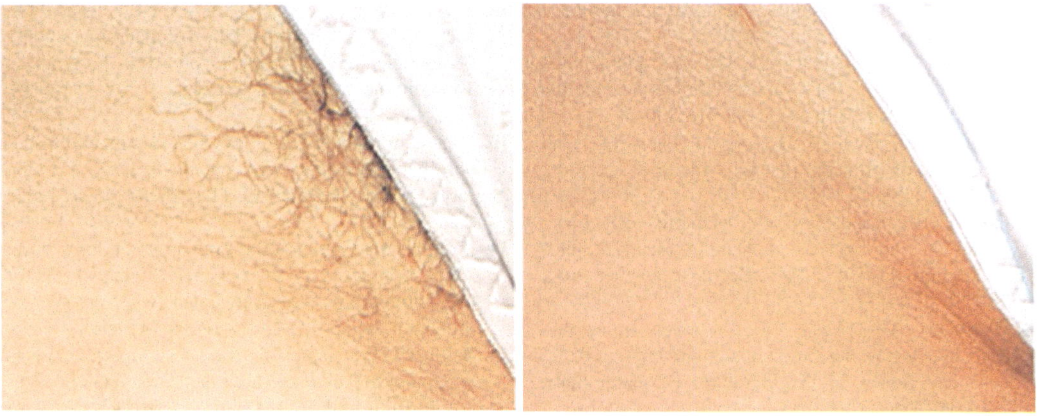

Case Study 5: A 36 year old woman was looking for a more effective, longer-lasting method for keeping her bikini line in check. She had previously tried shaving, waxing and sugaring and was only happy with the bikini line immediately after waxing or shaving. If shaved, she would have regrowth the following day, which would make the area itchy and uncomfortable. She found that waxing and sugaring provided a longer-lasting result, but the actual process was time consuming and painful. She would be happy with the results for a couple of weeks, but then suffered with ingrown hairs.

So her aim was to find a more permanent solution to maintain her bikini line—that wouldn't result in ingrown hairs or a shaving rash.

She was treated with Alexandrite laser, 12 mm spot size commencing at 20 J with a pulse width of 3 ms.

Patient noted a 75% reduction in hair growth after six treatments and complete resolution of ingrown hair.

References

1. Global Laser Hair Removal Market Report, https://www.marketwatch.com/press-release/at-170-cagr-laser-hair-removal-market-size-set-to-register-15468-million-usd-by-the-end-of-2025-2019-05-08
2. Haedersdal M, Wulf HC. Evidence-based review of hair removal using lasers and light sources. J Eur Acad Dermatol Venereol. 2006;20(1):9–20.
3. Zandi H, Lui H. Long-term removal of unwanted hair using light. Derm Clinics. 2013;31:179.
4. Slominski A, et al. Hair Foolical Pigmentation. J Invest Dermatol. 2005;124(1):13–21.
5. Caerwyn Ash et al Mathematical modeling of the optimum pulse structure for safe and effective photo epilation using broadband pulsed light, Journal of applied clinical medical physics, volume 13, number 5, 2012.
6. Lanigan SW. Incidence of side effects after laser hair removal. J Am Acad Dermatol. 2003;49:882–6.
7. Lim SP, Lannigan S. A review of the adverse effects of laser hair removal. Lasers Med Sci. 2006;21:121–5.
8. Alizadeh N, Aryoubi S, Naghipour R, et al. Can laser treatment improve quality of life of hirsute women. Int J Womans Health. n.d.;2017(9):777–80.
9. Lanigan S. Lasers in dermatology. London: Springer; 2000. p. 87.
10. Mintel. 2014. "The only way is smooth: half of Britains men feel the pressure to remove or groom their body hair." *www.mitel.com.* Accessed April 2015, 2015. www.mintel.com/press-centre/beauty-and-personal-care/the-only-way-is-smooth-half-of-britains-men-feel-the-pressure-to-remove-or-groom-their-body-hair.
11. Toosy S, Sodi R, Pappachan M. Lean polycystic ovary syndrome. J Diabetes Metabolic Disorders (Springer Nature). 2018;17:371.
12. Miletta NR, KIm S, Lezanski-Guida A, et al. Improving health related quality of life in wounded warriors: the promising benefits of laser hair removal to the residual limg-prosthetic ineterface. Dermatol Surg. 2016;42(10):1182–7.
13. Koch D, Pratsou P, Szczecinska W, Lanigan S, Abdullah A. The diverse application of laser hair removal therapy: a tertiary laser unit's experience with less common indications and a literature overview. Lasers Med Sci. 2015;30:453–67.
14. Lanzalaco A, Vanoosthuyze K, Stark C. A comparative clinical Study of diferent hair removal procedures

and their impact on asillary odor reduction in men. J Cosmet Dermatol. 2016;15:58–65.
15. Chicarilli ZN. Follicular occlusion triad: hidradenitis suppurativa, acne conglobata, and dissecting cellulitis of the scalp. Ann Plast Surg. 1987;18:230–4.
16. Schulze SM, Patel N, Hertzog D, Fares LG. 2nd Treatment of pilonidal disease with laser epilation. Am Surg. 2006;72:534–7.
17. Conroy FJ, Kandamany N, Mahaffey PJ. Laser depilation and hygiene: preventing recurrent pilonidal sinus disease. J Plast Reconstr Aesthet Surg. 2008;61:1069–72.
18. Benedetto AV, Lewis AT. Pilonidal sinus disease treated by depilation using an 800nm diode laser and review of the literature. Dermatol Surg. 2005;31:587–91.
19. Lavelle M, Jafri Z, Town G. Recurrent pilonidal sinus treated with epilation using a ruby laser. J Cosmet Laser Ther. 2002;4:45–7.
20. Downs AM, Palmer J. Laser hair removal for recurrent pilonidal sinus disease. J Cosmet Laser Ther. 2002;4:91.
21. Odili J, Gault D. Laser depilation of the natal cleft–an aid to healing the pilonidal sinus. Ann R Coll Surg Engl. 2002;84:29–32.
22. Landa N, Aller O, Landa-Gundin N, Torrontegui J, Azpiazu JL. Successful treatment of recurrent pilonidal sinus with laser epilation. Dermatol Surg. 2005;31:726–8.
23. Lukish JR, Kindelan T, Marmon LM, Pennington M, Norwood C. Laser epilation is a safe and effective therapy for teenagers with pilonidal disease. J Pediatr Surg. 2009;44:282–5.
24. Lukish JR, Kindelan T, Marmon LM, Pennington M, Norwood C. Laser epilation is a safe and effective therapy for teenagers with pilonidal disease. J Pediatr Surg. 2009;44:282–5.
25. Ghnnam WM, Hafez DM. Laser hair removal as adjunct to surgery for pilonidal sinus: our initial experience. J Cutan Aesthet Surg. 2011;4:192–5.
26. Ganjoo A. Laser hair reduction for pilonidal sinus-My experience. J Cutan Aesthet Surg. 2011;4:196.
27. Aleem S, Majid I. Unconventional uses of laser hair removal: a review. J Cutan Aesthet Surg. 2019;12(1):8–16.
28. Jain V, Jain A. Use of lasers for the management of refractory cases of hidradenitis suppurativa and pilonidal sinus. Cutan Aesthet Surg. 2012;5(3):190–2.
29. Tierney E, Mahmoud BH, Srivastava D, Ozog D, Kouba DJ. Treatment of surgical scars with nonablative fractional laser versus pulsed dye laser: a randomized controlled trial. Dermatol Surg. 2009;35:1172–80. [PubMed] [Google Scholar].
30. Highton L, Chan WY, Khwaja N, Laitung JK. Treatment of hidradenitis suppurativa with intense pulsed light: a prospective study. Plast Reconstr Surg. 2011;128:459–65.
31. Downs A. Smoothbeam laser treatment may help improve hidradenitis suppurativa but not hailey-hailey disease. J Cosmet Laser Ther. 2004;6:163–4.
32. Xu LY, Wright DR, Mahmoud BH, Ozog DM, Mehregan DA, Hamzavi IH. Histopathologic study of hidradenitis suppurativa following long-pulsed 1064-nm nd:YAG laser treatment. Arch Dermatol. 2011;147:21–8.
33. Yamauchi PS, Kelly AP, Lask GP. Treatment of pseudofolliculitis barbae with the diode laser. J Cutan Laser Ther. 1999;1:109–11. [PubMed] [Google Scholar].
34. Leheta TM. Comparative evaluation of long pulse Alexandrite laser and intense pulsed light systems for pseudofolliculitis barbae treatment with one year of follow up. Indian J Dermatol. 2009;54:364–8.
35. Smith EP, Winstanley D, Ross EV. Modified super-long pulse 810nm diode laser in the treatment of pseudofolliculitis barbae in skin types V and VI. Dermatol Surg. 2005;31:297–301.
36. Ross EV, Cooke LM, Overstreet KA, Buttolph GD, Blair MA. Treatment of pseudofolliculitis barbae in very dark skin with a long pulse nd:YAG laser. J Natl Med Assoc. 2002;94:888–93.
37. Rogers CJ, Glaser DA. Treatment of pseudofolliculitis barbae using the Q-switched nd:YAG laser with topical carbon suspension. Dermatol Surg. 2000;26:737–42.
38. Schulze R, Meehan KJ, Lopez A, Sweeney K, Winstanley D, Apruzzese W, et al. Low-fluence 1,064-nm laser hair reduction for pseudofolliculitis barbae in skin types IV, V, and VI. Dermatol Surg. 2009;35:98–107.
39. Boyd AS, Binhlam JQ. Use of an 800-nm pulsed-diode laser in the treatment of recalcitrant dissecting cellulitis of the scalp. Arch Dermatol. 2002;138:1291–3. [PubMed] [Google Scholar].
40. Krasner BD, Hamzavi FH, Murakawa GJ, Hamzavi IH. Dissecting cellulitis treated with the long-pulsed Nd:YAG Laser. Dermatol Surg. 2006;32:1039–44.
41. Parlette EC, Kroeger N, Ross EV. Nd:YAG laser treatment of recalcitrant folliculitis decalvans. Dermatol Surg. 2004;30: 1152–4. [PubMed] [Google Scholar].
42. Meesters AA, Van der Veen JP, Wolkerstorfer A. Long-term remission of folliculitis decalvans after treatment with the long-pulsed nd:YAG laser. J Dermatolog Treat. 2014;25:167–8.
43. Harowitz MR. Treatment of folliculitis decalvans with Nd: YAG laser. Surgical Cosmetic Dermatol. 2013;5:170–2.
44. Toosi S, Ehsani AH, Noormohammadpoor P, Esmaili N, Mirshams-Shahshahani M, Moineddin F. Treatment of trichostasis spinulosa with a 755-nm long-pulsed alexandrite laser. J Eur Acad Dermatol Venereol. 2010;24:470–3.
45. Badawi A, Kashmar M. Treatment of trichostasis spinulosa with 0.5-millisecond pulsed 755-nm Alexandrite laser. Lasers Med Sci. 2011;26:825–9.
46. Chavan DK, Chavan DD, Nikam BP, Kale MS, Jamale VP, Chavan SD. Efficacy of 800 nm diode laser to treat trichostasis spinulosa in Asian patients. Int J Trichol. 2018;10:21–3.

47. Moreno-Arias GA, Vilalta-Solsona A, Serra-Renom JM, Benito-Ruiz J, Ferrando J. Intense pulsed light for hairy grafts and flaps. Dermatol Surg. 2002;28:402–4.
48. Thomson KF, Sommer S, Sheehan-Dare RA. Terminal hair growth after full thickness skin graft: treatment with normal mode ruby laser. Lasers Surg Med. 2001;28:156–8.
49. Shim TN, Abdullah A, Lanigan S, Avery C. Hairy intraoral flap- an unusual indication for laser epilation. as series of 5 cases and review of the literature. Br J Oral Maxillofac Surg. 2011;49(7):50–2.
50. Shields BE, Moya MS, Bayon R, et al. A hairy siutation:laser hair removal after oral construction. Ann Otol Rhino Laryngol. 2018;127(3):205–8.
51. Toft K, Keller GS, Blackwell KE. Ectopic hair growth after flap reconstruction of the head and neck. Arch Facial Plast Surg. 2000;2:148–50.
52. Selvaggi G, Bellringer J. Gender reassignment surgery: an overview. Nat Rev Urol. 2011;8:274–82.
53. Bowman C, Goldberg JM. Care of the patient undergoing sex reassignment surgery. Int J Transgend. 2006;9:135–65.
54. Haedersdal M, Gøtzsche PC. Laser and photoepilation for unwanted hair growth. Cochrane Database Syst Rev. 2006:CD004684.
55. Görgü M, Aslan G, Aköz T, Erdoğan B. Comparison of alexandrite laser and electrolysis for hair removal. Dermatol Surg. 2000;26:37–41.
56. Zhang WR, Garrett GL, Arron ST, Garcia MM. Laser hair removal for genital gender affirming surgery. Transl Androl Urol. 2016;5:381–7.
57. Royston SL, Cole RP, Wright PA. Peristomal hair removal with an alexandrite laser. Colorectal Dis. 2013;15:1043–4. [PubMed] [Google Scholar.
58. Preston PW, Williams G, Abdullah A. Laser hair removal for peristomal skin. Clin Exp Dermatol. 2006;31:458.
59. Park HS, Kim JY, Choe YS, Han W, An JS, Seo KK. Alternative method for creating fine hairs with hair removal laser in hair transplantation for hairline correction. Ann Dermatol. 2015;27:21–5.
60. Desai S, Mahmoud BH, Bhatia AC, Hamzavi IH. Paradoxical hypertrichosis after laser therapy: a review. Dermatol Surg. 2010;36:291–8.
61. Moreno-Arias GA, Castelo-Branco C, Ferrando J. Side-effects after IPL photodepilation. Dermatol Surg. 2002;28(12):1131–4.
62. Town G, Bjerring P. Is paradoxical hair growth caused by low-level radiant exposure by home-use laser and intense pulsed light devices? J Cosmet Laser Ther. 2016;18(6):355–62.
63. Lolis MS, Marmur ES. Paradoxical effects of hair removal systems: a review. J Cosmet Dermatol. 2006;5:274–46.
64. Alajlan A, et al. Paradoxical hypertrichosis after laser epilation. J Am Acad Dermatol. 2005;53:85–8.
65. Moreno-Arias GA, Castel-Branco C, Ferrando J. Paradoxical effect after IPL photoepilation. Dermatol Surg. 2002;28:1013–6.
66. Willey A, Torrontegui J, Azpiazu J, et al. Hair stimulation following laser and intense pulsed light photoepilation: review of 543 cases and ways to manage it. Lasers Surg Med. 2007;39:297–301.
67. Radmanesh M, Azar-Beig M, Abtahian A, Naderi AH. Burning, paradoxical hypertrichosis, leukotrichia and folliculitis are four major complications of intense pulsed light hair removal therapy. J Dermatolog Treat. 2008;19(6):360–3.
68. Hélou J, Soutou B, Jamous R, Tomb R. Novel adverse effects of laser-assisted axillary hair removal. Annales de Dermatologie et de Venereologie. 2009;136(6-7):495–500.
69. Removal of unwanted hair: efficacy, tolerability, and safety of long-pulsed 755-nm alexandrite laser equipped with a sapphire handpiece. Lasers Med Sci. 2018, https://doi.org/10.1007/s10103-018-2503-z
70. Braun M. Comparison of high-fluence, single-pass diode laser to low-fluence, multiple-pass diode laser for aser hair reduction with 18 months of follow up. J Drugs Dermatol. 2011;10:62–5.
71. Barolet D. Low fluence–high repetition rate diode laser hair removal 12-month evaluation: reducing pain and risks while keeping clinical efficacy. Lasers Surg Med. 44:227–81.
72. Town G, Ash C. Are home-use intense pulsed light (IPL) devices safe? Lasers Med Sci. 2010; https://doi.org/10.1007/s10103-010-0809-6.
73. Alster TS, Tanzi EL. Effect of a novel, low-energy pulsed light device for home-use hair removal. Dermatol Surg. 2009;35:483–9.
74. Emerson R, Town G. Hair removal with a novel, low fluence, home-use intense pulsed light device: preliminary Results. J Cosmet Laser Ther. 2009;11(2):98–105.
75. Roosen G, Westgate G, Philpott M, Berretty P, Nuijs T, Bjerring P. Temporary hair removal by low fluence photoepilation: histological study on biopsies and cultured human hair follicles. Lasers Surg Med. 2008;40:520–8.

Ablative Lasers

5

Vishal Madan

Introduction

The term 'ablation' refers to removal of material from the surface of an object by vaporization, chipping, or other erosive processes. In the context of the skin, laser ablation can be achieved by heating the abundant water in the epidermis and dermis. The oldest laser device achieving this response was the continuous wave carbon dioxide laser (CO_2 laser) as the chromophore for CO_2 laser is water. Kumar Patel of Bell Labs invented the CO_2 laser in 1964-one of the first gas lasers to be invented [1]. However, the CO_2 laser does not meet the criteria for selective photothermolysis because its chromophore water exists uniformly in soft tissue. CO_2 laser surgery could, therefore, be described as tissue-selective. The absorption of water by the CO_2 laser makes it an ideal ablating and cutting laser and it remains one of the most essential and versatile surgical laser systems till date.

One of the main drawbacks of the traditional continuous wave CO_2 laser is the non-selective tissue damage resulting in scarring and dyspigmentation. The quest for precise tissue ablation and predictive results led to introduction of scanner assisted CO_2 laser and later to Er:Yag lasers [2]. Despite the advent of these technologies and more reproducible results, the aesthetically aware patients were keen to avoid the prolonged downtime that resulted from use of these devices.

Since the mid- 2000s, the concept of fractional laser technology has gained immense popularity. First conceptualised to be used with non-ablative systems, it was rapidly adapted for ablative laser devices. The result was an ablative system, with reduced downtime, lower risks of side effects at the expense of reduced efficacy.

Ablative Laser Devices

The CO_2 Laser

CO_2 laser emits energy at 10,600 nm which is in the far-infrared range. This wavelength is absorbed very well by water. By varying the parameters, the CO_2 laser can have varying biological effects on the skin. Focusing the beam to increase the power density allows the laser beam to incise the skin, defocusing the beam reduces the power density to coagulate tissue. One advantage of the CO_2 laser over 'cold steel' surgery is that the coagulation that is achieved results in haemostasis, so a relatively bloodless field is achieved. This particularly useful in reducing rhinophyma or excising hidradenitis suppurativa

V. Madan (✉)
Consultant Dermatologist, Laser and Mohs Surgeon, Salford Royal NHS Foundation Trust, Stott Lane, Salford, UK

Everything Skin Clinic, Haw Bank House, High Street, Stockport, UK
e-mail: vishal.madan@srft.nhs.uk

V. Madan (ed.), *Practical Introduction to Laser Dermatology*,
https://doi.org/10.1007/978-3-030-46451-6_5

nodules and sinuses, which are otherwise very vascular.

Besides the immediate visible effects of ablation, cutting and vaporisation, there are the invisible effects which result in many of the long term clinical effects of the CO_2 laser [1]. As the laser beam impacts the skin, this results in a photothermal reaction, raising temperatures to above 100 °C, resulting in ablation of the epidermis and dermis. From the point of initial impact, there is a reduction in the temperature gradient that results in coagulation (>60 °C), protein degradation (>55 °C) denaturation (40 °C) and cellular photobioactivation.

These biological effects are essential for collagen remodelling and neocollagenesis, which result in the desirable endpoints seen after CO_2 laser treatment of photoaging. On the flip side, excessive residual thermal damage (RTD) results in undesirable effects such as scarring and prolonged erythema. The amount of RTD which can be tolerated without scarring appears to be less than 300 μm.

This was the major drawback of the original continuous wave CO_2 lasers used in the dermatological setting. If however, the laser beam fired in trains of very short high peak power pulses within 1 ms (thermal relaxation time of skin), with very long interpulse intervals, there is a reduction in the residual thermal damage and consequently less risk of scarring. Such beam profiles were made possible by the use of scanners and oscillating mirrors which would generate superpulse and ultrapulse waveforms. These waveforms differ in their pulse widths and peak powers, with the ultrapulse mode generating very high peak powers in very short pulse widths resulting precise ablation with minimal RTD [1, 3].

Despite the reduction in RTD with ultrapulse and superpulse waveforms, the downtime after CO_2 laser treatment was still considered unacceptable by most patients.

The Erbium:YAG laser

The Erbium:YAG (Er:YAG) laser emits at 2940 nm, a wavelength that is much more strongly absorbed by water than the 10,600 nm of CO_2 laser (absorption coefficient 12,000 vs 800 cm^{-1} for CO_2). The RDT with Er:YAG is consequently reduced to less than 50 μm vs 150 μm observed with ultrapulse CO_2 laser [2].

The Er:YAG laser induced wounds re-epithelialize earlier than those formed after CO_2 laser. Comparative studies have convincingly demonstrated that Er:YAG laser treatment, at similar fluence per pulse and number of passes as CO_2 laser treatment, produces more superficial ablation, promotes faster healing with less post- treatment erythema, is less effective and results in inadequate haemostasis. By increasing the number of Er:YAG laser passes (≥5), the depth of injury can be increased to mimic the results of standard CO_2 laser resurfacing.

The differences between CO_2 and Er:YAG laser are listed in Table 5.1.

The Erbium: YSGG laser

The water absorption coefficient of Erbium: yttrium scandium gallium garnet (Er:YSGG) laser, which has a wavelength of 2790 nm, is between that of the Er:YAG laser and that of the CO_2 laser . It is therefore argued that Er:YSGG laser has an ideal wavelength, balancing the vaporization of the epidermis layer and the residual heating of the dermis layer. In other words, the Er:YSGG laser has advantages of both the CO_2 laser and the Er:YAG laser [3]. Despite the claims, this wavelength has not gained popularity and not many laser systems using this wavelength exist in dermatological practice.

Table 5.1 Differences between Carbon dioxide and Er:YAG lasers

PROPERTIES	CO_2	Er:YAG
Affinity for water	x	16 x
Per pass	20–60 μm	5–15 μm
RTD	150 μm	15 μm
Haemostasis	Yes	No
Healing	Slow	Fast(er)
Complications	More	Few

Table 5.2 Ablative laser indications in dermatology

Resurfacing mode	Superpulse mode	Cutting mode
Epidermal Naevi	Steatocystoma multiplex	Hidradenitis suppurutiva
Actinic keratoses	Sebaceous hyperplasia	Neurofibromas
Acne scarring	Colloid milium	Earlobe Keloids
Seborrhoeic keratoses	Comedones	
Bowen's disease	Dermatosis papulosa nigra	
Actinic cheilitis	Syringomata	
Rhinophyma	Angiofibromas	
Rhytides	Milia	
Darier's disease	Angiolymphoid hyperplasia	
Hailey Hailey disease	Hidrocystomas	
Neurofibroma		
Warts		
Eyeliner tattoos		
Zoon's balanitis		
Balanitis xerotica		
Lymphangioma circumscriptum		
Porokeratosis		
Nodular amyloidosis		
Xanthelasma		
Syringocystadenoma		
Granuloma faciale		
Trichoepitheliomas		
Pemphigus vegetans		
Melanoma metastases		
Superficial BCC		

Ablative Laser Technique and Indications

Ablative lasers can be used in resurfacing (coagulative), or cutting modes. Besides, high fluence, superpulse waveform of the CO_2 laser can be used for destruction of benign skin lesions (Table 5.2).

Preparation

A detailed medical history and thorough dermatological examination are essential prerequisites before any laser procedure. Especially with fully ablative laser treatments, it is important to spend time with the patient to ensure they understand the potential risks of the treatments. Showing patients immediate post-treatment photographs should help them decide on whether they would be able to cope with the healing phase and downtime of ablative laser treatment. Patients with history of herpes simplex infection should commence on oral anti herpetic tablets such as acyclovir on the day of the treatment and continue for 5–7 days. Strict sun protection measures should be employed for at least 4 weeks before the treatment and for 3–4 months following treatment to prevent post-treatment dyspigmentation. Recent oral isotretinoin treatment should preclude any laser resurfacing for at least 6 months.

Consent Ablative laser treatments carry significant risks of scarring, dyspigmentation and prolonged erythema. These risks should be clearly documented in the consent forms and in any pre-treatment information that is provided to the patients.

Anaesthetic Considerations Resurfacing procedures using the CO_2 and Er:YAG lasers require local/infiltration or general anaesthesia. Where possible, nerve blocks should be used to provide adequate anaesthesia without distorting the field of treatment with local infiltration. Such techniques are instrumental in the treatment of acne scars and rhinophyma.

When operating on small superficial skin lesions, e.g. milia, topical anaesthesia alone may be sufficient.

Pre-treatment Preparation Once adequate anaesthesia is achieved, the skin surface should be cleaned with saline and care should be taken to wipe the skin surface dry before laser treatment is initiated.

Laser Precautions Before laser treatment is initiated, the operator should ensure that adequate eye protection is in place for both the patient and the staff in the room. When operating in the periorbital zone, one should exercise extreme caution and use metal corneal shields to prevent corneal burns. Burning and singeing of the airway is a possibility if operating too close to the endotracheal tubes. A good practice is to secure the endotracheal tube and to wrap the exposed part with wet saline gauze.

Ablative laser treatments result in generation of the plume in which active viral DNA has been identified that can pose respiratory infection and potential carcinogenic risk. Adequate protection with specially made laser filtration masks and laser plume extraction devices should be used in all cases.

Post-ablative Laser Treatment Care
Ablative laser treatments result in superficial burns. These exudative wounds are best covered with absorbent (foam) dressings for 24–48 h following treatment. After this period the wounds should not be allowed to form dry crusts. This can be achieved by using bland emollients such as petrolatum jelly or aloe vera gel. Patients should be warned not to lift the crusts manually but to wash the wounds once daily with warm soapy water. For smaller areas and superficial treatments, the wounds can be left open from the outset.

Ablative lasers can be used in resurfacing (coagulative), or cutting modes. Besides, high fluence, superpulse waveform of the CO_2 laser can be used for destruction of small, benign skin lesions.

A. Resurfacing Mode Indications—when the continuous beam of the CO_2 laser is scanned to generate pulsed waveforms.

1. Acne Scarring Both the CO_2 and Er:Yag lasers can be used to improve acne scars. Not all acne scars can be treated with lasers and oftentimes, a multimodality approach is needed to achieve the desired outcomes. These could include ablative, non-ablative, fractional lasers, radiofrequency, subcision, punch excision, chemical peels and dermal fillers [4, 5]. Identifying the right candidate for laser resurfacing is often a challenge but the experienced operator should be able to choose the right candidate with appropriate scars of correct severity for the proposed laser treatment. Patients with active acne should have their acne adequately treated before being offered ablative laser treatments for the scarring.

Grouped box car scars and wider ice pick scars on a background of skin phototype 1–3 are best suited for ablative laser resurfacing (Fig. 5.1) . That said, patients with darker skin types may also be treated, but care should be taken to prevent post-treatment dyspigmentation. Hypertrophic scars also respond well to this approach (Fig. 5.2).

A laser patch test on a carefully selected representative site would be desirable, especially when treating darker skin types. An assessment should be undertaken at least 4 weeks later to ensure that desired response has been achieved.

Laser resurfacing for acne scarring comprises of shouldering the individual scars to ‘flatten’ the edges. This can be accomplished by 1–2 passes of the scanned CO_2 laser beam 3–4 mm spot at 12 Watts, equating to fluence of 5.5-6 J/cm^2.

Care should be taken to wipe the char formed following laser treatment before another pass is delivered. After shouldering the scars, the anatomical zone bearing the scars should be resurfaced. The edges of the treatment zone should be treated at a lower fluence (feathered) to achieve a similar effect. This would allow an even treatment zone without noticeable demarcation lines.

It is recommended to initiate treatments with the lowest ablative fluence and to advise patients that multiple sessions may be required to achieve the desired results. These sessions should be spaced at 3–6 monthly intervals.

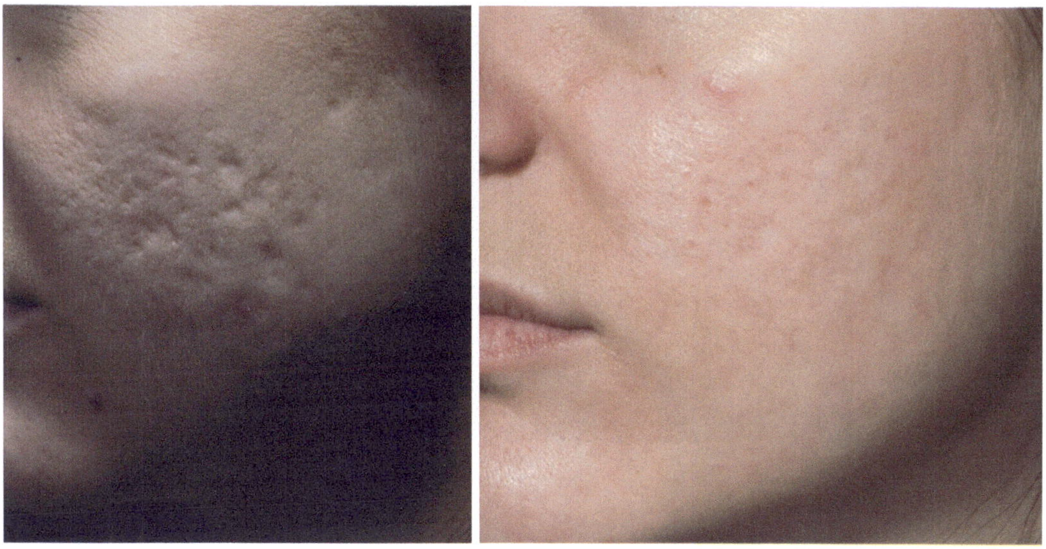

Fig. 5.1 Boxcar variant of acne scarring in a patient with skin phototype 2, before and after carbon dioxide laser resurfacing

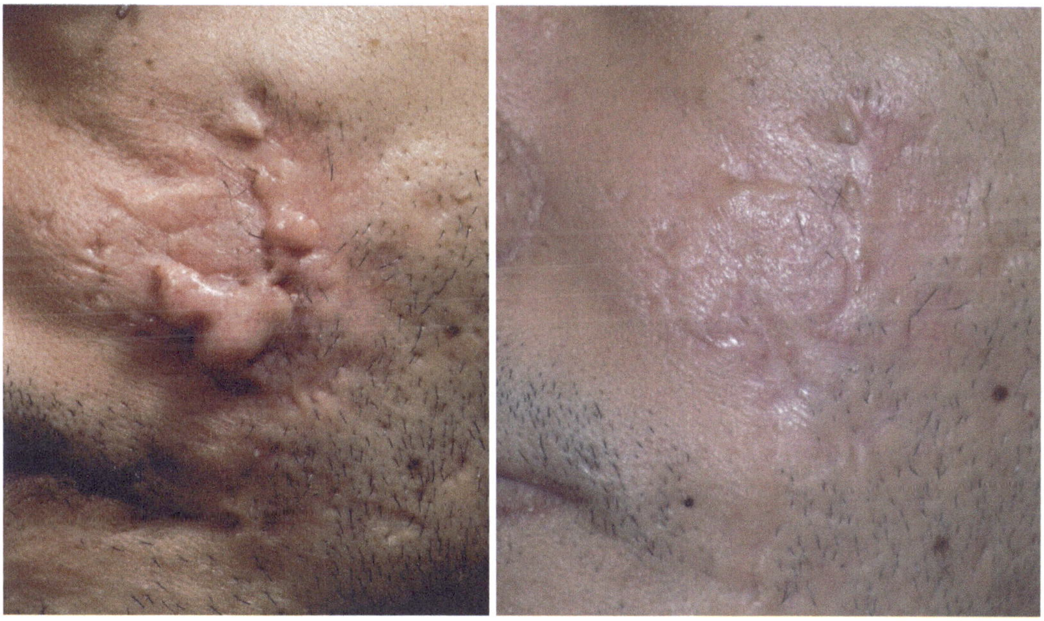

Fig. 5.2 Hypertrophic Acne scarring. Response to fully ablative Carbon dioxide laser resurfacing

2. **Rejuvenation/Rhytides** Both CO_2 and Er:YAG lasers are excellent devices for rejuvenation of the ageing skin. Ablative laser resurfacing can be used alone or in combination with non-laser modalities such as dermal fillers to achieve rejuvenation. While traditional fully ablative CO_2 laser resurfacing is considered the gold standard, the downtime associated is remarkably long and post laser sequel including prolonged erythema has made this form of treatment less popular. One added advantage of ablative laser treatment for facial rejuvenation is that superficial pigmentation, so commonly seen in photo-aged skin is also addressed by this modality [6] (Fig. 5.3).

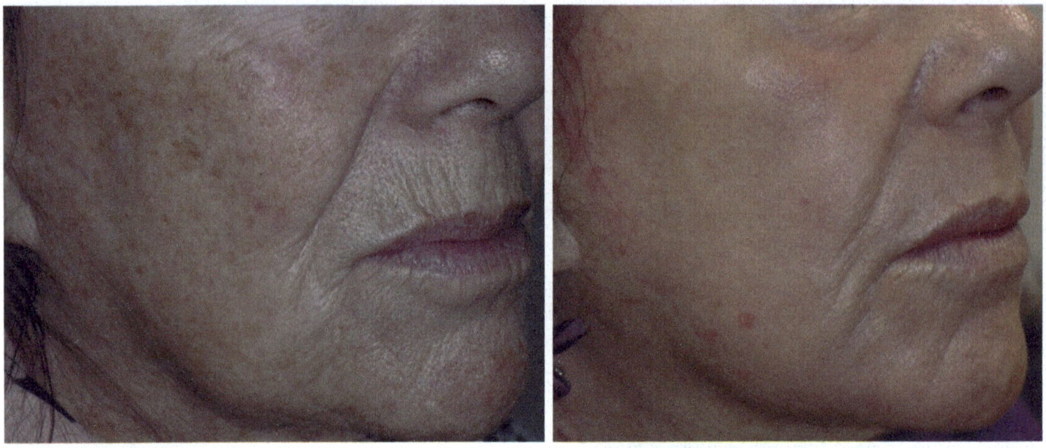

Fig. 5.3 Photoageing treated with fully ablative Carbon dioxide laser resurfacing (note the improvement in the solar lentigenes and perioral rhytides)

The number of passes depends upon the severity of the rhytides and photoaging. Pulse staking and aggressive treatment, especially around eyelids and perioral areas should be avoided.

Er:YAG laser resurfacing is particularly advantageous for resurfacing of perioral rhytides as the risk of post-treatment pallor is lower than with CO_2 laser resurfacing [2]. Care should be taken when treating the jaw line as risk of hypertrophic scarring is considered high at this site.

3. Rhinophyma The CO_2 laser has become the treatment of choice for moderate to severe rhinophyma [7]. The procedure is undertaken under local anaesthetic nerve blocks to the external nasal branch of the anterior ethmoidal nerve and infraorbital nerves. Once adequate anaesthesia is achieved, the phymatous tissue is debulked using high powered CO_2 laser in scanner mode (Figs. 5.4 and 5.5). The excessive tissue can be 'cut' by the using the laser in its continuous mode, however this approach can be dangerous as too much tissue can be inadvertently be excised resulting in scarring. Depending upon the thickness of the phymatous tissue to be ablated, the laser power required can range from 15–30 Watts. Care should be taken to avoid over treatment especially on nasal ala and dorsum. The risk of scarring is high at these sites. A good way of knowing the safe zone of treatment is to squeeze the tissue to ensure there is some sebaceous discharge. Presence of intact sebaceous glands would be required for reepithelialisation without scarring. The operative field is usually avascular, however; larger vessels may haemorrhage which can be controlled by defocusing the laser beam or using electrocautery.

4. Seborrhoeic Keratoses (Fig. 5.6) These stuck on lesions are easily removed using ablative lasers [8, 9]. The advantage of ablative lasers over other destructive techniques e.g. cryotherapy is the precision of the laser to avoid injury to normal skin and that multiple lesions can be treated in one sitting. The risk of hypopigmentation is also reduced with laser treatment. One to two passes of low fluence ablative laser beam followed by wiping the keratoses is all that is required for majority of seborrheic keratoses.

5. Actinic Cheilitis (Fig. 5.7) CO_2 laser treatment has long been considered the treatment of choice for actinic cheilitis but may have been superseded by photodynamic therapy. Before laser treatment, and in case of any doubt, a skin biopsy should be undertaken to rule out invasion as laser treatment would have no role in the treatment of squamous cell carcinoma. The laser is used in resurfacing mode to denude the actinically damaged mucosal epithelium [10, 11]. Pinpoint bleeding can be controlled by using the

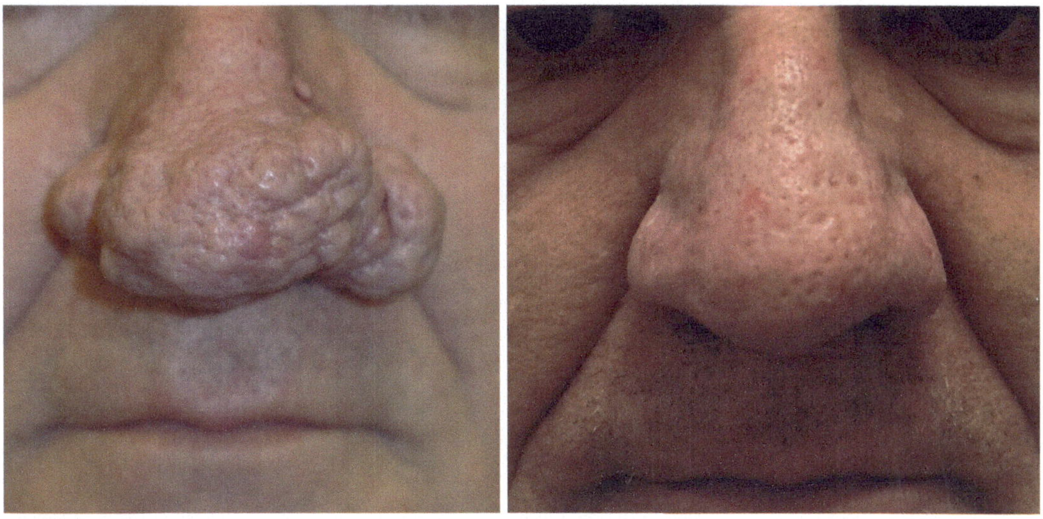

Fig. 5.4 Extensive Rhinophyma before and after carbon dioxide laser resurfacing-End on view

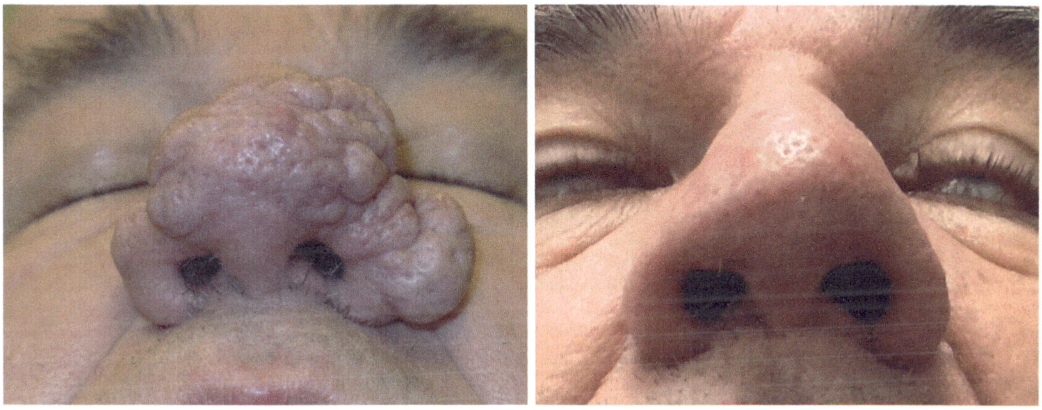

Fig. 5.5 Extensive Rhinophyma before and after carbon dioxide laser resurfacing-End on view

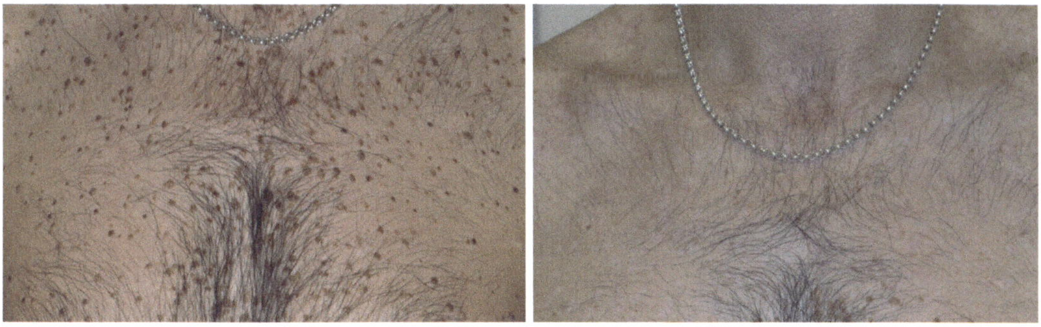

Fig. 5.6 Seborrhoeic keratoses before and after ablative laser treatment

laser in a defocussed mode. For persistent bleeding points, electrocoagulation may be necessary. Secondary intention healing with repeated applications of bland emollients is usually achieved in 1–2 weeks. Multiple sessions may be required.

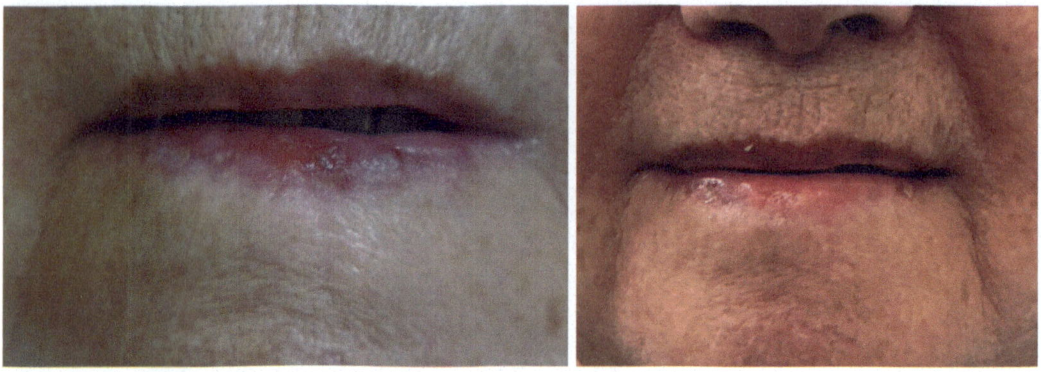

Fig. 5.7 Erosion on central lower mucosal lip was histologically confirmed as actinic cheilits with no evidence of invasion. Single session of carbon dioxide laser was undertaken with excellent results

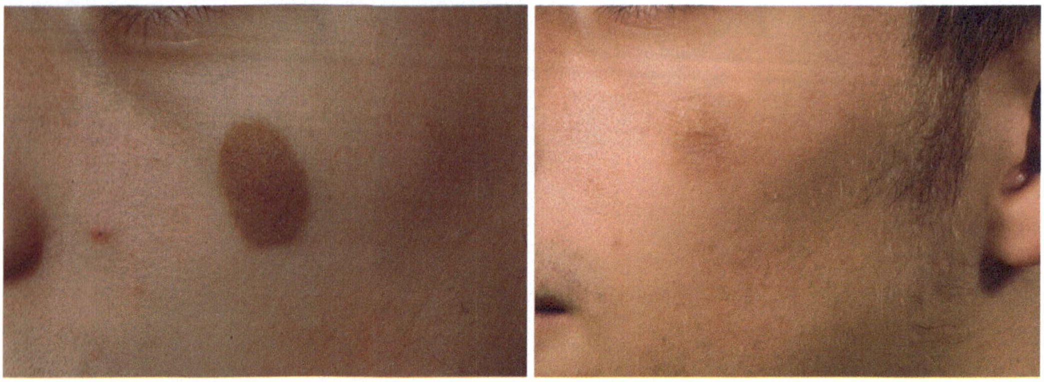

Fig. 5.8 Dark brown congenital melanocytic naevus on left cheek. Combination of carbon dioxide and QS 755 nm Alexandrite lasers, resulted in an acceptable cosmetic outcome. Patient had declined surgery

6. Actinic Keratoses and Bowen's Disease While destruction of the precancerous tissue can be readily accomplished with ablative lasers, the role of CO_2 and Er:YAG lasers in the management of actinic keratoses and Bowen's disease has been superseded by photodynamic therapy and topical treatments [11].

7. Epidermal and Congenital Melanocytic Naevi (Figs. 5.8 and 5.9) Small to medium-sized congenital melanocytic naevi and verrucous epidermal naevi can be ablated with CO_2 and Er:YAG lasers [12]. The risk of scarring with surgical excision should be weighed against the risk of recurrence and hypopigmentation with laser treatment. Similarly, given the small risk of progression of sebaceous naevi to basal cell carcinoma, where possible such lesions should be excised.

8. Darier's and Hailey-Hailey Disease (Fig. 5.10) The exact mechanism by which laser resurfacing the verrucous plaques and erosions of Darier's and Hailey-Hailey disease results in long term remission remains unknown [13, 14]. It is likely that the fibroplasia created by the laser prevents recurrence. As such, topical therapies form the treatment of choice and laser treatment should be offered for recalcitrant disease.

9. Neurofibromas Small neurofibromas can be ablated with the CO_2 laser. Larger lesions have a deep subcutaneous component which will invariably recur should the lesion only be resurfaced.

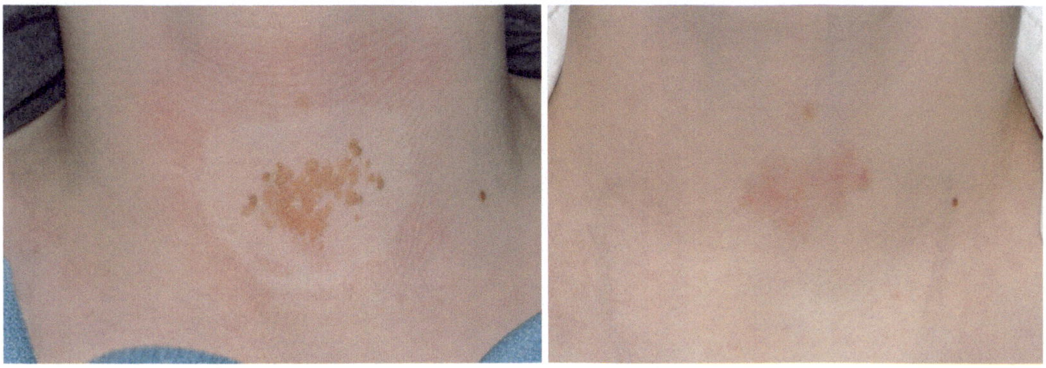

Fig. 5.9 Epidermal naevus on the neck of a young adult before and 3 months following ablative laser resurfacing using CO_2 laser

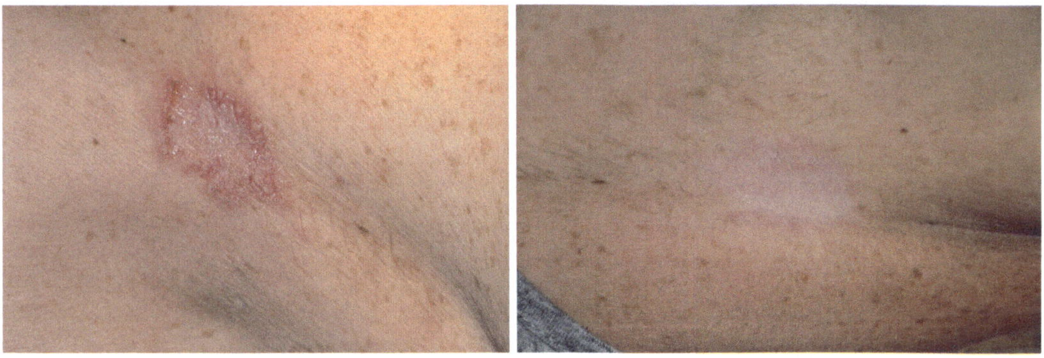

Fig. 5.10 Complete resolution of resistant Hailey-Hailey disease plaque with ablative laser resurfacing. Note the residual hypopigmentation following laser treatment

Such lesions need to be excised with the laser in its cutting mode. Post laser depigmentation is a frequent sequel of treatment of neurofibromas which should be explained to the patient before treatment [15] (Fig. 5.11).

10. Warts Cutaneous warts not responding to topical therapies or cryotherapy should be considered for laser treatment. The laser of choice for such warts would be the less invasive pulsed dye laser. However, multiple sessions are required and the treatment is not always guaranteed to bring about a cure. Patients with hyperkeratotic warts and those non-responsive to the pulsed dye laser may be offered CO_2 or Er: YAG laser resurfacing [14]. CO_2 laser treatment is also very effective for anogenital warts and for debulking the warty tissue before pulsed dye laser treatment (Fig. 5.12).

The laser can be used to excise the wart or to resurfacing the hyperkeratotic surface.

Immunosuppressed patients tend not to respond very well to laser treatment of warts given the high risk of recurrence following treatment.

11. Cylindromas and Other Benign Cutaneous Tumours (Figs. 5.13 and 5.14) Benign cutaneous lesions such as cylindromas, hydrocystomas, angiofibromas, trichoepitheliomas can be resurfaced with ablative lasers. This would be preferable to surgical excision especially for multiple lesions [16].

B. Superpulse Mode Indications

1. Steatocystoma Multiplex (Fig. 5.15) Patients with steatocystoma simplex have multiple small

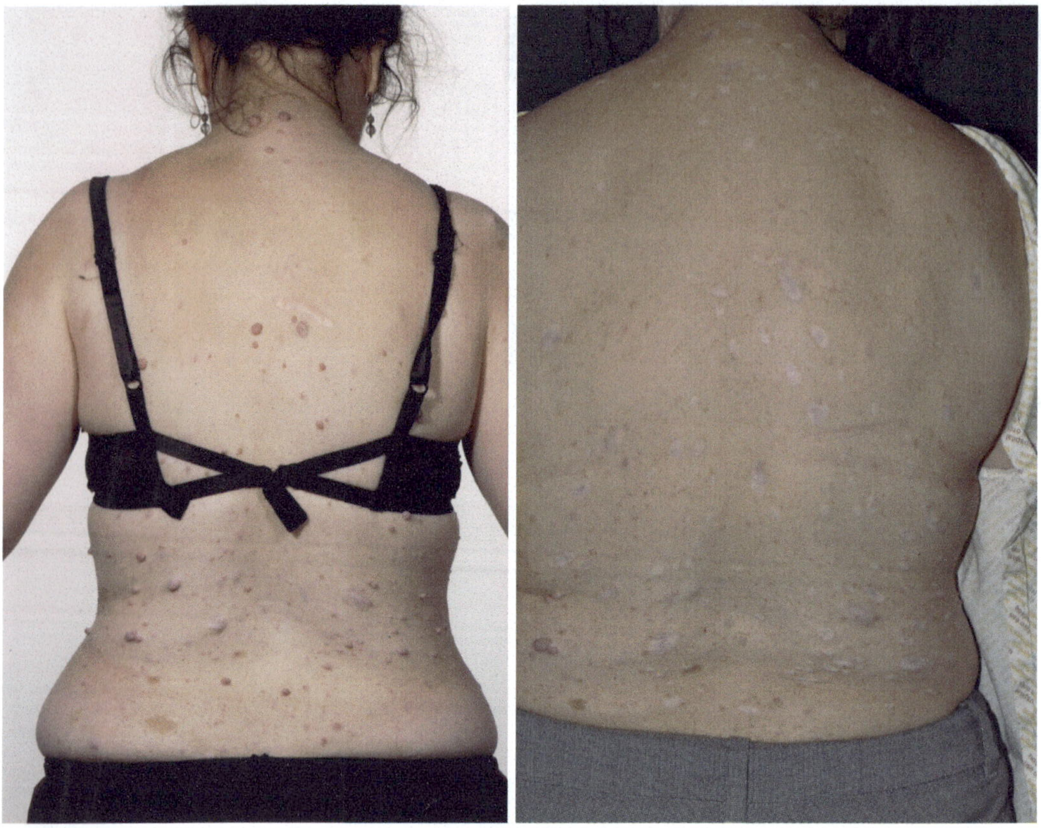

Fig. 5.11 Neurofibromatoses 1, before and after carbon dioxide laser resurfacing. Reduction in numbers of lesions can be seen at the expense of depigmented patches

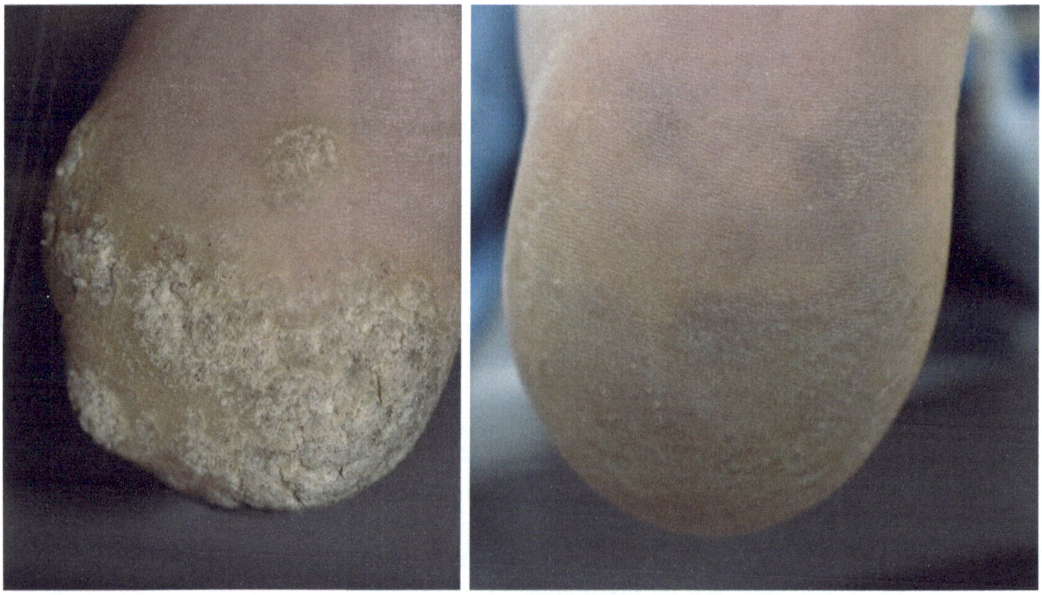

Fig. 5.12 Hyperkeratotic cryotherapy resistant plantar verruca vulgaris before and after ablative laser followed by pulsed dye laser. Results after 6 combination laser treatment sessions

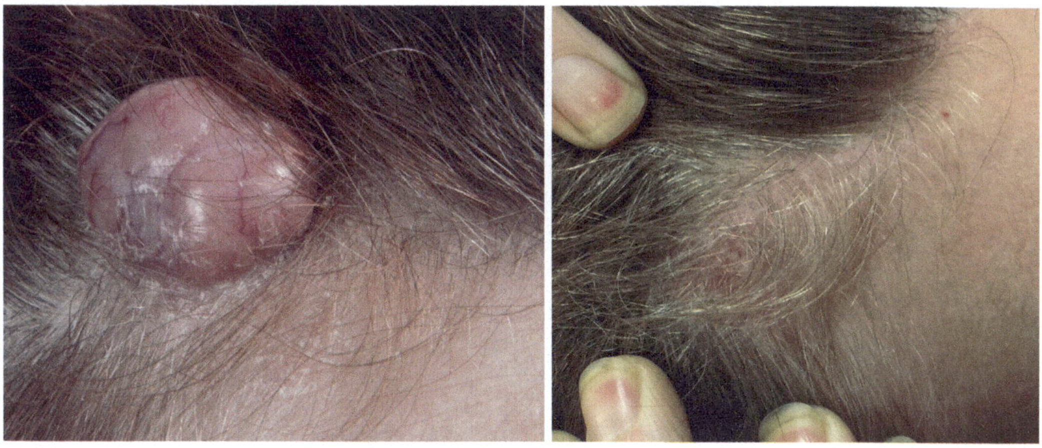

Fig. 5.13 Benign cutaneous lesions such as Cylindroma shown here respond very well tto ablative laser resurfacing

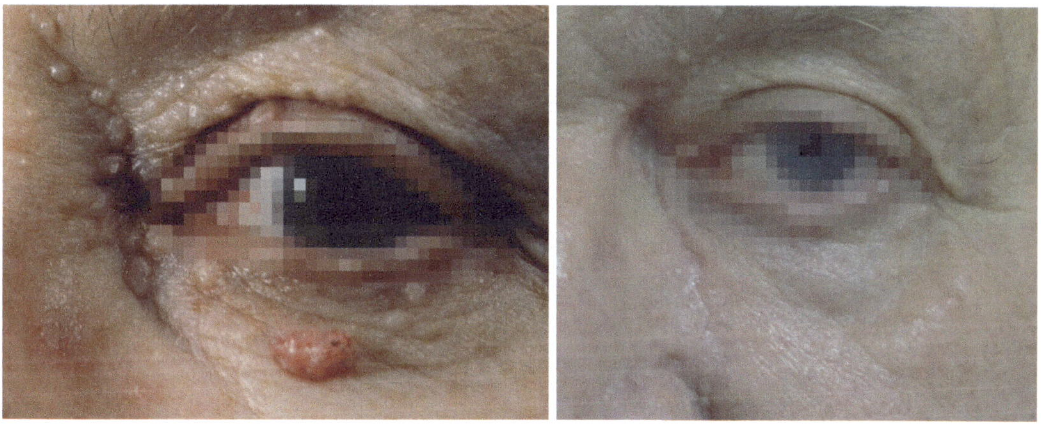

Fig. 5.14 Smaller benign lesions such as tricholetheliomas respond favourably to laser ablation

to large cysts. Excision of these cysts will result in scarring which is unacceptable to most patients. An alternative to excision is the perforation of the cysts with the superpulse mode of CO_2 laser followed by extirpation of cyst contents and cyst wall using a small chalazion curette introduced through the laser created puncture [17].

Once the cyst wall is extirpated, the risk of recurrence is considerably reduced and the small laser puncture heals secondarily to leave minimally visible scars.

2. Sebaceous Gland Hyperplasia (Fig. 5.16) In the superpulse mode the CO_2 laser is an excellent tool for superficial ablation of the rim of sebaceous gland hyperplasia [14]. This eliminates the need for resurfacing and consequently risks of scarring and dyspigmentation. With superpulse treatment, the downtime is reduced to 3–4 days. For larger lesions, either CO_2 or Er:YAG lasers may be used in fully ablative modes to resurface the lesions. Lower fluence is required to achieve this response.

3. Comedones Closed acne comedones or solar comedones seen in Favre Racouchot Syndrome can be superficially ablated or resurfaced. Occasionally it may be necessary to 'scoop' the solar comedonal contents [18].

4. Dermatosis Papulosa Nigra (Fig. 5.17) Dermatosis paulosa nigra are small seborrheic kera-

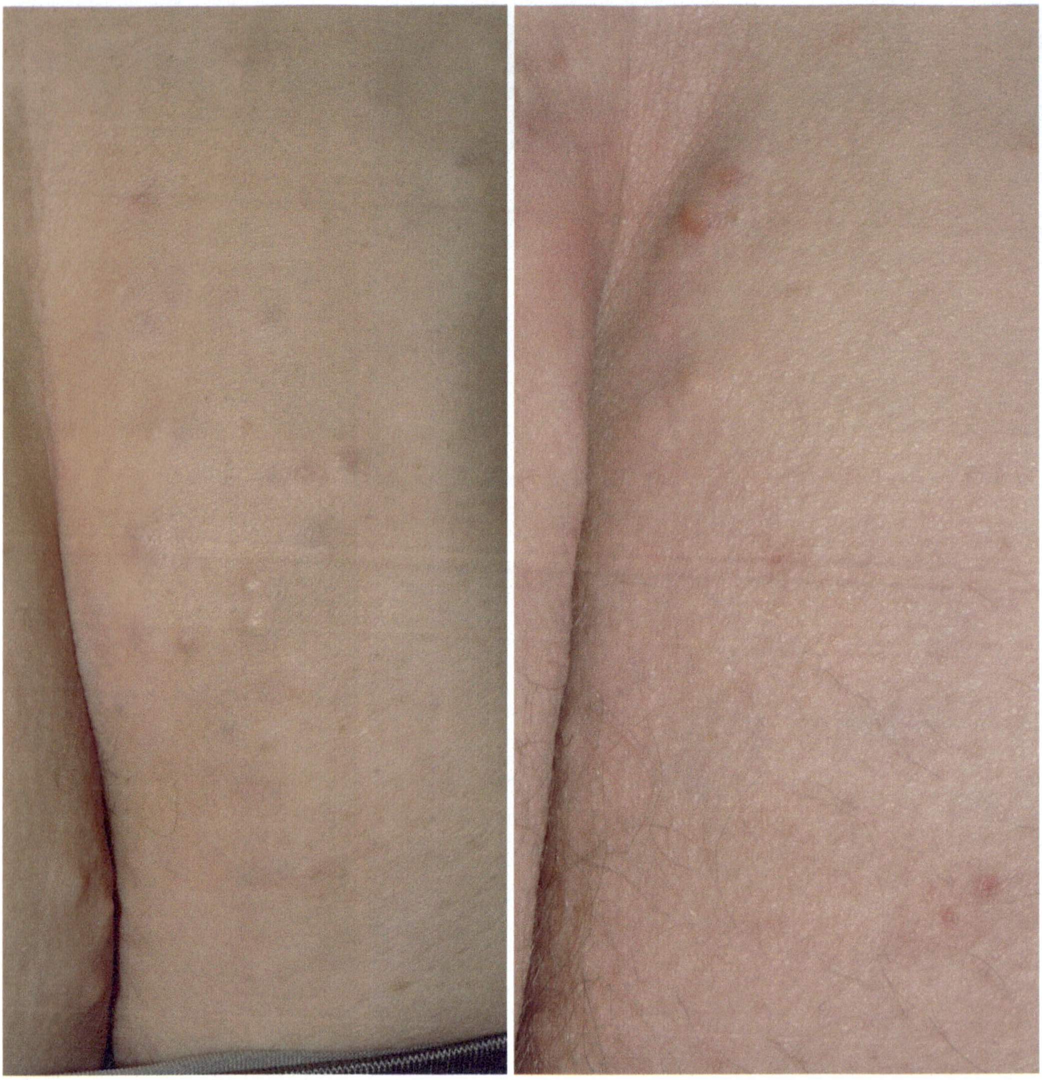

Fig. 5.15 Steatocystoma multiplex on buttock after perforation and extirpation

tosis like papules predominantly seen on the face and neck of darker skin patients. They can be ablated using the superpulse mode of the CO_2 laser [19]. Risks of scarring and dyspigmentation can be substantially reduced as laser energy is deposited superficially.

5. Syringomas Periorbital syringomas are very difficult to treat as the lesions are deep sited and complete ablation will invariably result in pitted scars. To avoid this, superficial ablation may be a better approach, albeit, associated with a higher recurrence rate.

6. Milia Small keratinous cysts can be punctured with the CO_2 laser, and the contents of the cysts can be wiped or extracted with ease.

C. Cutting Mode

1. Hidradenitis Suppurativa (Fig. 5.18) Hidradenitis suppurativa is a disabling condition which may be resistant to topical and systemic therapy. For localised, Hurley 2–3 disease with recurrent non healing nodules or sinuses, CO_2 laser can be used in continuous cutting mode to excise the diseased tissue.

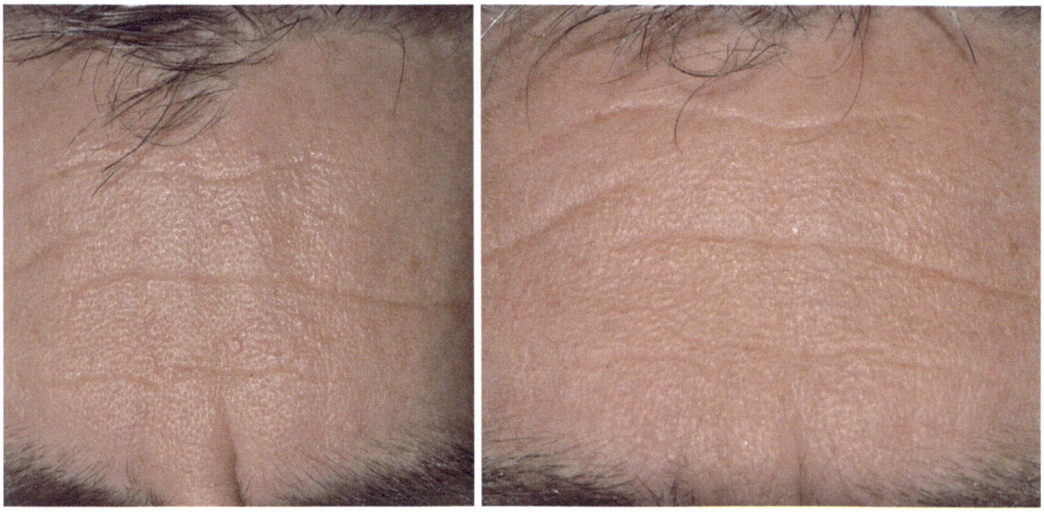

Fig. 5.16 Sebaceous gland hyperplasia on forehead treated with superpulse mode carbon dioxide laser

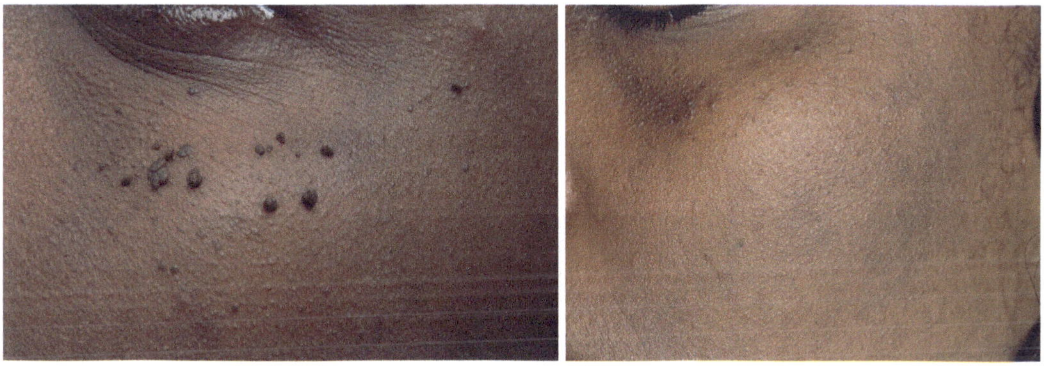

Fig. 5.17 Dermatosis papulosa nigra before and after superpulse mode carbon dioxide laser treatment

The resultant defect is left to heal secondarily or sutured for primary closure. The relatively bloodless field that is achieved is a particular advantage over scalpel surgery [20, 21].

2. Neurofibromas Small neurofibromas (less than 1 cm) can be readily ablated. Larger lesions are best excised as the dumbbell subcutaneous extension of the lesions, if left in situ will invariably result in recurrence [15]. Smaller defects can be left to heal secondarily where are larger defects will require suturing.

3. Ear keloids (Fig. 5.19) Excision of ear keloids is an effective modality, especially when combined with intralesional triamcinolone. Ear keloids differ from keloids on other locations as they are more responsive to this form of treatment. In the author's experience, intralesional triamcinolone 10–40 mg/ml is required every 4 weeks for 12 weeks to achieve remission.

Post-treatment Care

Bland products such as petrolatum-jelly or non-perfumed aloe vera gel are recommended over topical antibiotics. Care should be given to post-treatment use of petrolatum jelly and patients should be warned of fire risk, so they should refrain from smoking. Occasionally, acneiform eruption or folliculitis may develop from over enthusiastic use of occlusive products.

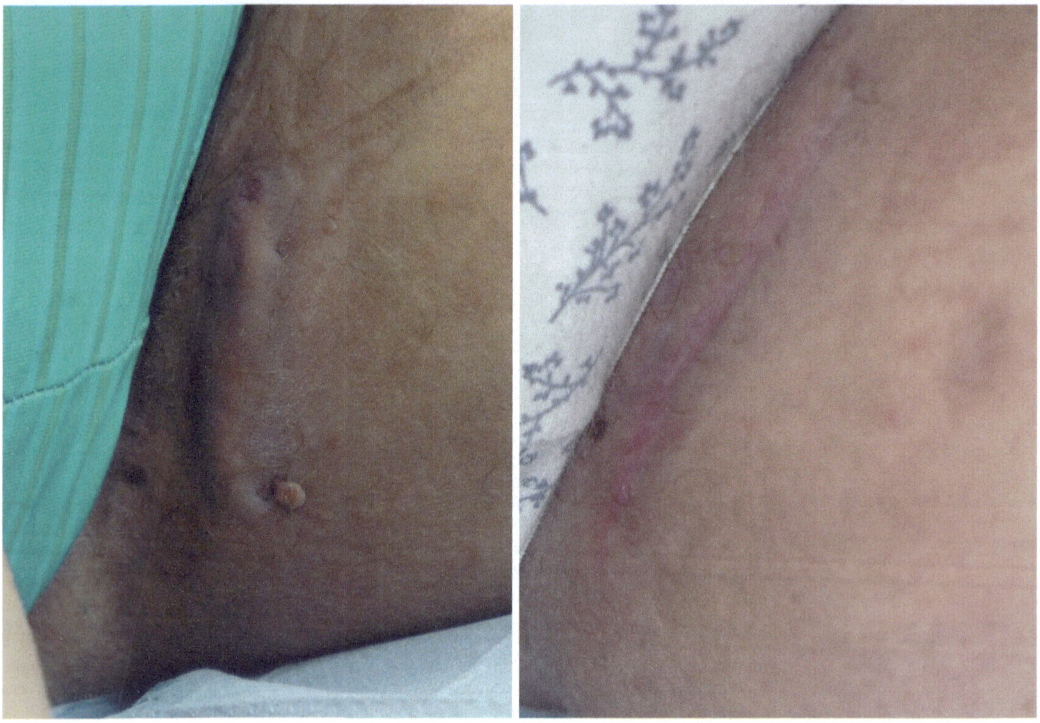

Fig. 5.18 A recalcitrant, recurrent linear plaque of hidradenitis suppurativa before and after excision with continuous mode carbon dioxide laser

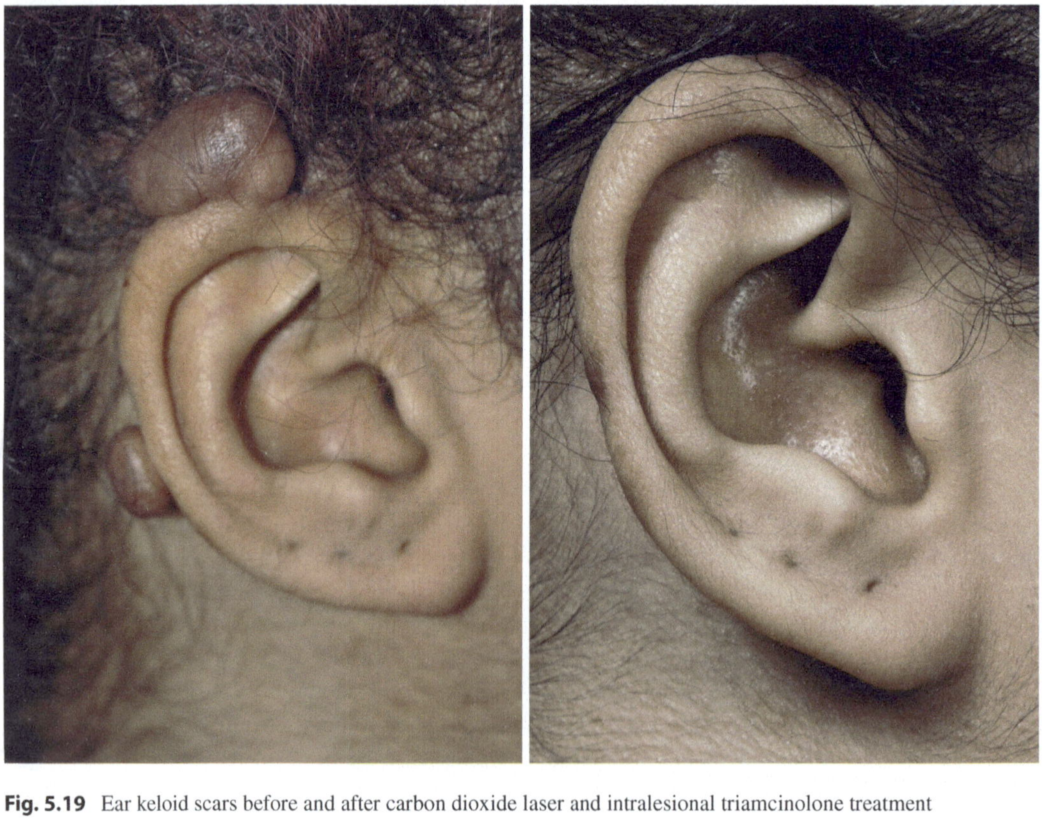

Fig. 5.19 Ear keloid scars before and after carbon dioxide laser and intralesional triamcinolone treatment

A post-treatment aftercare leaflet should be provided to all patients. After care advice should be tailored dependent on the extent and mode of treatment, as patients undergoing superpulse treatment tend to have a lower downtime than those treated using the resurfacing or cutting modes.

Complications of Ablative Lasers

Any laser procedure has a potential to cause undesirable effects. Unlike other laser procedures, ablative laser treatments carry a higher risk of complications; hence these should be undertaken cautiously. Some reactions to laser treatments are unpredictable, while most are avoidable. The most common causes of complications following laser procedures can be attributed to operator or patient factors.

Operator Factors

Inadequate training—A robust laser training programme, which imparts clear understanding of ablative lasers and their effects on the skin should be mandatory for anyone contemplating ablative laser treatments. Under no circumstances should the practitioner undertake these laser procedures without adequate training and ablative laser training programmes should only be available to medically qualified personnel such as dermatologists.

Inexperience—Most mistakes are likely to be made by inexperienced practitioners. Cautious and judicious use of these devices under direct supervision of an experienced practitioner is advised especially early in one's career.

Overzealous treatments—overcorrection and over treatment with ablative laser treatment should be avoided. Heat induced scarring is inevitable if one is not careful especially when resurfacing on nasal ala, jaw line and perioral areas.

Patient Factors

Scarring tendency—patients with keloidal tendency should be treated with caution. Careful test patches should be undertaken before embarking on full treatments.

Dysmorphophobia—patients displaying signs of dysmorphophobia should be treated with caution. Signs of dysmorphophobia can be subtle and may only become obvious after treatment, which is why the practitioner should evaluate the patient carefully during the initial consultation. Corrective treatments for minor issues when offered, should prompt evaluation of non-invasive, non-ablative treatments which should be offered before ablative laser treatments.

Complications

Erythema—post-treatment erythema lasting 1–2 weeks is not uncommon after ablative laser treatments. Occasionally, the erythema may be prolonged and can last 3–6 months. Reasons for such prolonged erythema may not always be obvious, some reasons include, higher fluence, multiple passes and possible candidal infection. If the latter is suspected, one should undertake skin scrapes for microscopy and culture. Pulsed dye laser help in dampening reactive, non-infective erythema (Fig. 5.20).

Infection—Bacterial infections are uncommon after ablative laser treatments. Impetiginisation can however occur and can be treated effectively

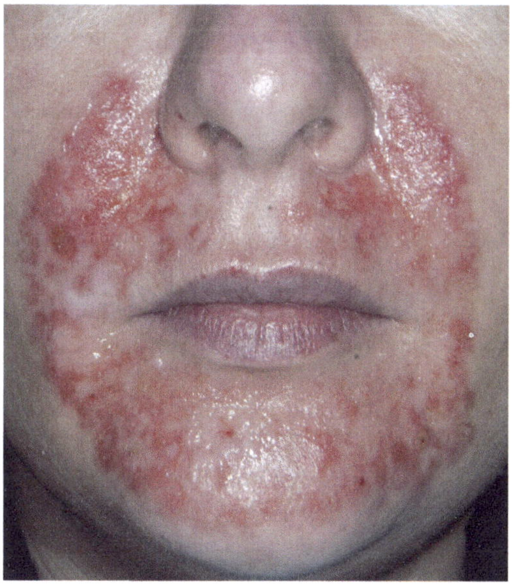

Fig. 5.20 Prolonged erythema lasting >12 weeks following ablative laser treatment

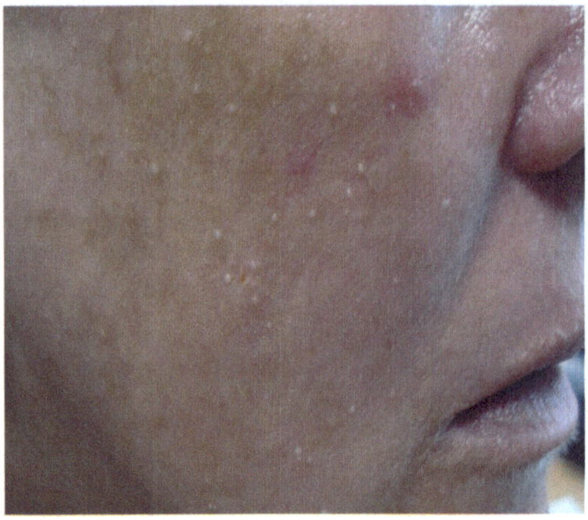

Fig. 5.21 Milia after ablative laser resurfacing for acne scarring. Overuse of occlusive emollients was implicated in this case

with topical and oral antibiotics. There is no role of prophylactic antibiotics in ablative laser treatments. Candidial infections are very rare and may present as prolonged erythema and pruritus. As herpes simplex can complicate facial laser resurfacing procedures, oral antiherpetic treatments such as acyclovir should be used prophylactically especially in patients prone to developing herpes labialis.

Milia—occlusive ointments and thermal energy from ablative lasers can result in occlusion of sweat glands, and consequently milia (Fig. 5.21). This is a temporary phenomenon and complete resolution is usually achieved by swapping the occlusive ointments to water based creams.

Contact dermatitis—While contact dermatitis to topical treatments is uncommon, a high index of suspicion would be required necessitating appropriate treatment including the withdrawal of the offending topical treatment.

Dyspigmentation—Both hyperpigmentation and hypopigmentation are recognised complications of ablative laser treatments. While hyperpigmentation tends to improve either spontaneously, or with skin bleaching agents such as hydroquinone and adequate sun protection, hypopigmentation and depigmentation caused by thermal destruction of melanocytes is more difficult to treat and can be permanent (Fig. 5.22).

Scarring—ablative laser treatments can result in hypertrophic or atrophic scarring. Care should be taken to avoid aggressive treatments on sites

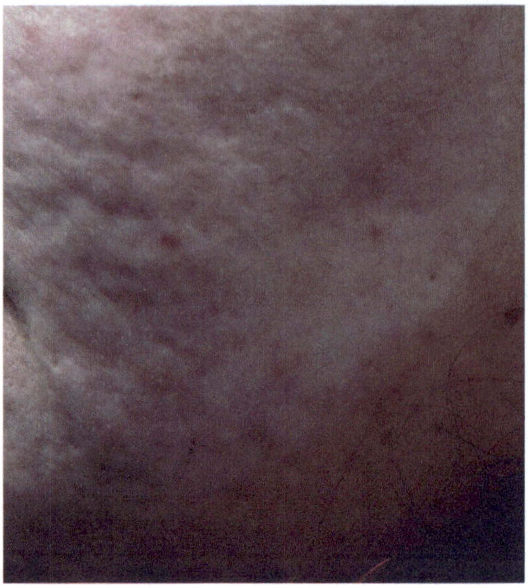

Fig. 5.22 Ablative laser resurfacing for acne scarring resulting in depigmentation

prone to scarring such as the jaw line and nasal ala. It is better to err on side of caution and use lower fluence and if needed repeat the procedure in 2–3 months (Fig. 5.23).

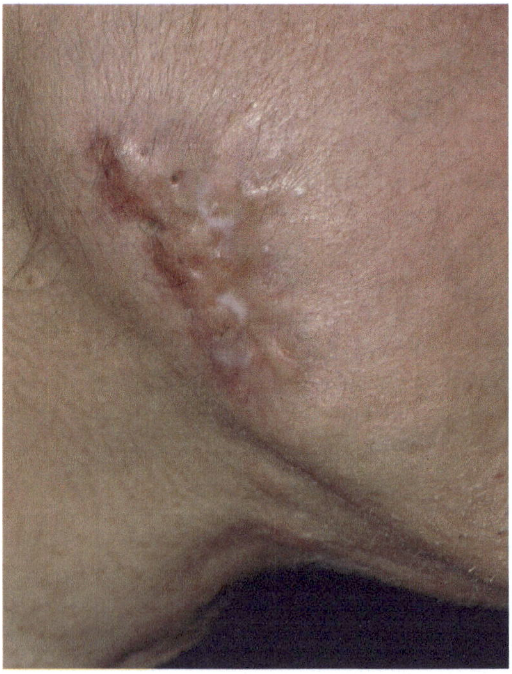

Fig. 5.23 Hypertrophic scarring is a rare adverse effect of ablative laser treatment. In this case, the cause of scarring was high fluence delivered on transitional skin of jaw line

Case Studies

1. Acne scarring (Fig. 5.24)

   A 35 year old year man presented with severe acne scarring. He had been to the local salon and undergone 4 sessions of microneedling with 2.5 mm depth needles. Minimal improvement was reported. He was seeking laser resurfacing for his acne scarring.

   On examination, he had skin phototype 2 and grouped boxcar and hypertrophic scars on both cheeks.

   He was offered CO_2 laser resurfacing under local anaesthetic. Risks of permanent hypopigmentation, long standing redness, and scarring were discussed. He was prescribed oral acyclovir, 400 mg bd for 5 days.

   A 4 mm spot on 12 W was used to shoulder the scar edges. Following this, the CO_2 laser was used at 18 W, 8 mm spot two passes to resurface the entire subunit. Post treatment, a proprietary healing gel was applied and patient was advised to use petrolatum jelly 4 times a day to the laser treatment sites. Sun avoidance advice was provided.

   Post treatment; follow up at 3 months showed a good improvement in the profile of the scars.

2. Rhinophyma (Fig. 5.25)

   A 65 year old man had noticed a gradually worsening thickening of skin of nose. He was seeking an improvement in the profile of the nose. He was counselled to the effects of laser resurfacing, downtime of 3–4 weeks and risks of prolonged redness, and permanent pallor. Nerve blocks were administered to anaesthetise the external nasal branch of anterior ethmoidal nerve and infraorbital nerves. The CO_2 laser was used in fully ablative mode at 25 W on a 5 mm spot, to debulk the phymatous tissue. Multiple passes were required to sculpt the nose, with repeated wiping of the charred tissue. Presence of sebaceous discharge on squeezing the phymatous tissue ensures treatment is in safe zone, prevents overheating of tissue and consequent scarring.

3. Sebaceous gland hyperplasia (Fig. 5.26)

   A 40-year-old with multiple skin coloured to yellowish papules on background of sebaceous quality skin was diagnosed as having sebaceous gland hyperplasia. Carbon dioxide laser was offered under topical anaesthetic. The laser was used in superpulse mode 1–1.5 W to ablate the peripheral edges of the hyperplastic sebaceous glands. Very good

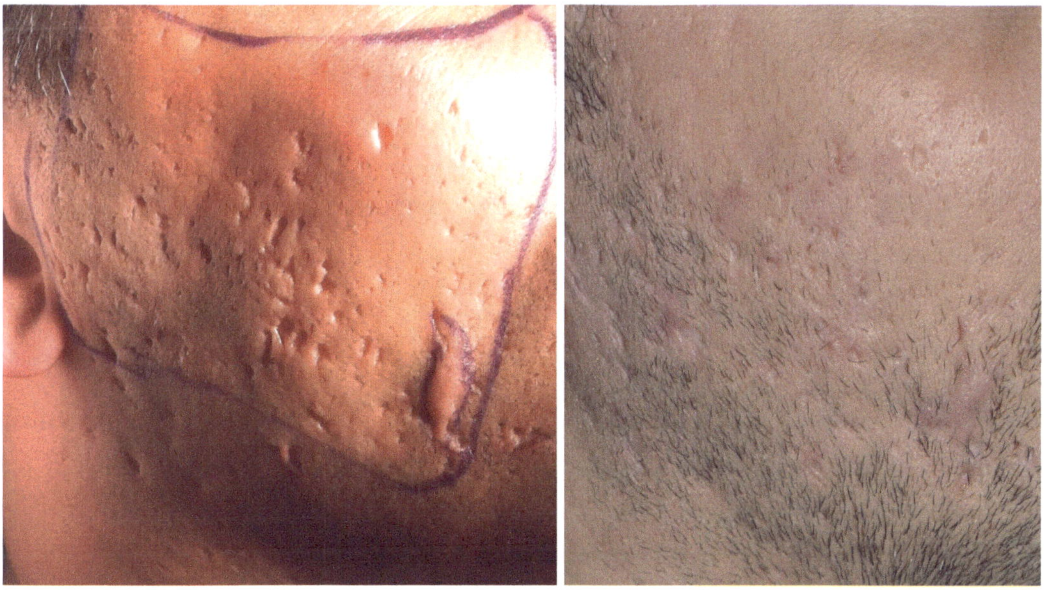

Fig. 5.24 Case 1

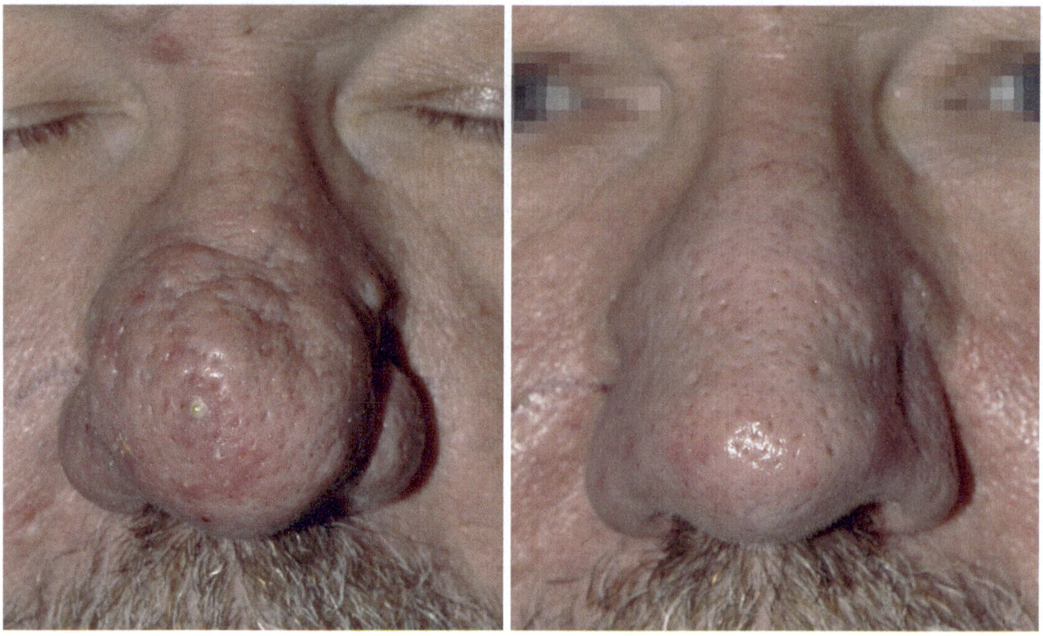

Fig. 5.25 Case 2

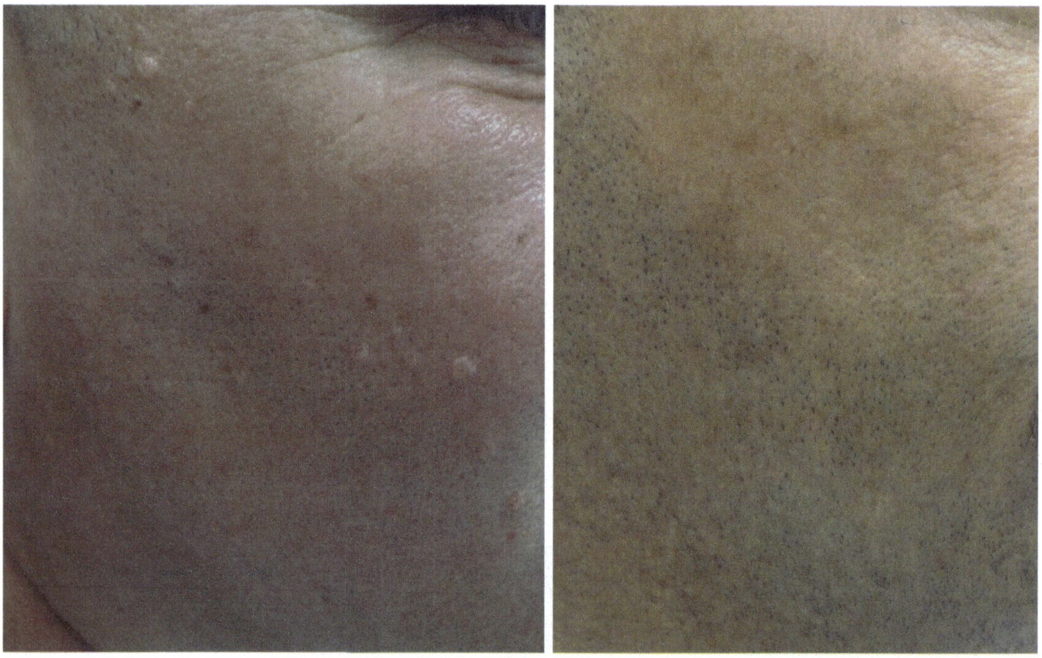

Fig. 5.26 Case 3

improvement was noted after 2 sessions. Patient was counselled regarding recurrence of the lesions which could be reduced by low dose oral isotretinoin.

4. Steatocystoma multiplex (Fig. 5.27)
   Multiple skin coloured sebaceous cysts of varying sizes are seen in this genetic disorder. Excision is reasonable for few symptomatic

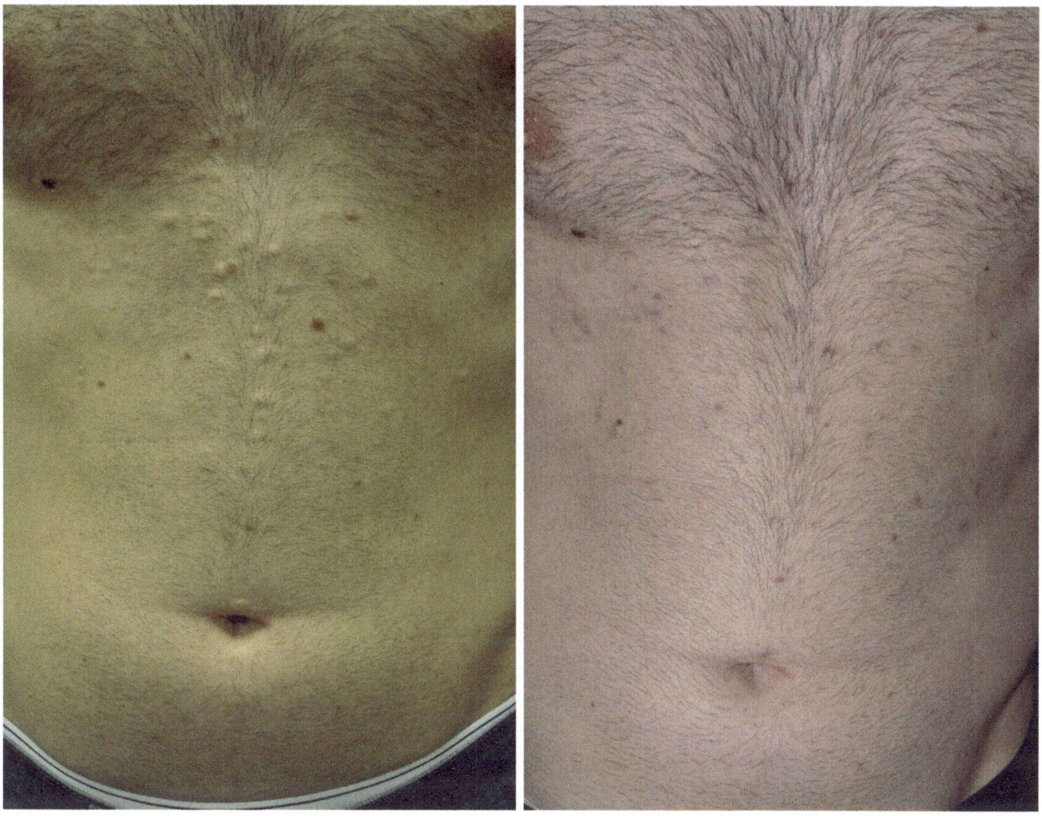

Fig. 5.27 Case 4

lesions, however, for multiple lesions, this would be impractical. The CO_2 laser perforation and extirpation technique offers a suitable alternative to excision, with the advantage of multiple lesions treated in a single session and reduced scarring.

The procedure was under local anaesthetic. Each lesion was 'perforated' using the CO_2 laser at 2 W superpulse mode. A chalazion curette is then inserted from the perforation to scoop out the contents of the cyst and the cyst wall. The resulting wound was then left to heal secondarily.

References

1. Omi T, Numano K. The role of the CO2 laser and fractional CO2 laser in dermatology. Laser Ther. 2014;23(1):49–60.
2. Khatri KA, Ross V, Grevelink JM, Magro CM, Anderson RR. Comparison of erbium:YAG and carbon dioxide lasers in resurfacing of facial rhytides. Arch Dermatol. 1999;135(4):391–7.
3. Rhie JW, Shim JS, Choi WS. A pilot study of skin resurfacing using the 2,790-nm erbium:YSGG laser system. Arch Plast Surg. 2015;42(1):52–8.
4. Rivera AE. Acne scarring: a review and current treatment modalities. J Am Acad Dermatol. 2008;59(4):659–76.
5. Deirdre Connolly, Ha Linh Vu, Kavita Mariwalla, Nazanin Saedi, Acne Scarring pathogenesis, evaluation, and treatment options. J Clin Aesthet Dermatol. 2017;10(9):12–23.
6. Janik JP, Markus JL, Al-Dujaili Z, Markus RF. Laser resurfacing. Semin Plast Surg. 2007;21(3):139–46.
7. Madan V, Ferguson JE, August PJ. Carbon dioxide laser treatment of rhinophyma: a review of 124 patients. Br J Dermatol. 2009;161:814–8.
8. Wollina U. Seborrheic Keratoses – The Most Common Benign Skin Tumor of Humans. Clinical presentation and an update on pathogenesis and treatment options. Open Access Maced J Med Sci. 2018;6(11):2270–5.
9. Fitzpatrick RE, Goldman MP, Ruiz-Esparza J. Clinical advantage of the CO2 laser superpulsed mode: treatment of verruca vulgaris, seborrheic keratoses, lentigines, and actinic cheilitis. J Dermatol Surg Oncol. 1994;20(7):449–56.

10. Whitaker DC. Microscopically proven cure of actinic cheilitis by CO_2 laser. Lasers Surg Med. 1987;7(6):520–3.
11. Trimas SJ, Ellis DAF, Metz RD. The carbon dioxide laser: an alternative for the treatment of actinically damaged skin. Dermatol Surg. 1997;23(10):885–9.
12. Hohenleutner U, Wlotzke U, Konz B, Landthaler M. Carbon dioxide laser therapy of a widespread epidermal nevus. Lasers Surg Med. 1995;16(3):288–91.
13. Ortiz AE, Zachary CB. Laser therapy for Hailey-Hailey disease: review of the literature and a case report. Dermatol Reports. 2011;3(2):e28.
14. Madan V. Dermatological applications of carbon dioxide laser. J Cutan Aesthet Surg. 2013;6(4):175–7.
15. Yi Zhen Chiang, Firas Al-Niaimi, Janice Ferguson, Paul Jeffrey August, Vishal Madan. Carbon dioxide laser treatment of cutaneous neurofibromas. Dermatol Ther (Heidelb) 2012;2(1):7.
16. Martins C, Bártolo E. Brooke-Spiegler syndrome: treatment of cylindromas with CO_2 laser. Dermatol Surg. 2000;26(9):877–81.
17. Madan V, August PJ. Perforation and extirpation of steatocystoma multiplex. Int J Dermatol. 2009;48:329–30.
18. Rai S, Madan V, August PJ, Ferguson JE. Favre Racouchot syndrome; a novel two-step treatment approach using the carbon dioxide laser. Br J Dermatol. 2014;170:657–60.
19. Ali FR, Bakkour W, Ferguson JE, Madan V. Carbon dioxide laser ablation of dermatosis papulosa nigra: high satisfaction and few complications in patients with pigmented skin. Lasers Med Sci. 2016;31:593–5.
20. Hazen PG, Hazen BP. Hidradenitis suppurativa: successful treatment using carbon dioxide laser excision and marsupialization. Dermatol Surg. 2010;36(2):208–13.
21. Madan V, Hindle E, Hussain W, August PJ. Outcomes of treatment of nine cases of recalcitrant severe hidradenitis suppurativa with carbon dioxide laser. Br J Dermatol. 2008;159(6):1309–14.

Fractional Laser Technology

6

Sarah Felton and Vishal Madan

Introduction

Despite the excellent efficacy of the fully ablative carbon dioxide (CO_2) and Erbium:YAG (E:YAG) resurfacing lasers, the significant downtime associated with such treatments deters many patients. This prompted the development of fractional laser devices, the first of which was the Fraxel™ device [Reliant Technologies Inc., now Solta Medical], which was launched in USA 2004. Whilst water in the epidermis and dermis remains the target chromophore for fractional ablative lasers, the laser beam, as the name suggests, is fractionated into thousands of regularly-spaced 'micro-beams', each delivering a microthermal treatment zone (MTZ) into the skin (Fig. 6.1) [1].

Within each MTZ, the skin begins its repair process with transepidermal extrusion within around 7 days of necrotic tissue termed Microscopic Epidermal Necrotic Debris (MEND) [2]. MEND consist of coagulated melanin, elastin and dermal contents, accounting for improved pigmentation and subsequent skin tightening. The depth and diameter of the MTZ varies according to both clinical indication and laser device, but is usually around 300–700 microns deep and 100–400 microns wide. Since overall between around 5% and 50% of skin is treated per session (usually around 20% at 2000 MTZ/cm^2), the untreated

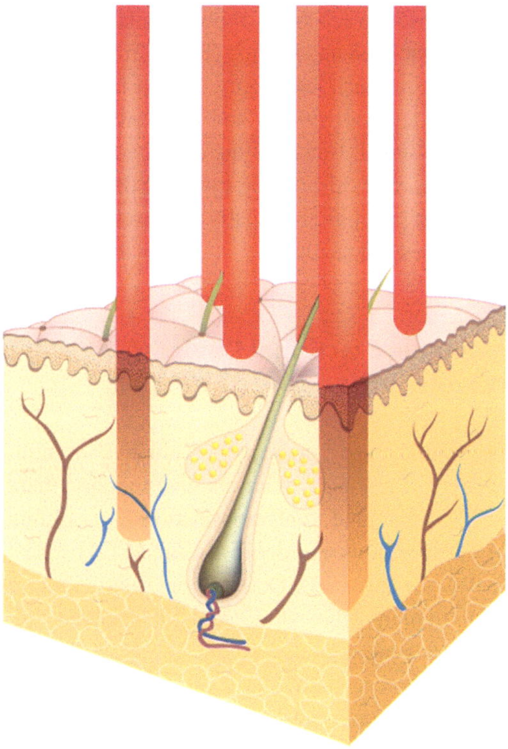

Fig. 6.1 Multiple fractional laser beams create arrays of superheated thermal wounds that extend from the epidermis down to the reticular dermis (up to 1000 μm)

S. Felton
Department of Dermtatology Churchill Hospital Old Road Headington, Oxford, Oxfordshire, UK
e-mail: sarah.felton@nhs.net

V. Madan (✉)
Consultant Dermatologist, Laser and Mohs Surgeon, Salford Royal NHS Foundation Trust, Stott Lane, Salford, UK
e-mail: vishal.madan@srft.nhs.uk

V. Madan (ed.), *Practical Introduction to Laser Dermatology*,
https://doi.org/10.1007/978-3-030-46451-6_6

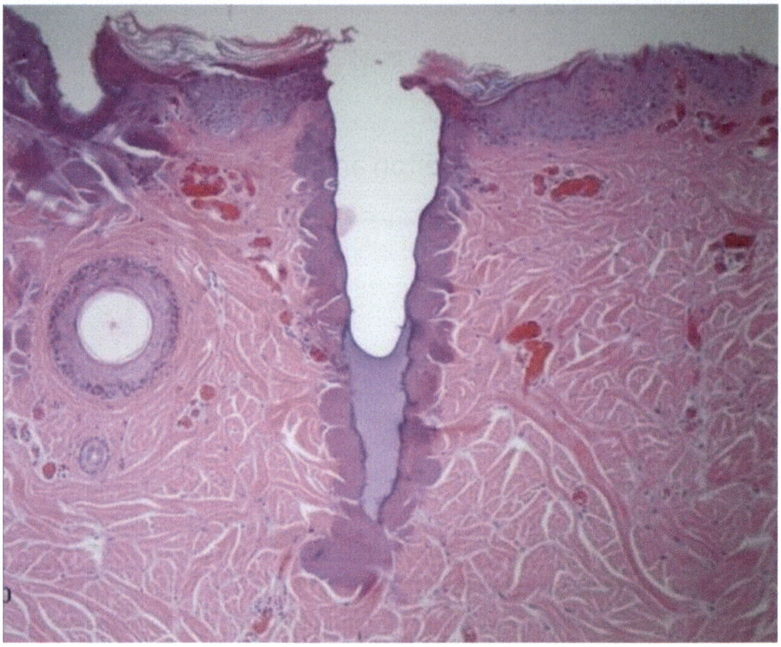

Fig. 6.2 Histology of skin treated with fractional ablative CO_2 laser. Ablative Width < 300 μm and Necrosis 30–100 μm

skin between each MTZ remains intact, so supporting rapid wound healing (Fig. 6.2). Downtime is therefore much less than with non-fractionated devices, and side effects and risks are concomitantly lessened. However, the efficacy from a single treatment is also lower, meaning that multiple treatment sessions are usually required to achieve overall desired results.

Available Fractional Devices/Wavelengths

Fractional laser can be either ablative or non-ablative (Table 6.1). With ablative therapy, there is immediate and total vaporisation of a column of the epidermis and dermis in the MTZ by heat (>100 °C) (Fig. 6.3). Dermal/epidermal contraction tightens the skin, and subsequent re-epithelialisation by day 7, and fibroblast-derived neocollagenesis particularly of collagen III from around 1 month post-treatment, improve skin texture and appearance. Non-ablative lasers, in contrast, deliver less thermal injury, causing photocoagulation and heat shock protein-induced activation of skin stem cells in the basal epidermis and dermis without ablating the epidermis. The skin barrier thus remains intact as the *stratum corneum* is spared. This accounts for the variation in indications and efficacy of ablative versus non-ablative devices.

An ever-increasing number of laser devices are becoming available that use this fractionated technology, and they now tend to be classified as non-ablative (such as Fraxel re:store [1550 nm] by Reliant, Fraxel re:fine [1410 nm] by Reliant and Affirm [1440 nm] from Cynosure, as microablative (including Active FX by Lumenis, Fraxel re:pair by Reliant and Affirm CO_2 by Cynosure) or as deep dermal ablative (such as Deep FX by Lumenis or Pearl by Cutera; Table 6.1). An appraisal of each individual device is beyond the scope of this chapter. However, as Fraxel™ was the first to be released, there is an abundance of evidence in the literature supporting its efficacy. As there are many fractional devices now available, differing in their injury patterns and energy/intensity delivered, and thus optimal indications, it is the responsibility of the operator to choose a machine for which they are familiar with the settings and anticipated outcomes.

Fractionated Laser Indications

The original US Food and Drug Administration (FDA) approval for Fraxel™ devices included the treatment of fine lines and wrinkles, pig-

Table 6.1 Comparison of fractional ablative and non-ablative devices

	Ablative	Non-ablative
Wavelengths	2790 nm 2940 nm 10,600 nm	1410 nm 1440 nm 1540 nm 1550 nm 1565 nm
Chromophore	H_2O	H_2O
Mechanism of action	Microthermal treatment zones	Microthermal treatment zones; stratum corneum remains intact
Depth of ablation	Microablative: <750 microns Deep ablative (>750 microns)	–
Return to work	3–5 days	0–2 days
Recovery	2–4 weeks	3–10 days
Noticeable improvement	Immediate on skin healing	Improvement over months
Key indications	Photorejuvenation Scarring Pigmentation	Photorejuvenation Scarring Pigmentation
Risks	Less suitable for pigmentary disorders/darker skin types due to risk hyper or hypopigmentation. Greater risk of complications, especially infection and scarring; risks increase with deeper ablative treatments	Incidence of side effects lower than for ablative
Usual treatment course-dependant on indication	1–3 sessions	4 to 6 treatments

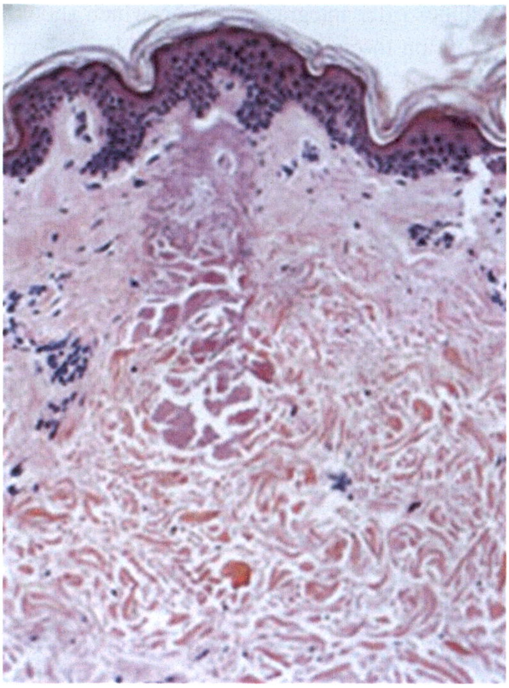

Fig. 6.3 Histology of skin treated with Fractional Non Ablative device. Note that epidermis is not involved

mented lesions including melasma, acne and surgical scars, skin lesions such as actinic/seborrheic keratoses, and skin rejuvenation and resurfacing [3]. Since then, as the market has expanded, there have been many case reports/case series describing their usage in a variety of indications, from granuloma annulare and epidermolysis bullosa to disseminated superficial actinic porokeratosis, but their mainstay of treatment currently remains in skin aesthetics. Laser assisted drug delivery is also emerging as an area of immense interest.

Pre-treatment Preparation and Precautions

Pre-treatment assessment includes a review of the patient's medical history, both current and past, including their medications, previous cosmetic treatments and any tendency for abnormal pigmentation or scarring. Vitiligo or other koebnerising skin conditions would be considered relative contraindications due to the propensity for disease to develop at treated sites, and in those with connective tissue diseases, careful consideration should be given as to how these may affect the healing process. Skin should not be treated where there are any signs of cutaneous infection (e.g. impetigo or herpes simplex) or active disease such as eczema or psoriasis, so these would need addressing appropriately beforehand. If pregnant or breastfeeding, then treatment should be postponed.

The intended treatment area should be examined to confirm suitability and the patient's individual concerns and realistic treatment expectations should be addressed. If body dysmorphic disorder is suspected, psychological evaluation prior to treatment would be prudent. Photographs should also be taken at the preoperative visit. Aftercare instructions should be given in advance so that patients are fully prepared.

It is important that the skin is not tanned at the time of treatment due to the risk of dyspigmentation post-recovery. Consequently, a broad-spectrum sunscreen should be worn daily and sun exposure (i.e. tanning) avoided for about 2 months pre-treatment and in the post-treatment healing phase. Other treatments that can sensitise the skin such as waxing, microdermabrasion, peels/harsh scrubs should also be avoided in the weeks preceding treatment. If there is a history of Herpes virus infection, antiviral medication is started pre-treatment and continued until around 7 days post-therapy. It is generally recommended to avoid topical retinoids for around 2 weeks and oral retinoids for 6 months pre-treatment due to earlier reports of an increased risk of keloid or atypical scarring following ablative procedures [4, 5]. If possible, anticoagulants/anti-platelet medications such as aspirin, fish oils or ibuprofen, and photosensitising medications should be stopped in advance. If melasma is to be treated, some practitioners advocate depigmenting regimens (such as topical hydroquinone 2–4 weeks pre-procedure).

Test patches prior to first treatment are of paramount importance, and the practitioner should be alerted to any changes in medication or medical history between these time points that would warrant a repeated test patch.

Laser Technique

Written informed consent should be taken prior to commencing treatment. Treatments are commonly performed under topical anaesthesia, though some practitioners also provide an anxiolytic (such as diazepam or lorazepam orally), particularly prior to full-face ablative fractional resurfacing. If this is the case, then the patient should not drive or consume alcohol until the effects have fully worn off. Skin should be thoroughly cleansed and dried prior to treatment. Safety eyewear appropriate to the laser's wavelength should be worn by patient (lead goggles), operator and assistants throughout and, particularly for ablative therapy, medical staff should utilise a laser-plume face mask and plume extractor.

Laser devices from the various manufacturers have tips of differing shapes and sizes, often square, some with changeable dot patterns and certain devices also employ automatic skin surface motion scanning, whereby a computerised handpiece tracks the operator's movement over the skin surface, firing only when in motion, thus protecting the skin and optimising results. Most machines offer integrated cooling which should be kept on throughout during non-ablative laser resurfacing. Cooling is not mandatory with ablative fractional ablative resurfacing devices.

Working in a stepwise process, for instance laterally to medially, from superior to inferior on the right side then left, the skin surface should be systematically covered with minimal overlap (Fig. 6.4). As settings (fluence) will

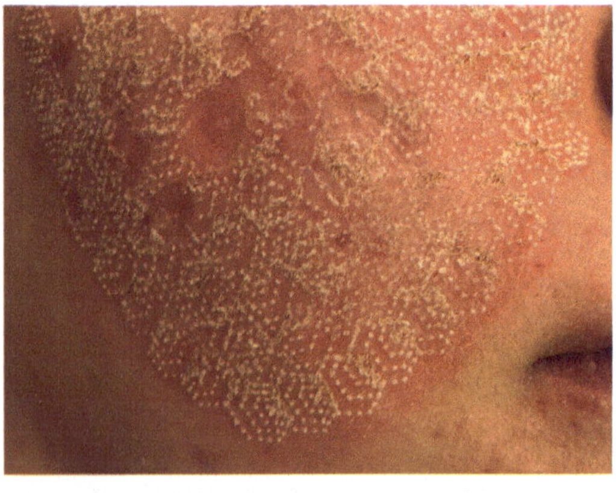

Fig. 6.4 Fractional CO_2 laser treatment of acne scarring

need to be changed at different sites and for differing indications, such as acne scarring, some practitioners choose to treat full right side then the left, whilst others perform the same site bilaterally prior to changing. Although the treatment is generally well-tolerated as a pin-prick heat sensation, sensitivities across the face can vary. Therefore, it is common to begin on the cheek area, before moving to chin, forehead and nose. With practice, laser surgeons develop their own individual approach. When the entire site has been covered, one should visually check over to ensure that no area has been inadvertently missed, in which case it should now be treated.

Settings vary according to test patch results, device used and clinical indication, and it is of paramount importance that the operator is familiar with and fully trained in these prior to usage, otherwise complications, particularly scarring may occur. Settings will also need to be varied according to such factors as patient skin phototype, previous response and anatomical site, and it is imperative to fully and accurately document the settings used in the patient's record, particularly if a treatment course is being planned. Guidance settings for Erbium:YAG fractionated laser are available [6]. At the end of treatment, further prolonged cooling is required, post-procedure gel applied and aftercare advice given.

Post Treatment Care

Immediately after treatment, there is cutaneous erythema and a mild sunburn sensation for 1–3 h. Application of ice for 5–10 min each hour for the first 5 h post-treatment can help diminish this. For the following 3–5 days, the skin may have a pinkish hue, accompanied by minimal oedema for 2–3 days. Sleeping in a more elevated position may reduce this.

Within 24 h, as the epidermis regenerates, the skin assumes a bronze appearance that can last up to 2 weeks. Flaking may also occur as the treated skin is shed; this can be treated with emollient therapy but 'picking' should be avoided.

This transient bronzing of the skin and exfoliation are the manifestation of MEND extrusion.

In most cases, patients can return to work directly after treatments or the following day, depending upon their skin condition and treatment. If necessary, gentle shaving and application of make-up can also restart the following day. Whilst showers can be taken, hot water (steam, saunas) and direct shower spray should be avoided for 3 days, and strenuous activity (particularly head-down activities) should also be avoided for 48–72 h.

Whilst the skin remains sensitive, for the first week or so, it should be washed with a gentle cleanser (i.e. no salicylic/lactic/glycolic acids, retinol or alcohol ingredients) and moisturised with a non-comedogenic emollient.

As ablative therapy is more aggressive, recovery is longer and redness, swelling and peeling more pronounced; this should be gently aided with tap water, petrolatum and gauze once or twice daily. Vinegar soaks are often recommended after ablative resurfacing procedures due to their antiseptic/antibacterial activity to aid wound healing: gauze soaked in vinegar water (1 tablespoon of white vinegar mixed in a cup of water) is draped on face for around 5 min 2–4 times a day for 3 days.

During the healing phase and for several months after treatment, the area should continue to be protected with a sunblock, preferably a physical blocker with zinc oxide or titanium dioxide; protective clothing and wide-brimmed hats would also help in this.

Complications of Fractional Laser Treatments and How to Treat and Avoid Them

Complications of fractional laser treatments are similar to those of non-fractionated CO_2 or Erbium:YAG devices, but the risks are theoretically lessened by the fractional technology. Nevertheless, careful patient selection, pre-procedure education and good technique are paramount, and prompt reaction to complications can help to minimise most problems.

Early Complications in the Immediate Post-Procedure Period [7, 8]

Infection

Infection is a risk following any cutaneous intervention and results in delayed and potentially unpredictable wound healing, with concomitant increased risk of scarring. Although incidence of infection is small, and much lower than with non-fractional counterparts, patients should still be counselled regarding hand hygiene and wound care to minimise its occurrence. If infection is suspected, swabs should be taken for culture and broad-spectrum (including activity against *Pseudomonas Aeruginosa*) empiric antibiotics started, pending culture results. Consideration is also give pre-operatively to prophylactic oral antibiotics and intranasal mupirocin ointment to reduce *Staphylococcal* colonisation and post-operative acetic acid soaks, particularly where there is a significant risk of bacterial infection during recovery such as full face resurfacing or if acne-prone.

Viral infection with Herpes simplex presents with pain or a tingling sensation followed by an eruption of vesicles, usually around the time of re-epithelialisation. As described above, patients should be screened for a history of herpes simplex at the pre-operative visit and, if present, or if undergoing perioral laser treatment, a prophylactic course of antiviral therapy (acyclovir or valcyclovir) commencing day of and continuing for around 5–7 days post-treatment is usually recommended. If an outbreak occurs, antiviral treatment should be escalated to a treatment rather than prophylactic dose.

Rarer causes of infection include Mycoplasma, presenting with granulomas, and fungal infection with Candida, presenting with subtle signs such as prolonged erythema and pruritus.

Acneiform Eruptions

Acneiform outbreaks may develop, particularly following usage of greasy petrolatum emollients. Switching to less occlusive moisturisers usually suffices, otherwise oral antibiotics may be warranted. If acne is active, treatment should be delayed. Milia are another complication of the application of thick creams to the skin during re-epithelialisation. If bothersome to the patient, they can be removed by needle extraction or electrodessication.

Contact Dermatitis

Post-operative allergic or irritant contact dermatitis is also possible, whilst integrity of the skin barrier is disrupted. It is therefore important to avoid usage of topical agents containing common allergens such as topical antibiotics, fragrances and preservatives during this time-period. Presentation is non-specific with potential erythema, oedema, pruritus and flaking, and should be treated with topical corticosteroids and allergen avoidance.

Prolonged Erythema

Prolonged erythema is that lasting beyond 4 days in non-ablative, or 1 month following ablative therapy. It is more likely when higher fluences or pulse stacking are employed, and rosacea patients undergoing resurfacing seem particularly at-risk. Post-operative cooling may help diminish it, possibly with mild topical corticosteroid, but it usually fades itself with extra time. 590 nm Light Emitting Diode may expedite recovery by 24–48 h, and topical ascorbic acid (vitamin C) can also be helpful.

Other complications include marked oedema, particularly of periorbital skin, diminished by sleeping in a more elevated position, excessive desquamation and crusting and development of petechiae/pupura usually secondary to use of NSAIDs/blood thinners and high fluences, which settle spontaneously.

Late/Delayed Complications [7, 8]

Dyspigmentation

Post-inflammatory hyperpigmentation is more common in darker skin types (skin phototype III or above), particularly following ablative procedures, the treatment of melasma or in those with a personal history of abnormal pigmentation. Higher fluency/lower density settings and longer treatment intervals may decrease the risk; tanned skin should not be treated and the importance of strict photoprotection post-procedure must also be emphasised to the patient. Delayed hypopigmentation (beyond 6 months post-procedure) is fortunately a rare outcome but remains a possibility, even in lighter skin types, particularly around the neck or chest area. Whilst hypopigmentation, caused by thermal injury to melanocytes, may be permanent, post-inflammatory hyperpigmentation often spontaneously resolves. This may be assisted by depigmenting agents such as hydroquinone, alpha-hydroxy acid, retinoic acid and kojic acid, or more interventional procedures such as Intensed Pulsed Light and gentle chemical peels.

Scarring

Scarring and, in particular, hypertrophic scarring is a feared complication of laser treatment. A history of abnormal scarring should be screened for at the preoperative visit. The neck is particularly prone to scarring, and for this reason excessive fluence should be avoided, particularly in this area. Strict wound care and prompt treatment of suspected infection should reduce its incidence. Treatment options should scarring occur include topical silicone and/or corticosteroids, and PDL, although none are guaranteed to work.

Scarring ectropion is rare but can occur after periorbital laser treatment. Therefore, excessive treatment of lower eyelid skin should be avoided, particularly if the patient has lower eyelid laxity or has previously undergone lower lid blepharoplasty. Treatment options include steroids, massage and PDL but, if significant, surgical correction is usually needed.

Koebnerisation

Theoretically, any dermatosis capable of koebnerisation can develop at the site of laser treatment regardless of technique, including vitiligo and psoriasis. Eruptive keratoacanthomas have also been described [9].

Overall, risks of laser treatment are higher with more aggressive or ablative treatments, particularly on the neck and in darker skin types. In general, to minimise complications do not pulse stack, do not treat recently tanned skin, and use fewer passes and/or lower density at scar-prone areas such as the neck, chest, mandible or infraorbital skin [10].

What's on the Horizon?

Uses of fractionated lasers are continually being extended beyond the original indications, to include the treatment of fibrosing conditions and foreign body removal. Particularly good efficacy has been seen for the treatment of traumatic and burn scars, with measurable functional and cosmetic improvements. Home-use devices are also being introduced, such as the "Age Defying Laser" by Tria®, designed with lower outputs so as to be used more frequently for skin rejuvenation. Fractional technology has also been introduced to bipolar radiofrequency systems, for sublative rejuvenation [11].

Laser-assisted Drug Delivery

Perhaps the most exciting of developments is in the usage of fractionated lasers for laser-assisted drug delivery (LADD), a process which takes advantage of the MTZ: The fractional ablative laser (CO_2 or Erbium:YAG) provides microscopic channels of specific diameter and depth through the epidermis and dermis, through which topically-applied molecules can be delivered, so bypassing the repellent *stratum corneum* [12]. By combining cutaneous drug application with laser treatment, depth of penetration is controlled and permeability is enhanced, with local cutaneous and potential systemic effects dependent upon resultant dose.

The use of LADD has been explored for varied indications including corticosteroids and methotrexate for inflammatory disorders, 5-aminolaevulinic acid, imiquimod and 5-fluorouracil for actinic keratosis/Bowen's disease, tranexamic acid for hyperpigmentation and vitamin C for collagen stimulation [13, 14].

This is an exciting avenue for the future, opening a number of possibilities for expanding our array of treatment options in dermatology, once further studies have evaluated dosing schedules, side effects and efficacy.

Case Studies

1. This 64 year old woman was seeking improvement of her facial pigmentation and rejuvenation. While QS 532 laser could have been very

effective for her solar lentigenes, she was treated with non-ablative Fractional 1550 and 1927 nm (Fraxel Dual) laser as she wanted to address photoaging as well. An improvement in her facial pigmentation is visible after 3 sessions.

1550 nm 25 mJ, 15% coverage, 4 passes

1927 nm 15 mJ, 40% coverage, 4 passes (Fig. 6.5).

2. Fractional ablative treatments are now more popular for treatment of superficial box car acne scarring. This patient has darker skin tone and fully ablative laser resurfacing would have resulted in high risk of post inflammatory pigmentation. Prolonged erythema is an additional risk.

   Fractional CO_2 laser was used to treat these scars 5.6 J/cm^2, 6 mm spot, 25% coverage. Three sessions over 9 months with pre and post procedure sun avoidance resulted in good improvement in the scars (Fig. 6.6).

3. Perioral rhytides are a common cosmetic concern. Whilst Er: YAG or CO_2 laser resurfacing

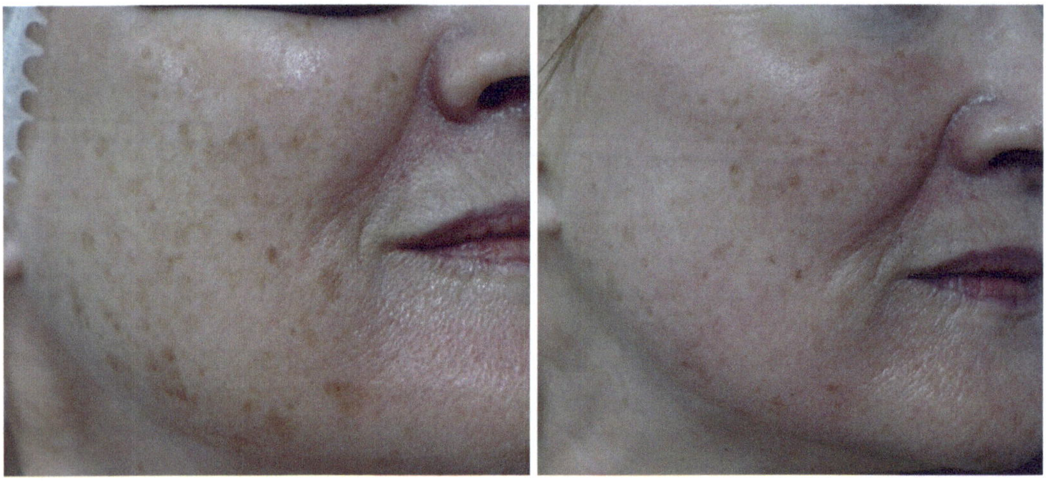

Fig. 6.5 Case 1

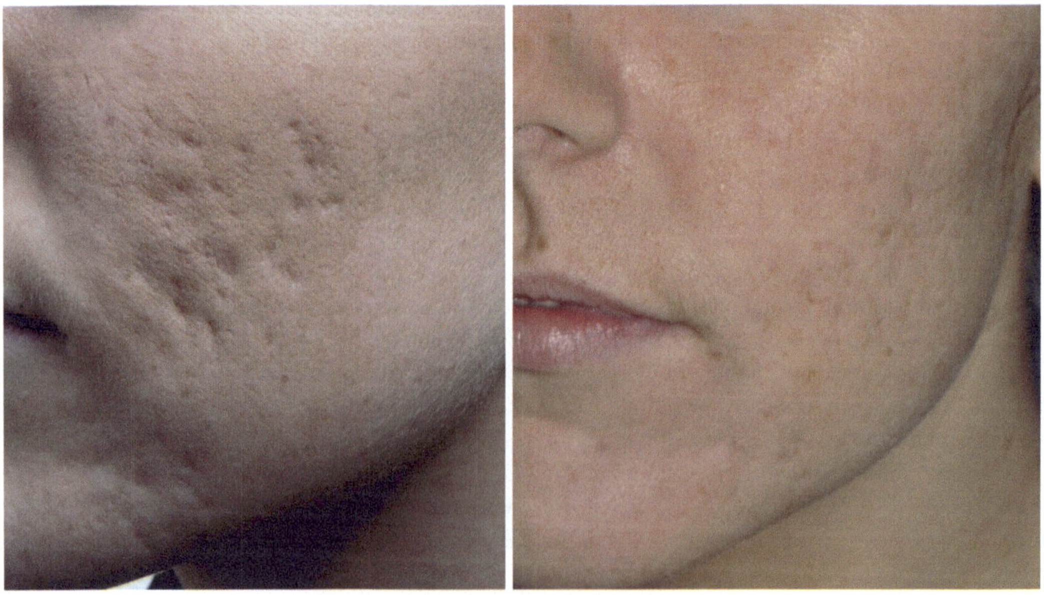

Fig. 6.6 Case 2

would be perfectly acceptable modalities, the post treatment hypopigmentation with these modalities is irreversible. For this reason, we opted to treat this patient with fractional CO_2 laser 6 J/cm^2, 30% coverage, 6 mm spot. Results 4 weeks after single session (Fig. 6.7).

4. Surgical scars such as this one after Mohs surgery for Basal cell carcinoma and subsequent reconstruction using cheek interpolation flap, resulted in a trap door deformity. This was easily corrected using fractional ablative CO_2 laser resurfacing of the flap. 8 J/cm^2 6 mm spot, 30% coverage (Fig. 6.8).
5. Open pores are difficult to correct. There are no good treatment options especially in skin phototypes 4+. This patient with skin phototype 6 underwent 5 non ablative fractional laser treatments with 1550 nm device. 10–20 mJ, 20–30% coverage, 8 passes (Fig. 6.9).

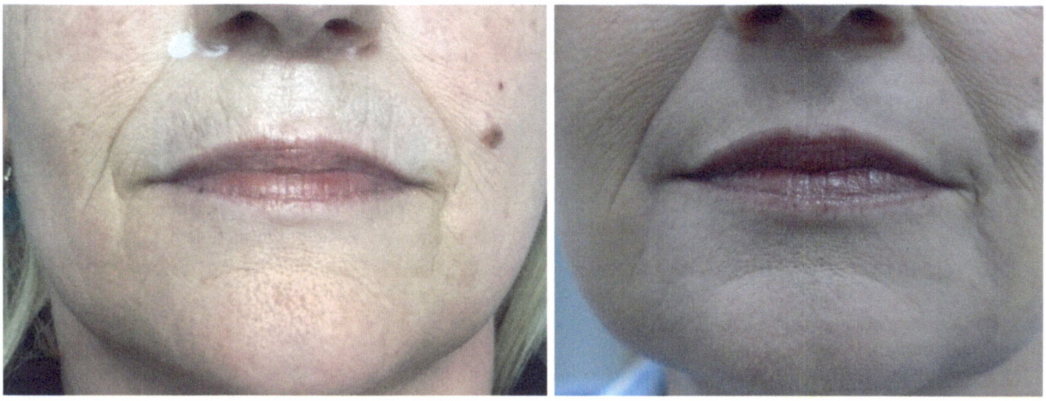

Fig. 6.7 Case 3

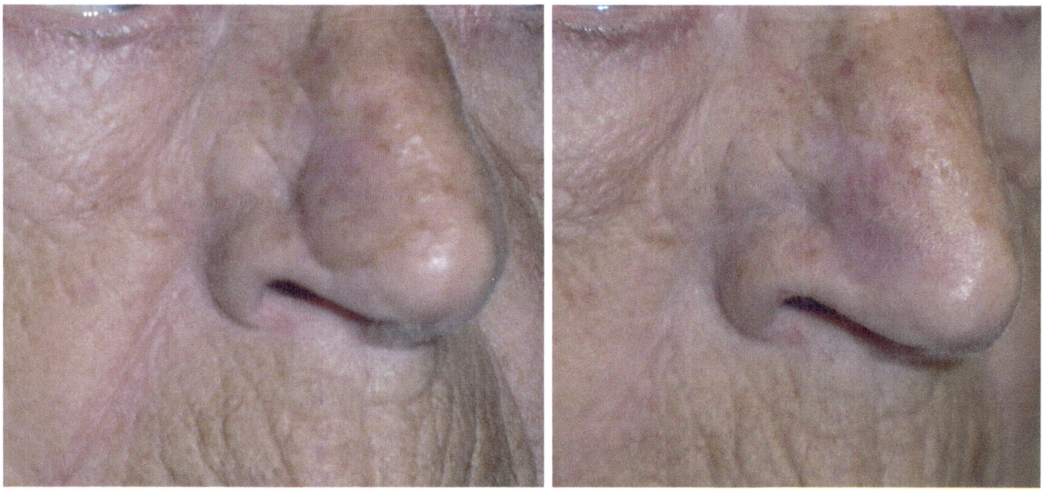

Fig. 6.8 Case 4

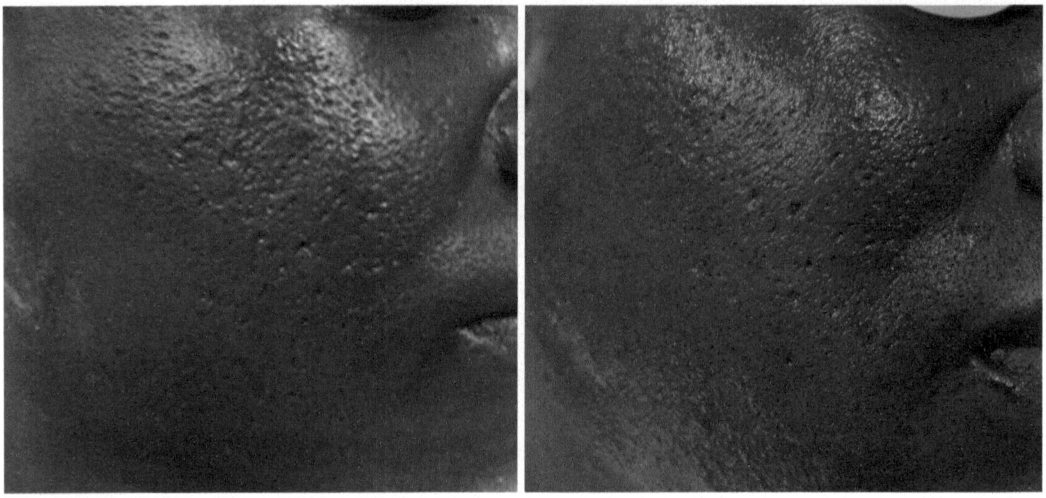

Fig. 6.9 Case 5

References

1. Manstein D, Herron GS, Sink RK, Tanner H, Anderson RR. Fractional photothermolysis: a new concept for cutaneous remodeling using microscopic patterns of thermal injury. Lasers Surg Med. 2004;34:426–38.
2. Laubach HJ, Tannous Z, Anderson RR, Manstein D. Skin responses to fractional photothermolysis. Lasers Surg Med. 2006;38(2):142–9.
3. US Food & Drug Administration 08/09/2015. https://www.accessdata.fda.gov/cdrh_docs/pdf8/K080915.pdf. Accessed 25/02/2019.
4. Rubenstein R, Roenigk HH Jr, Stegman SJ, Hanke CW. A typical keloids after dermabrasion of patients taking isotretinoin. J Am Acad Dermatol. 1986;15:280–5.
5. Katz BE, Mac Farlane DF. Atypical facial scarring after isotretinoin therapy in a patient with previous dermabrasion. J Am Acad Dermatol. 1994;30:852–3.
6. Sherling M, Friedman PM, Adrian R, et al. Consensus recommendations on the use of an erbium-doped 1,550-nm fractionated laser and its applications in dermatologic laser surgery. Dermatol Surg. 2010;36(4):461–9.
7. Graber EM, Tanzi EL, Alster TS. Side effects and complications of fractional laser photothermolysis: experience with 961 treatments. Dermatol Surg. 2008;34:301–7.
8. Metelitsa AI, Alster TS. Fractionated laser skin resurfacing treatment complications: a review. Dermatol Surg. 2010;36:299–306.
9. Mamelak AJ, Goldberg LH, Marquez D, Hosler GA, Hinckley MR, Friedman PM. Eruptive keratoacanthomas on the legs after fractional photothermolysis: report of two cases. Dermatol Surg. 2009;35(3):513–8.
10. Alster TS, Khoury R. Treatment of laser complications. Facial Plast Surg. 2009;25:316–23.
11. Hruza G, Taub AF, Collier SL, Mulholland SR. Skin rejuvenation and wrinkle reduction using a fractional radiofrequency system. J Drugs Dermatol. 2009;8(3):259–65.
12. Lee WR, Shen SC, Lai HH, Hu CH, Fang JY. Transdermal drug delivery enhanced and controlled by erbium:YAG laser: a comparative study of lipophilic and hydrophilic drugs. J Control Release. 2001;75(1–2):155–66.
13. Waibel JS, Rudnick A, Shagalov DR, Nicolazzo DM. Update of ablative fractionated lasers to enhance cutaneous topical drug delivery. Adv Ther. 2017;34(8):1840–9.
14. Zaleski-larsen LA, Fabi SG. Laser-assisted drug delivery. Dermatol Surg. 2016;42(8):919–31.

7 Radiofrequency Devices Including Fractional Radiofrequency

Ileana Afroditi Kleidona, Ali M. Ghanem, and Nicholas J. Lowe

Introduction

Electromagnetic Radiation The electromagnetic (EM) spectrum consists of radiation in the form of waves. Preliminary studies performed by Maxwell and later confirmed by Hertz, predicted that these waves encompass oscillation of electrical and magnetic fields carrying energy, which in air and free space travel at the speed of light. Typically, the EM waves are classified in seven regions by their frequency (number of cycles per second, reported in Hz) and their relative wavelength (distance between consecutive peaks, reported in m). Frequency and wavelength are inversely proportional (Fig. 7.1). The energy carried by the EM waves is higher with increasing frequency [1]. The Institute of Electrical and Electronics Engineers Inc. (IEEE) defines radio waves the part of the spectrum with frequency range of 3 kHz–300 GHz. Radiofrequency (RF) has various applications including in communication, industry and healthcare. In the medical field RF is used for diagnostic purposes (MRI), therapeutic diathermy, electrosurgery or tissue ablation. RF waves do not have enough energy to cause ionization of biological systems. Primarily, the effects are thought to be secondary to thermal mechanisms [2]. It can be delivered in continued, burst or pulsed mode. RF medical devices conduct electric current to tissues in repetitive pulses. The energy delivered causes oscillation and vibration of charged particles against tissue's resistance (impedance). This kinetic energy is converted to thermal energy [3]. As per Ohm's law, tissue impedance and ultimately generates heat. The Joule's first law determines the power of heat generated by an electric current through a resistive conductor, such as skin, at a given time: $P = I^2R$ (P: Power in watts, I: Electric current in amperes, R: Resistance in ohms). Tissues with high impedance, for example subcutaneous tissue, generate greater amount of heat.

Skin Thermal Interactions In the 1940s, Henriques performed experimental studies to elucidate the effects of thermal energy to tissues. It this report, it became apparent that time-temperature relationship of heat determines the characteristics of response [4]. At 44 °C, irreversible damage is reached after 7 h. Conversely, at 70 °C trans-epidermal necrosis results in less than 1 s. In middle temperatures, 44–51 °C,

I. A. Kleidona
Department of Dermatology, 1st University Clinic of Dermatology-Venerology, Athens, Greece

A. M. Ghanem
Cranley Clinic, London, UK

College of Medicine and Dentistry, Birmingham, UK
e-mail: drghanem@cranleyclinic.com

N. J. Lowe (✉)
Cranley Clinic, London, UK

UCLA, Los Angeles, California, USA
e-mail: Drlowe@cranleyclinic.com

V. Madan (ed.), *Practical Introduction to Laser Dermatology*,
https://doi.org/10.1007/978-3-030-46451-6_7

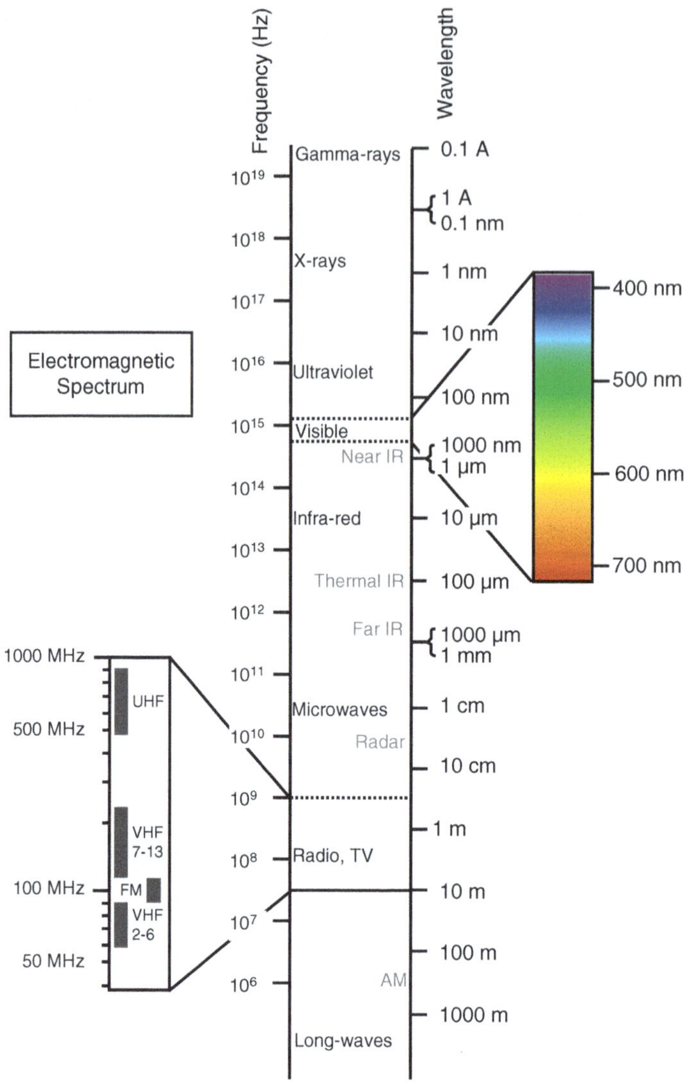

Fig. 7.1 The electromagnetic spectrum

injury doubles for each degree rise. Obviously, besides time and temperature exposure, the behaviour varies with differences in tissue composition. It has been established that up to 40 °C cells are able to resist heat; denaturation of proteins occurs at 65–70 °C in most tissues. Above 100 °C vaporisation, carbonisation and thermoablation is observed. Near critical sub-lethal temperatures there is rapid tissue coagulation [5–7]. Typically, in the connective tissue fibrils of type I collagen denaturate at about 65 °C with subsequent tissue shrinkage. The triple helix "unwinds" due to destruction of intermolecular links and undergoes transformation to a gel-like structure. In addition, a wound healing response initiates with fibroblast activation and new collagen synthesis. Recent studies concentrate on the importance of proteins activated upon thermal stimulus, named heat shock proteins (HSP), produced to protect the skin. For instance, thermal energy upregulates HSP47, a procollagen type I promoter, which stimulates collagen biosynthesis. Additionally, HSP70 binds to peptides of denaturated proteins to prevent aggregation and precipitation [8, 9]. The biologic and histologic effects of heat are postulated to be beneficial in

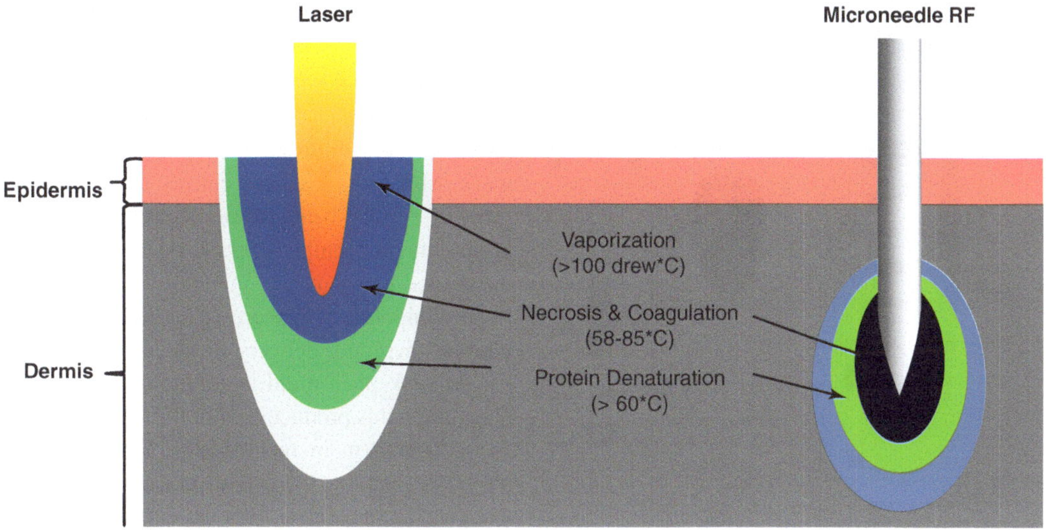

Fig. 7.2 Schematic representation of laser and fractional radiofrequency thermal effects [11]

the treatment of pathologic and aesthetic concerns. Because RF is not selectively absorbed by chromophores is safer in darker skin than some laser wavelengths. Radiofrequency (RF) and light-based devices are used for thermal modification of tissues for therapeutic and cosmetic purposes [10] (Fig. 7.2).

Radiofrequency in Aesthetic Medicine Since the development of the first electrocautery device by Cushing and Bovie in 1928, RF energy has been applied for cardiac (e.g. atrial ablation), oncological (e.g. liver resection), arthroscopic (e.g. capsular tightening) or cosmetic indications. Usually, RF systems consist of a generator and a handheld applicator with electrodes. Device's parameters (e.g. frequency, mode, power/pulse settings, size/configuration of delivery tip) and tissue's characteristics (e.g. hydration, temperature) are significant variables of the thermal effects. Various types of this technique have gained popularity in the cosmetic field targeting the dermis or the subcutaneous fat. It is presumed that heat causes initial collagen contraction and subsequent new collagen synthesis through long-term repair processes, resulting in dermal remodelling and skin tightening [12, 13]. Also, studies on adipose tissue indicate alterations of adipocyte's morphology and increased rate of apoptosis [14].

Available Radiofreqeuncy Systems

Monopolar Radiofrequency

Mechanism of Action Monopolar radiofrequency systems apply electrical current to the skin via a circuit, where one pole is located on the delivery handpiece placed on the skin and the other on a remote "passive" ground pad (Fig. 7.3). Increasing distance between the two poles and larger surface area of the grounding pad, concentrates the amount of thermal energy close to the active electrode. In this way, heat can be delivered with the possibility of high penetration through the mechanism of capacitive coupling.

Available Devices and Technique of Administration In 2002, the Food and Drug Administration (FDA) approved the first monopolar RF device Thermage Thermacool TC (Solta Medical Inc., Hayward, Calif., USA) for the treatment of periorbital wrinkles (Fig. 7.3). This product generates heat in the dermis at 65–75° and contains a cooling component to protect the epidermis keeping the superficial temperature at 35–45°. Generally, the depth of heating is 3–6 mm. Initial studies associated this treatment with significant discomfort and fat atrophy. Since then, various devices have been introduced to the market and techniques evolved aiming to opti-

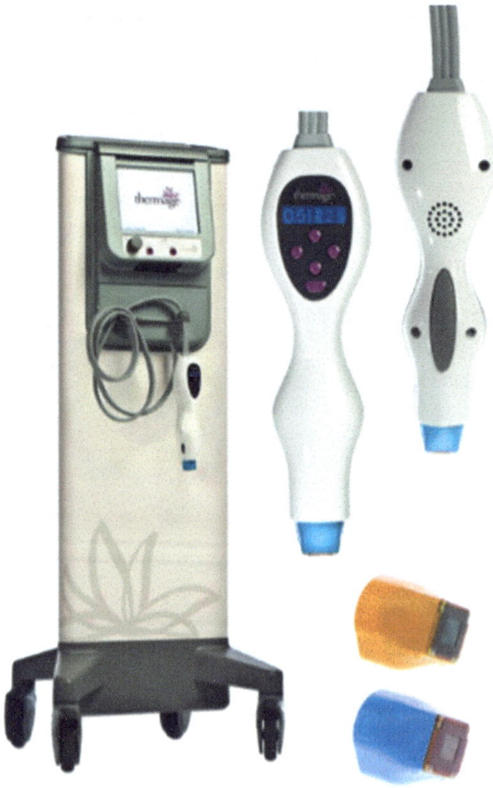

Fig. 7.3 Example of monopolar radiofrequency system

mize outcomes and limit side effects. In this view, larger tips allowed faster treatment of larger areas and multiple passes with lower energy levels decreased discomfort. RF technology was also cleared for full face (2004) and off-face treatments (2006). Other monopolar devices are the ThermaCool NXT system with specific tips for different anatomic areas, the Thermage Comfort Plus Technology with a vibrating and post-RF pulse cooling handpiece to reduce discomfort, the Exillis (BTL Aesthetics, Prague, Czech Republic) and the Pellevé Wrinkle Reduction System (Ellman International Inc., Oceanside, NY) [15, 16].

The technique of administration differs depending on the device employed. For example, Thermage CPT is delivered with a stamping method along a ruled grid, while other devices, such as Exilis and Pellevé, administer RF with a continuous movement of the handpiece. Some providers use a cryogen cooling unit and an infrared thermometer to monitor the temperature.

Unipolar Radiofrequency

Mechanism of Action Unipolar radiofrequency systems deliver energy in a different mode compared to the traditional monopolar and bipolar ways. Monopolar devices convey energy in the form of current between an electrode tip and a grounding pad, while in bipolar systems energy is distributed between two points of the handpiece. In the unipolar form there is a single electrode without involving delivery of electric current. It should be kept in mind that, alternating electromagnetic fields produce heat in the biological tissues via two main mechanisms. Practically, at lower frequencies there is displacement of ions and production of heat by ionic current, whereas at higher frequencies electromagnetic oscillations result in rapid rotational movements of water molecules dissipating heat into the tissues. Through the single electrode of a unipolar device, electromagnetic radiation at high frequencies (30–40 MHz) is emitted, in a mode analogous to a radio tower. Such high frequency waves cause rapid rotation of water molecules, resulting in dielectric heating of biological tissues. The heating is observed along the central axis of the delivery electrode and can penetrate to 15–20 mm depth [17]. This technology is applied in body contouring, skin tightening and cellulites.

Available Devices and Technique of Administration An example is the Accent RF System (Alma Lasers, Inc., Buffalo Grove, USA). The Accent RF System (Alma Lasers, Inc., Buffalo Grove, USA) uses a unipolar applicator with cooling to deliver thermal energy to the subcutaneous tissues in a continuous mobile manner. The device has also a second handpiece delivering bipolar RF, theoretically for more superficial heating of the dermis. There are different tips available, such as an eye tip, a unilarge tip and cellulite tip.

Bipolar Radiofrequency

Mechanism of Action In bipolar radiofrequency systems, the current passes through the skin between 2 or more electrodes. These are usually placed into the handpiece at a specific fixed distance. With this configuration the distribution of energy can be controlled, and current flow is limited in the tissue between the two electrodes. Generally, it is thought that the maximum depth of penetration is half the distance between the electrodes. Compared to monopolar devices, in the bipolar configuration distribution of heat is better controlled but less penetrating [17].

Available Devices and Technique of Administration In order to overcome the issue of penetration depth, more complex systems were designed. In this view, bipolar RF has been combined to light (IPL: Aurora SR, Syneron, Yokkneam, Israel) or laser (Polaris WRA, Syneron Medical Inc., Yokneam, Israel) for synergistic electro-optical effects in a technology termed ***ELOS*** (electro-optical synergy). The light energy precedes RF to pre-heat the target by photothermolysis and lower its impedance, aiming to achieve better results with lower levels of energy. These devices have been proposed for the treatment of rhytides, acne, unwanted hair, vascular and pigmented lesions. Further, vacuum has been used in RF systems ***FACES*** (Functional Aspiration Controlled Electrothermal Stimulation) (Aluma System Lumenis, Inc., Santa Clara, Ca, USA) to fold the skin and allow penetration in a controlled, maximised, pre-determined depth and to enhance lymphatic drainage. Combination of bipolar RF, infrared light, vacuum and mechanical rollers have been used for face and body contouring (VelaShape, VelaSmooth, Syneron Medical Ltd) [18].

Also, there are ***tripolar systems*** (Pollogen, 2011), which have one positive and two negative electrodes, and the ***multipolar RF*** (Venous Freeze, 2011-Venous Legacy, 2013). The concept of the latter technology was to allow change of direction of the electromagnetic field while moving the handpiece and warranty uniform and dense heat matrix.

Fractional Radiofrequency

Mechanism of Action Fractional photothermolysis was introduced as an intermediate approach between ablative and non-ablative lasers to minimise the risks of delayed healing, dyspigmentation and scarring without compromising efficacy. The concept was to produce microscopic thermal zones (MTZ) of injury surrounded by unaffected skin which would enable quicker healing [19]. This notion was applied in the development of fractionated radiofrequency (FRF) which recently has gained traction combining efficacy and safety. This technique uses minimally invasive microneedles or electrode pins to achieve targeted dermal injury with minimal superficial involvement (Fig. 7.4). The thermal injury results in denaturated fibrils of collagen and initiates a wound healing response [16].

In 2009, Hantash et al. developed the first microneedle therapy system (MTS) through which bipolar radiofrequency was introduced into the skin. In this way, he generated fractional radiofrequency thermal zones (RFTZ) in the dermis. These zones were separated by areas of spared skin, aiming to combine the thermal effects of denaturated collagen to a more efficient wound healing reaction. Using immunohistochemistry and PCR studies, he observed dermal remodelling with new collagen and elastin deposition up to 10 weeks after the treatment. The intention was to associate targeted dermal injury with minimal superficial involvement [21]. It is hypothesised that global enhancement of skin quality could be achieved through signalling processes of wound healing spreading in the dermis and the overlying epidermis [22]. Similar changes have been reported with microneedling. This technique creates controlled injury by micropunctures in the skin and initiates a healing cascade [23].

One of the differences between the two fractionated techniques is that lasers produce uniform columns of thermal injury, while FRF creates "pyramid-shaped" areas wider superficially. There is mild epidermal ablation and bulk of thermal effect in the dermis. The term "sublation" was introduced in the device lexicon to indicate the greater effect in the deeper layers of the skin [24]. In microneedle RF, the tip distributes energy via either non-insulated-electrode-microneedles or insulated-microneedles where part of the needle is non-conductive and the energy flows through the tip causing a "sphere" of thermal injury.

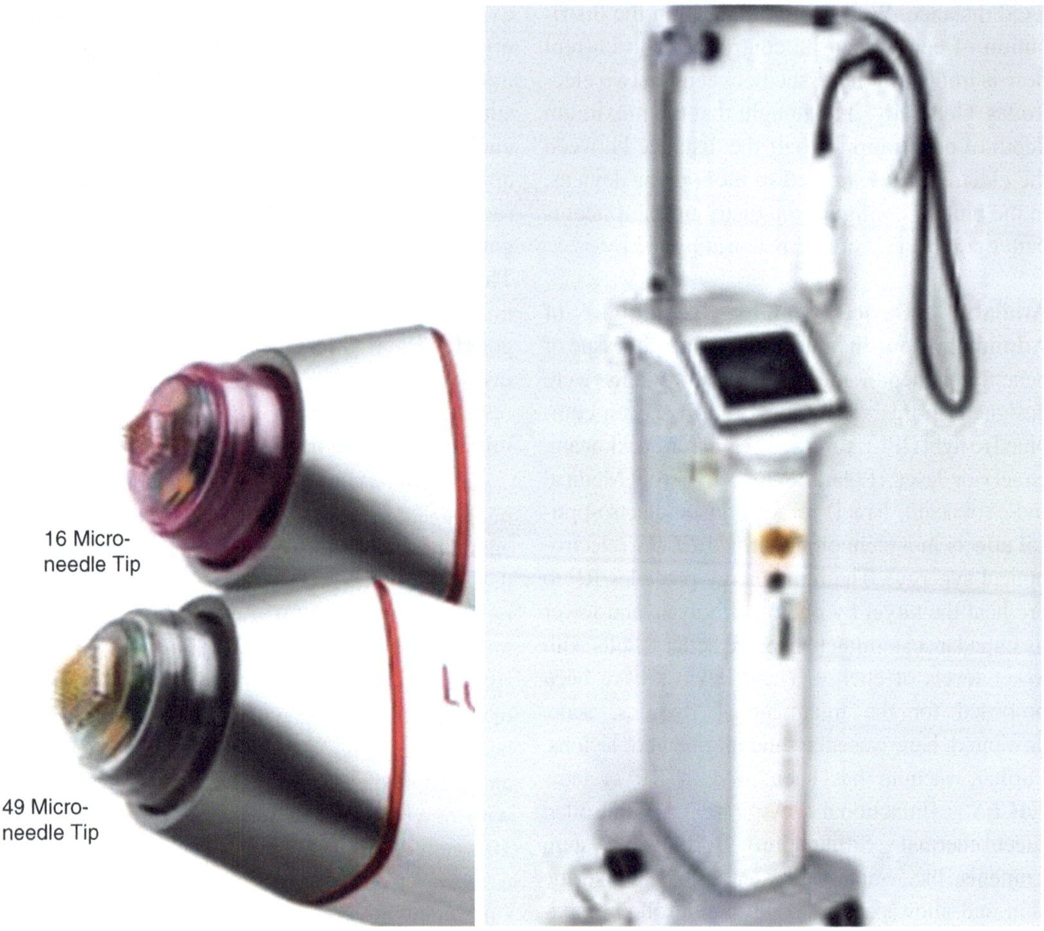

Fig. 7.4 Example of Microneedle Radiofrequency System [20]

Available Devices and Technique of Administration There are various commercially available devices with different specifications in terms of size of the tip, number of microneedles, frequency, pulses and energy delivered (Table 7.1). Some examples of microneedling RF systems are the Infini (Lutronic, Korea), the INTRAcel (Jeysis, Korea), the Scarlet (Viol, Korea) and the ePrime (Syneron-Candela, Israel). RF devices with electrode pins include the eMatrix and the MatrixRF (Syneron-Candela, Israel).

The procedure usually starts by selecting the tip and mode technique based on location, depth of microneedles (where available) and intensity. The handpiece tip is applied on the skin and pulse switch is triggered to deliver RF energy. The microneedles penetrate the skin automatically within the set time and then retract. Some techniques involve spacing between pulses and additional passes with adjustment of settings.

Advantages and Disadvantages

Monopolar Radiofrequency The monopolar system delivers volumetric heating to tissues with deep penetration but could result in significant discomfort. RF does not target melanin and is often described as "colour blind" and safer for all skin types. The downside is the significant discomfort that could result with the procedure. Besides, some cases of subcutaneous fat atrophy has been reported, especially with high energies [25].

Table 7.1 Examples of microneedle radiofrequency devices

Device	System specifications
INFINI™ LUTRONIC	Mode: Microneedle radiofrequency—49 insulated microneedle 0.5–3.5 mm 1 Hz, 10 ms–1000 ms, max power 50 W (up to level 20)
FRACTORA™ INMODE	Mode: Microneedle radiofrequency—60/24/24 coated pins 600 µ/3000 µ/3000 µ 1 Hz, max energy: 62 mJ/pin at 75 W, repetition rate: Up to 2pps
INTENSIF EndyMed	Mode: Microneedle radiofrequency—PRO up to 5 mm needles/ PURE 2.0 up to 3.5 mm needles 25 microneedles
VIVACE™ Aesthetics biomedical	Mode: Microneedle radiofrequency, 36 insulated or non-insulated microneedles, 0.5–3.5 mm P = 30–70 W, pulse = 100–800 ms,
INTRAcel SmartMed	Mode: Microneedle radiofrequency 49 insulated microneedles, 0.5–2 mm

Unipolar Radiofrequency This is a deeply penetrating technology targeting the reticular dermis and subcutaneous tissue. Can reach a depth of 15–20 mm and can target fibrous septa and irregularities of cellulitis. Also, can be combined with bipolar RF, the latter targets more superficial tissues, theoretically combining improvement of laxity and fine rhytides.

Bipolar Radiofrequency Bipolar technology offers better control of the RF energy delivered to tissues which is applied via two electrodes in close proximity. This results in less energy density and reduced risk of complications. The target tissues are heated in an almost symmetrical manner. Compared to monopolar devices, in the bipolar configuration distribution of heat is better controlled but less penetrating [17].

Fractional Radiofrequency Fractional devices were developed to achieve precise, focal, targeted, high energy treatment zones within the dermis with minimal epidermal injury. This results in lower risks of complications and short downtime. The procedure is well tolerated with local anaesthetic and is proposed to have a safe profile even in darker skin type patients. The disadvantage is the need for repeated sessions and the lack of clear protocols with a large variability of RF delivery parameters. The aesthetic results are not visible immediately but there is progressive improvement up to few months after treatment. Treatments with RF devices are minimally invasive and post-procedure patients can return to their routine [26].

Indications

There use of Radiofrequency technology has been reported for various indications. The are some considerations to be taken into account when treating different areas.

The periorbital area has a delicate morphology and function. The formation of wrinkles mainly results from a combination of photodamage and muscle contraction. Monopolar RF was used to treat this area in different studies (Fig. 7.5).

Skin ageing results from the cumulative effects of genetic-associated modifications and other exogenous factors such as repetitive exposure to ultraviolet radiation, smoking, diet and air pollution. Clinically there is often xerosis, rhytides, loss of tone, elastosis, dyspigmentation and telangiectasia. In the midface, the manifestations of ageing are multifactorial, mainly related to volume loss and laxity. Moreover, there is reduction of dermal thickness and alterations of the overall skin envelope. The lower face ageing is largely dominated by changes in the perioral region and the jawline. Monopolar RF has been demonstrated useful in the treatment of these complex issues.

The ageing of the dorsal surface of the hands is characterised by thin, translucent epidermis, decreased collagen and elastin, conferring a skeletonised appearance. In clinical practice, different strategies have been proposed for hand rejuvenation, such as topical therapies or energy based devices as monotherapy or in combination.

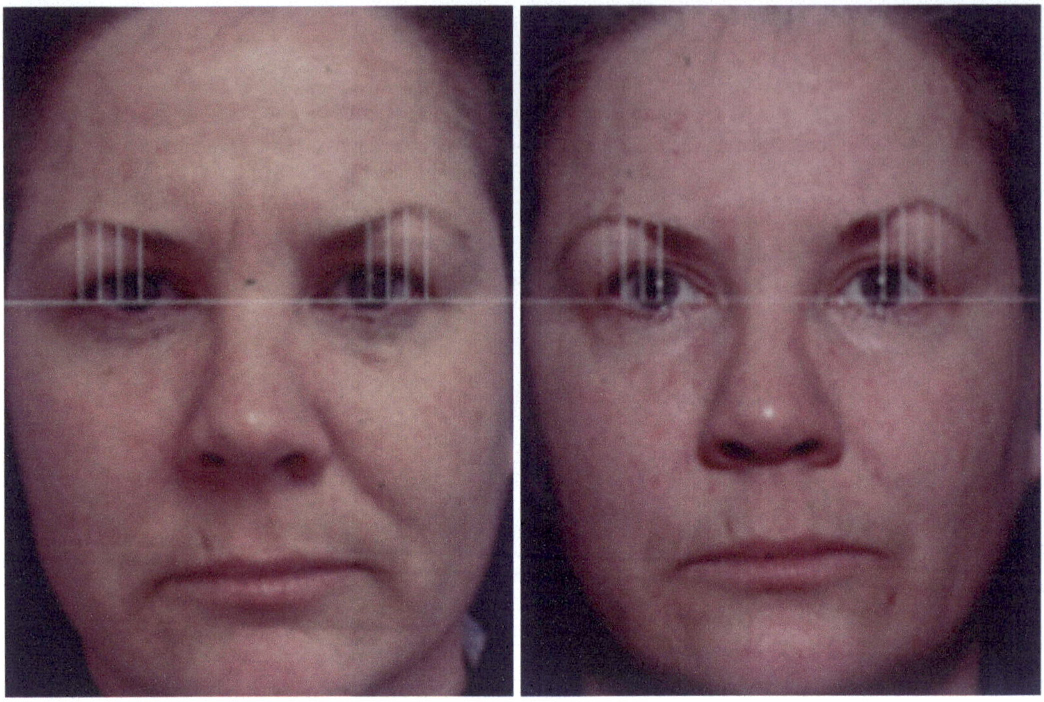

Fig. 7.5 Example of eyebrow lift following Radiofrequency treatment. Left pre-treatment; Right post-treatment. (from Fitzpatrick et al. 2003)

Acne vulgaris is a common inflammatory condition of multifactorial pathogenesis. Clinically presents with comedones, papules, pustules and nodules or cysts in serious cases. Furthermore, can be complicated by scarring causing additional psychological distress. Conventional treatments include antibiotics and retinoids. More recently, minimally invasive procedures such as RF are proposed for the treatment of acne vulgaris and its consequences (Fig. 7.6). Acne scarring and acne has a substantial socio-psychological impact on patients. Atrophic acne scars are typically classified in icepick, rolling and boxcar scars. Often these are associated with large pores, poor skin quality and discolouration. Various dermatosurgical methods are currently employed such as lasers, dermabrasion, chemical peels, surgical excision and lately fractional RF.

Cellulite is a multifactorial condition of unknown exact pathophysiology. It is largely believed, that fat lobules of metabolically stable adipocytes herniate through the dermo-hypodermal junction surrounded by fibrosed collagen septa. Consequently, shortening and retraction of the septa appear as the characteristic depressions of cellulites. It is common in post-pubertal women and is mainly located in lower body, abdomen, femoral and gluteal areas with the characteristic orange-peel appearance. Therapeutic approaches range from topical agents to energy based devices. Radiofrequency is used to deliver targeted collagen remodelling and lipolysis (Fig. 7.7).

The décolletage is a particularly delicate area of skin which is highly exposed to the sun and prone to damage. Visible changes are laxity, rhytides and dyspigmentation and treatment is challenging.

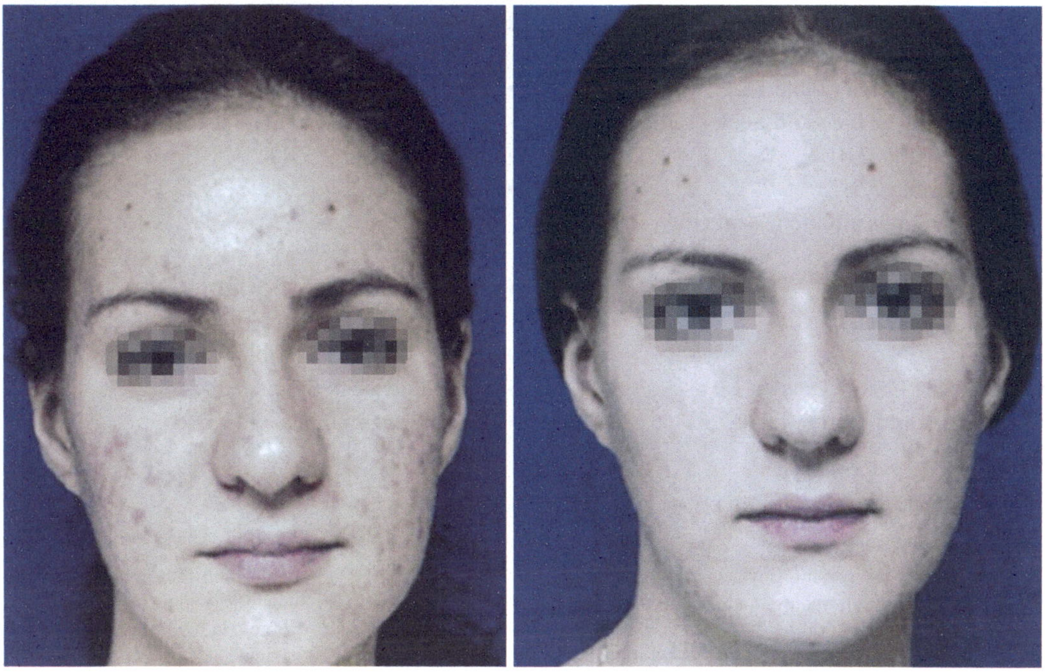

Fig. 7.6 Example of patient with acne treated with Radiofreqeuncy. Left pre-treatment; Right post-treatment. (from Ruiz-Esperanza et al. 2003)

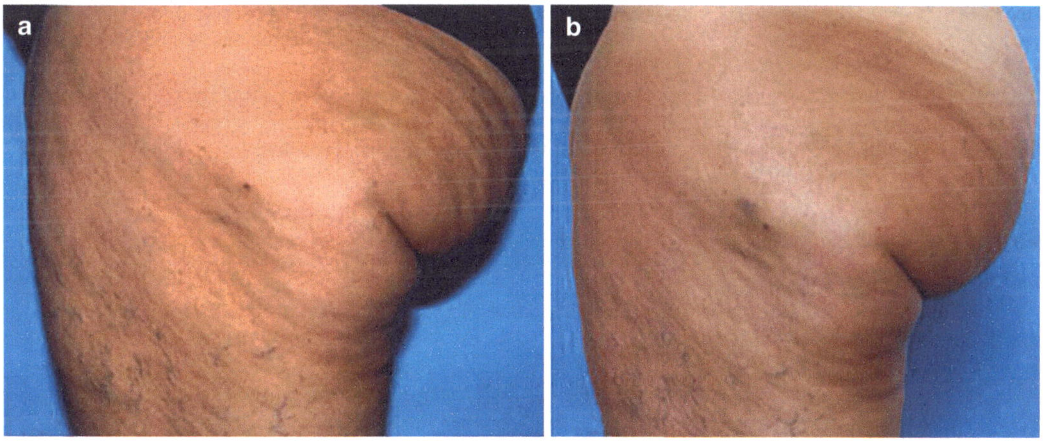

Fig. 7.7 Example of patient with cellulite treated with Radiofrequency. A: Pre-treatment; B: Before 12th treatment session. (Van Der Lugt et al. 2009)

Striae distensae or "stretch marks" are lesions in the dermis which at early stages appear as erythematous (striae rubrae) and at a later chronic stage become atrophic and hypopigmented (striae albae). Histologically, there is elastolysis and thickening of collagen fibres in the dermis, while the epidermis is gradually atrophied. SD are very difficult to eradicate and various modalities are advocated such as topicals, lipolysis and energy based strategies including radiofrequency.

Monopolar Devices

- **Periorbital area** (Table 7.2)
- **Middle-lower face and neck** (Table 7.3)
- **Hands** (Table 7.4)
- **Body** (Table 7.5)
- **Acne vulgaris and acne scarring** (Table 7.6)

Unipolar Devices

- **Cellulite** (Table 7.7)
- **Rhytides and laxity** (Table 7.8)

Bipolar Devices

- **Skin rejuvenation** (See Table 7.9)
- **Acne vulgaris and acne scars** (See Table 7.10)
- **Cellulite** (Table 7.11)
- **Hair removal** (Table 7.12)

Fractional Radiofrequency

- **Periorbital area** (Table 7.13)
- **Face and neck** (Table 7.14)
- **Décolletage** (Table 7.15)

Table 7.2 Studies of monopolar RF in the treatment of the periorbital area

Study	Outcomes
Fitzpatrick [27]	86 patient, single session of monopolar RF (ThermaCool TC), 6 months multicentre, blinded trial. Achieved at least one-point FWCS (Fitzpatrick wrinkle classification system) improvement of periorbital wrinkles in most patients and 0.5 mm lifting of the eyebrow in 62% of cases. Adverse effects were mild-moderate pain, oedema, erythema, 0.36% incidence of second degree burns and residual scarring in 3 patients
Nahm [28]	10 patients, split-face study with ThermaCool TC. Observed statistically significant elevation of the brow and the superior palpebral crease. Adverse reactions limited to swelling and mild bruising post-treatment
Han [29]	70 Korean patients with periorbital wrinkles treated with monopolar RF. Reported 15% improvement ratio at 1 month. The pain was tolerable and mild erythema was the only adverse effect
Bassichis [30]	Prospective controlled study in the upper third of the face. Described measurable brow elevation with asymmetry and difficult to predict effects post-treatment. Also, the majority of patients did not perceive the benefit, although were satisfied with the non-invasivity of the procedure

Table 7.3 Studies of monopolar RF in the treatment of middle-lower face and neck

Study	Characteristics and outcomes
Jacobson [31]	Monopolar RF in 24 patients. Demonstrated improvement in nasolabial folds, marionette lines and jowls. Reported further tightening with subsequent treatments at 3 months after last treatment
Alster [32]	Monopolar RF in the treatment of skin laxity. A single treatment resulted in significant improvement of nasolabial folds and tightening of the cheek and neck. Patients experienced moderate discomfort during the procedure with limited and transient side effects
Alhaddad [33]	Randomized, split-face trial, compared two non-invasive modalities for skin tightening: Monopolar RF and microfocused ultrasound with visualization. Six months follow-up of 20 patients with mild-moderate skin laxity revealed significant improvement with no statistical difference between the two techniques
Chipps [34]	Pellevé in the face and neck of 49 subjects. Clinical efficacy based on GAIS (global aesthetic improvement scale) showed more than 80% improvement in skin laxity, wrinkles and overall skin texture with high patient satisfaction
Weiss [35]	Retrospective review of more than 600 patients to establish the degree and rate of adverse events when monopolar RF was used to treat lower face laxity. Most commonly, oedema and erythema were described. In a small number of cases were reported acneiform erythematous papules, superficial crust, erythematous subcutaneous nodules, slight depression of the cheek skin and neck tenderness. All reactions were transient and self-limited
de Felippe [36]	Investigated retrospectively the safety of monopolar RF in 759 treatments. Concluded that these were associated with low incidence oedema and erythema. Less frequently, headache, scarring and fat atrophy were reported. However, second degree burns occurred in 2.7% of cases

Table 7.4 Studies of monopolar RF in the treatment of hands

Study	Outcomes
Vega [37]	A multicentre, randomized study to evaluate effectiveness of monopolar radiofrequency in the treatment of aging hands. 31 patients received 3 sessions at 2-weekly intervals and the response was assessed using GAIS (global aesthetic improvement scale). In 89% of patients there was visible improvement and no side effects other than mild to moderate discomfort during treatment

Table 7.5 Studies of monopolar RF in body treatments

Study	Characteristics and outcomes
Zelickson [38]	TermaCool TC radiofrequency was to two volunteers prior to elective abdominoplasty. Performed biopsies pre-treatment, immediately after and 8 weeks post-treatment. Electron microscopy of the specimens demonstrated increased diameter of collagen fibrils with loss of distinct borders and northern blot analysis showed elevation of collagen type I messenger RNA
Anolik [39]	ThermaCool TC device with Thermage multiplex tip in 12 patients undergoing body shaping. Follow-up visits revealed decrease of waist circumference and laxity score at 1, 2, 4, and 6 months

Table 7.6 Studies of monopolar RF in the treatment of acne and acne scarring

Study	Characteristics and outcomes
Ruiz-Esperanza [40]	22 patients with moderate to severe active acne vulgaris with or without concomitant scarring, treated with 1 or 2 sessions of monopolar RF, followed up to 8 months. Excellent response was achieved in the majority of cases (82%), the treatment was tolerated well, and no adverse events were identified

Table 7.7 Studies of unipolar RF in the treatment of cellulite

Study	Characteristics and outcomes
De Pino [41]	2 sessions of unipolar RF to 26 patients with grade 1–3 cellulitis on the thighs and/or buttocks. Evaluation with real-time ultrasound 15 days after the last treatment showed 20% volumetric contraction between the stratum corneum and the Camper's fascia in 68% of cases
Goldberg [42]	6 sessions of unipolar RF to 30 patients with grade III–IV cellulite of the upper thigh and followed them up to 6 months. There was a mean decrease in leg circumference of 2.45 cm with histologic evidence of dermal fibrosis in the upper dermis and no MRI evidence alterations in the pannicular layer. The contraction between the stratum corneum and the Camper's fascia was postulated to be secondary to transient deep tightening
Alexiades-Armenakas [43]	Randomized, blinded, comparative study of 10 subjects with minimum grade 2 cellulitis of the thighs. Favourable clinical outcomes but not statistically significant were reported

- **Acne scars and acne vulgaris** (Table 7.16)
- **Axillary hyperhidrosis** (Table 7.17)
- **Cellulite** (Table 7.18)
- **Striae distensae** (Table 7.19)

Pre-Treatment Preparation and Precautions

The clinician should counsel the patient, obtain informed consent and ensure clear documentation and standardised photographs are taken before and after every session. Patients should be treated if expectations and desired outcomes are realistic. Appropriate patient selection is paramount in order to increase efficacy and minimise complications. Detailed medical history including previous cosmetic procedures should be taken and the procedure should not be undertaken if there are contraindications, such as connective tissue disease, history of keloids, autoimmune disease, severe renal, cardiac or liver disorders, pregnancy, pacemaker, metal implants, breast feeding, previous allergic reactions with the pro-

Table 7.8 Studies of unipolar RF in the treatment of rhytides and laxity

Study	Characteristics and outcomes
Aelxiades-Armenakas [44]	Evaluated the efficacy of unipolar RF versus bipolar RF in the treatment of facial rhytides and laxity. Performed 4 weekly sessions in 10 patients and concluded that, although there was improvement with both modalities, statistical significance was not achieved. Side effects were limited to minimal transient erythema

Table 7.9 Studies of bipolar RF in skin rejuvenation

Study	Characteristics and outcomes
Sadick [45]	Evaluated the outcomes of combined optical and RF energies using the system Aurora for full face skin rejuvenation. Series of 108 patients applied 5 treatments every 3 weeks and achieved overall skin improvement of 75.3% including skin texture, wrinkles, laxity, pore size, dyspigmentation and telangiectasias. High rate of patient satisfaction >90% and low rate of minor complications were also reported. One patient treated with high optical fluence for resistant telangiectasia developed a nasal scar
Yu [46]	The combination of IL (infrared light) and bipolar RF (ReFirm ST applicator) was used in 19 Chinese volunteers. At 3 months follow-up they showed general mild to moderate improvement of wrinkles and laxity. Less satisfactory results were obtained in the neck and periorbital area
Choi [47]	Compared the efficacy and safety of Polaris WRA (diode laser and RF) and ReFirm ST (infrared and RF) in 14 Korean subjects. Both techniques demonstrated comparative clinical and histological outcomes except for patient satisfaction which was superior in the Polaris cohort.
Gold [48]	56 patients with combined infrared light and bipolar RF followed by fractional bipolar RF. Follow-up at 6 months after treatment showed 85% improvement rate based on investigator-directed outcomes using GAI while subjects rated results even higher (91%). Only minor transient complications such as oedema and erythema were reported
Verner [49]	Compared the use of combined IPL and RF versus IPL alone in the aging hands. Concluded that combination therapy resulted in superior outcomes in terms of skin laxity and hyperpigmentation
El-Domyati [50]	The histological changes following electro-optical therapies were examined by El-Domyati et al. combination of IPL and RF was applied in the peri-orbital area of 6 patients and punch biopsies were performed for histology and immunohistochemical assessment. There was increase in epidermal thickness, 53% decrease in elastin, enhanced expression of type I, III, VII collagen and new collagen synthesis which continued to improve 3 months after the last session.
Gold [51]	The FACES technology was used to treat 46 adults with facial skin aging. Achieved progressive improvement of wrinkles and elastosis which persisted 6 months after a course of 8 treatments. Adverse events included oedema, erythema, purpura, burn/blistering in 15 cases and hyperpigmentation in 1 case but all resolved within 2–4 weeks

Table 7.10 Studies of bipolar RF in acne vulgaris and acne scars

Study	Characteristics and outcomes
Prieto [52]	Combination of pulsed light and radiofrequency (Aurora AC) was employed in 32 subjects with moderate papulo-pustular acne who received twice weekly sessions for 4 weeks. Reported 47% average reduction in lesion count and "good" overall improvement in 32% of patient-directed assessments. Biopsies were performed in four subjects with inflamed non-comedonal lesions and showed decrease in the size of sebaceous glands and reduced perifolliculitis
Camelli [53]	Compared factional laser alone with combined fractional laser/RF. Used combination fractional CO_2 laser and bipolar radiofrequency (SmartXide2, DEKA M.E.L.A., Catanzaro, Italy) to treat six patients with superficial boxcar/rolling acne scars and four patients with photoaging. Combination therapy demonstrated better results in terms of tissue remodelling and depth of scars with lower side effects and quicker healing
Min [54]	Showed superior efficacy of Er:YAG laser compared to Polaris in a single-blind, randomized, split-face study of 24 patients with mild to moderate acne scars. Treatment with Er:YAG resulted in thicker and denser collagen deposition and significantly higher patient satisfaction

Table 7.11 Studies on bipolar RF in the treatment of cellulite

Study	Characteristics and outcomes
Van Der Lugt [55]	The ThermaLipo RF device (Thermamedic ltd., Alicante, Spain) was used to treat 50 patients with cellulite. He showed improvement in the shape of buttocks and skin texture
Nootheti [56]	Compared the VelaSmooth (infrared light and RF) with the TriActive (diode laser, suction and massage). Both systems provided improvement of cellulitis and reduction of thigh circumference with no significant statistical difference between them
Sadick and Mullholland [57]	The VelaSmooth device was used in a preliminary two-Centre study. After 16 treatments they achieved 0.8 inches mean decrease of thigh circumference. Some patients reported minimal discomfort and there was transient swelling
Romero [58]	Results of combination infrared light and RF were compared to no treatment in small trial. Twice weekly sessions over a period of 12 weeks resulted in improvement of cellulite based on photography and profilometry
Hexsel [59]	The efficacy and safety of Velashape was investigated in 9 females with cellulite. Results showed improvement of cellulite severity grading on the buttocks and hips circumference. However, no statistically significant difference was observed on the thighs

Table 7.12 Studies of bipolar RF in hair removal

Study	Characteristics and outcomes
Sadick and Shaoul [60]	Examined the effect of combined IPL and RF in photoepilation of various colours of hairs and skin types. Hair density decreased by 75% on average on all body areas at 18 months follow-up with maximum results on the axillae and legs. Histology revealed vacuolar degeneration of hair follicles. Interestingly, there was no dependence on skin colour but dark hair showed better clearance. The only reported adverse event was temporary erythema
Sadick [61]	Performed photoepilation of white and blond hair with combined IPL and RF showed 52% removal of blond hair versus 44% of white hair
Goldberg [62]	Used combined IPL and RF on non-pigmented hair and concluded that it could be useful on terminal white hair (35% removal at 6 months) with better results when pre-treated with aminolevulinic acid. Conversely, vellus white hair did not respond to treatment

Table 7.13 Studies of fractional RF in the peri-orbital area

Study	Characteristics and outcomes
Jeon [63]	Compared the efficacy of microneedle RF with BoNT/A. showed that, despite the rapid and better results of BoNT/A at 3 and 6 weeks, the radiofrequency microneedling group had superior gradual improvement at 18 weeks. Additionally, they performed skin biopsy to one patient and described increased expression of elastin and procollagen-3 in immunohistochemistry but no difference in collagen-4 and procollagen-1 at 18 weeks follow-up
Kim [64]	11 darker-skin subjects were treated with 3 sessions of FRF and were subsequently evaluated at 3 months. Following photographic blinded assessment using FWCS, statistically significant improvement of wrinkles and patient satisfaction were reported
Lee [11]	Small study of 20 Korean patients with variable degrees of wrinkles, performed 3 sessions of microneedle radiofrequency to treat the periorbital area. The outcome measurements included WAS by blinded dermatologists based on standardised photos, patient's satisfaction and adverse events. Significant clinical improvement and participant's satisfaction was described in all cases at 6 months follow-up. In terms of side effects, there were 2 cases of hyperpigmentation in Fitzpatrick photo-type III-IV which resolved spontaneously after 4 weeks
Shin [65]	Treated lower eyelid fat bulging with 2 types insulated microneedling RF in 22 volunteers. Using 3D photogrammetry and Investigator's global assessment showed statistically significant decrease of fat bulging up to 12 weeks after treatment
Roh [66]	Treated 70 Korean patients with crow's feet and demonstrated 20% decrease of wrinkles using digital skin photo-analyser for quantitative analysis
Lolis and Goldberg [26]	80% of patients demonstrated improvement of periorbital wrinkles

Table 7.14 Studies of fractional RF in the face and neck

Study	Outcomes
Calderhead [67]	Reported results from five geographically separated study centres, which treated 499 patients with a wide range of Fitzpatrick skin type. Although outcome measurements were not clearly reported from individual centres, it appears that clinicians achieved significant overall skin rejuvenation in the majority of patients
Alexiades [68]	Randomised blinded trial to compare the efficacy of a single session RF microneedling with surgical face lift in patients with similar baseline laxity. Assessed skin laxity with quantitative grading and demonstrated better results with surgery. However, they suggested that the minimally invasive treatment could be an important option
Alexiades [22]	Multicentre open-label trial of 100 subjects with mild to severe wrinkles or laxity evaluated the efficacy of microneedle RF. It was noted 24% improvement of rhytids at 3 months and 25.6% at 6 months. Similarly, laxity scores decreased by 22.3% at 3 months and by 24.1% at 6 months
Lu [69]	Randomized, double-blind, split-face study performed by Lu et al. concluded that microneedle RF is effective in treating skin laxity with superior outcomes when applied to the deep dermis compared to the superficial approach
Seo [70]	Investigated the efficacy of microneedle RF in Asian skin. Treated 25 females and showed greater than 50% clinical improvement of pores, wrinkles and overall skin appearance in most patients. Of note, skin hydration measured with Corneometer and skin roughness measured by Visiometer, showed significant enhancement ($p < 0.05$). Conversely, mean melanin index and erythema index, measured by Mexameter, were not significantly improved
Park [71]	Large multicentre study which enroled 204 Korean patients. Following photographic blinded assessment with a 5-point global aesthetic improvement score, they described grade 3 or 4 improvement in 140 patients
Gold [72]	Multicentre trial of 53 patients of various ages. Performed 3 sessions of microneedle RF using protocols based on anatomic areas. The assessment included blinded evaluation by dermatologists using the Fitzpatrick scoring, patient's satisfaction and side effects. Showed statistically significant reduction of wrinkles at 1 month, with continued improvement up to 3 months after the last treatment. Noted improvement in GAIS and skin tightening in the mid and lower face
Hruza [73]	Prospective multicentre study to evaluate the efficacy of fractional RF in facial rhytides and skin texture. The participants were assessed based on the Fitzpatrick classification and were selected if they had minimum two areas of score 2–6 wrinkles and elastosis. The authors used a 5-point grading scale and noted that the majority of patients had more than 40% improvement in wrinkling, smoothness, brightness and tightness, 1 month after the last treatment. They noticed some improvement in elastosis, mainly in the periorbital area, although the change was not statistically significant
Akita [74]	Reported statistically significant improvement of wrinkles, mainly in the lateral canthus and the lower eyelid and little effect in the forehead. Also, the majority of patients reported moderate to very good improvement of the nasolabial folds but of unclear statistical significance
Jiang [75]	22 subjects with face wrinkles and laxity in the lower face. Reported improvement after 2–3 sessions, suggesting that multiple treatments were necessary to achieve satisfactory results

Table 7.15 Studies of fractional RF in décolletage

Lyons [76]	The treatment of rhytides and skin laxity in the décolletage was studied by Lyons et al. in 12 patients. Demonstrated 80% overall patient satisfaction and improvement of GAIS in 67% of cases

Table 7.16 Studies of fractional RF in acne scars and acne vulgaris

Cho [77]	Investigated the efficacy of fractional microneedle RF in acne scars and large pores. They enrolled 30 patients and achieved more that 70% improvement in all cases. Described increase of the dermal matrix with minimal change in the function of the epidermal barrier
Gold and Biron [78]	Acne scars severity improved significantly in a study done by Gold and Biron. Interestingly, patients reported also enhancement of skin texture and reduction of wrinkles and pigmentation
Dai [79]	Dai and al performed a metanalysis to compare fractional RF and fractional lasers in Asian patients with acne scars. They concluded that results were similar with both modalities but adverse events such duration of erythema and PIH was lower with fractional RF
Kaminaka [80]	In a series of 8 subjects, Kaminaka et al. achieved long term improvement of mild atrophic acne scars and mild-moderate acne
Phothong [81]	Phothong et al. performed a split-face, double-blinded, randomized study to explore how the outcomes are related to amount of energy used when treating acne scars with fractional RF. Despite the superiority of high energy settings at 1 month, later evaluation at 3 and 6 months showed comparable results between higher and lower energy levels. Additionally, high energies were associated with more side effects
Kravvas and Al-Naimi [82]	A recent systematic review on acne scarring done by Kravvas and Al-Naimi, concluded that fractional RF manifest good outcomes but slightly inferior to that of fractional lasers. However, fractional RF appeared to have better safety profile in terms of pain, downtime and hyperpigmentation

Table 7.17 Table of fractional RF in axillary hyperhidrosis

Abtahi-Naeini [83]	Microneedle RF to treat 25 patients with severe primary axillary hyperhidrosis in a comparative study and achieved reduced sweating. Finally, there was relapse in 45.9% and no-relapse in 41.6% of cases at 12 months follow-up
Schick [84]	Reported decrease of the hyperhidrosis disease severity scale (HDSS) from 3.4 to 2.1, improved dermatology life quality index from 16 to 7 and 72% reduction of sweating. Side effects were mild and transient
Kim [85]	Pilot study showed clinical improvement using HDSS and histological evidence of reduction in size and number of apocrine and eccrine sweat glands

Table 7.18 Table of fractional RF in cellulite

Alexiades [86]	A multicentre clinical trial evaluated the efficacy of microneedle RF (profound, Syneron, Israel) in the treatment of 50 patients with Muller grade II/III cellulite. The overall improvement was 88% and 86% in both thighs at 3 and 6 months respectively. Patients reported mild discomfort during the procedure and were satisfied with outcomes in 75% of cases. There were no adverse reactions

Table 7.19 Table of studies in striae distensae

Harmelin [87]	Comparative study on the treatment of 384 abdominal stretch marks. The abdomen was divided in 4 quadrants and the following treatments were randomised: RF with IR light, fractional RF, RF with IR followed by fractional RF and no treatment. The striae depth but not the width decreased in the arm treated with combined RF/IR followed by fractional RF

Table 7.20 Risk factors and contraindications

History of keloids	Pregnancy	Allergic reactions	Implanted devices (pacemaker)
Connective tissue disease	Breastfeeding	Bleeding disorders	Immunosuppression
Autoimmune disease	Metal implants	Anticoagulants	Impaired wound healing
Serious renal, cardiac, liver disorders	Breast feeding	Thrombolytics	Active infection

cedure or topical anaesthetics. Some drugs, such as anticoagulants, anti-inflammatories, certain herbal remedies that could increase bleeding is advisable to be stopped few days before and after treatment (Table 7.20).

The pre-procedure preparation generally includes mild cleansing and topical anaesthetic 30–60 min prior to the intervention to alleviate discomfort. It has been reported that concomitant use of vibration devices can ease pain. In some cases additional intradermal anaesthetic and epinephrine is employed. Antiviral prophylaxis could be considered if there is history of Herpes Simplex Virus infection. Patient's characteristics, degree of skin damage and specific treatment area should guide meticulous selection of procedure's specifications.

Example of information and consent form for Intracel- Fractional RF Microneedling used at the senior author's clinic:

- What happens during the procedure?

Prior to the treatment the area to be treated should be cleansed and ready for pre treatment photographs to be taken (if you are having your face treated, please remove your makeup at least 15 min prior to your appointment time). You will need to remove contact lenses if you wear them. Local anaesthetic cream is applied and left on for up to 1 h to numb the area however it will not completely numb the area and some discomfort may be felt.

The INTRAcel treatment twill take approximately 30 minutes (depending on the extend of the area to be treated). You may be advised to stay at the clinic for observation for approximately 30 min after the treatment. Additional time may be required for post treatment photographs so please allow a total time of 2 h at the clinic.

- What will I notice after the procedure?

Immediately following the INTRAcel treatment there will be mild to moderate erythema (redness) and mild puffiness. You may also see tiny little needle marks which can appear as purple dots. The following 1–3 days after treatment erythema (redness), swelling and a hot feeling will be experienced, this is a normal sign that your skin is healing. 3–5 after treatment skin usually becomes dry and flakey for approximately 5 days. You may wish to sleep with your head slightly elevated for the first 24 h following your treatment to help reduce swelling.

- What are the possible risks?

Bacterial infection: Even though the needles are sterilized and are for single use only, bacteria from your skin can cause infection.

Folliculitis: This can be caused due to the temporary sudden increase in sebum in the sebaceous gland. A topical steroid ointment or antibiotics may be prescribed to prevent or reduce this.

Skin scaling: This may occur over the first 2–5 days—often worse around your mouth.

Acne: This can be worsened temporarily because pores can be blocked by the skin reaction to the treatment. This is a normal reaction to after the treatment. Antibiotics may be prescribed to prevent this.

Bruising: In some cases, the treatment may cause bruising which typically dissipates within several days.

Bleeding: The treated area will experience pinpoint bleeding which usually stops as the treatment finishes.

Post-Treatment Care Advice and Plan

The post-procedure care generally involves moisturiser, sunscreen and sun avoidance. In come cases skin cooling with ice masks or cooling devices are applied. Rarely, topical antibiotics are advised.

Complications and Pitfalls and How to Identify and Avoid Them

Traditionally, skin rejuvenation with energy devices has been associated with risk of scarring and dyspigmentation. Fractional laser is considered one of the resurfacing modalities with relatively safe profile but not without complications. These complications are clasified into mild (erythema, purpura, acne, superficial erosions), moderate (infection, dyspigmentation, eruptive keratoacanthomas) and severe (scarring, disseminated infection, ectropion). Radiofrequency has been proposed as a safer technique in all types skin. The electromagnetic radiation generates a thermal effect and hypothetically there is risk of burns, scarring, post-inflammatory hyperpigmentation, dysesthesia, prolonged erythema, oedema, haematomas, skin irregularities or unsatisfactory results.

Although complications potentially vary between different devices, generally mild adverse events, such as pain, erythema and oedema, commonly occur but usually resolve within few hours. Occasionally, last longer up to few weeks. Mild complications do not require any treatment in most cases. It always useful to inform patients regarding side effects prior to the procedure to avoid disappointment. If there is a problem, it should be acknowledged and explained. The possibility to contact the clinic for further support and help should be offered. Bruising may result, this typically resolves within several days. Cold compresses or arnica medication could help to resolve quicker. The electromagnetic radiation generates a thermal effect and there is risk of burns, scarring, post-inflammatory hyperpigmentation, dysesthesia, prolonged erythema, oedema, haematomas, skin irregularities or unsatisfactory results [11]. In case of prolonged oedema non steroidal anti-inflammatory drugs may be useful. Avoidance of strenuous exercise, consumption of alcohol and hot food should be advised to prevent vasodilatation. Hyperpigmentation could persist for few months or even require skin lightening therapies.

What's on the Horizon

Throughout history people have researched "beauty", although standardisation and definition remain elusive. Efforts to improve attractiveness and desire for youthfulness, appear to be motivated by intention to increase self-esteem [88]. Based on data released from the American Society of Plastic Surgeons (ASPS), during the last decade there has been a substantial increase of cosmetic interventions with a trend towards non-surgical techniques. In particular, minimally-invasive cosmetic procedures showed a growth of 186% from 2000 to 2017 [89]. The development of new technologies and techniques is rapidly growing to meet requirements for facia rejuvenation with optimal, quick efficacy and minimal side effects. Procedures using devices for non-surgical "skin tightening" increased by 9% in just 1 year (2016–2017) according to ASPS statistics. Fractional radiofrequency appears promising with encouraging efficacy and safety profile. In the recent years, there has been evolution of technology and development of new devices with a trend to combination techniques. For example the Morpheus 8 (InMode Aesthetic Solutions, Lake Forest, CA) is the modification of Fractora, with 24 coated needles, adjustable settings and penetration depth [90]. Efforts should be directed to deliver appropriate amount of radiofrequency effects to precise anatomic areas. In the era of Evidence Based Medicine, clinicians should apply the best, reliable and valid evidence to decide patients' management. Unfortunately, often the cosmetic practice depends on individual mentorship and training. The principles of EBM should be applied in aesthetic medicine and standardised evaluation systems could aim to overcome limitations regarding efficacy and safety. Recently, Kleidona et al. published a systematic review of the current literature and created a protocol for minimally invasive radiofrequency in skin rejuvenation [91]. Furthermore, there is need for well high quality studies and development of clear guidelines.

Case Studies in Each Indication

Periorbital Rejuvenation A clinical case of the senior author's experience with Thermage application in the upper eyelids and forehead is illustrated in Fig. 7.5. Correspondingly, decrease of laxity score was achieved in the lower eyelids from 7.358 to 2.317, as measured by VISIA skin analysis system (Figs. 7.8 and 7.9).

Body Treatments Laxity of abdominal skin post-partum was treated by NJ Lowe with two sessions of Thermage, large treatment tip, 600 pulses, level 4. The results are illustrated in Fig. 7.10.

Fractional Radiofrequency

Facial rejuvenation: The INTRAcell fractional Radiofrequency device leads to fractional thermal injury and new collagenesis (Fig. 7.11). This system was used for facial rejuvenation. The outcomes were assessed after 5 sessions using VISIA skin analysis, and demonstrated improvement of wrinkles (10.5–6.5), skin texture (2.2–1.2) and pores (1.3–0.7). Each area treated at energy settings4, 5 and 6 with 0.8 mm, 1.5 mm 2 mm depth (Fig. 7.12).

Rejuvenation of the lower face and neck was achieved with microneedle radiofrequency. Examples of three cases are illustrated in Figs. 7.13, 7.14, and 7.15.

Poat-traumatic Scars The same author combined microneedle radiofrequency with botulinum toxin and IPL (Intense Pulsed Light) post-traumatic scars and photodamage in the upper face (Fig. 7.16).

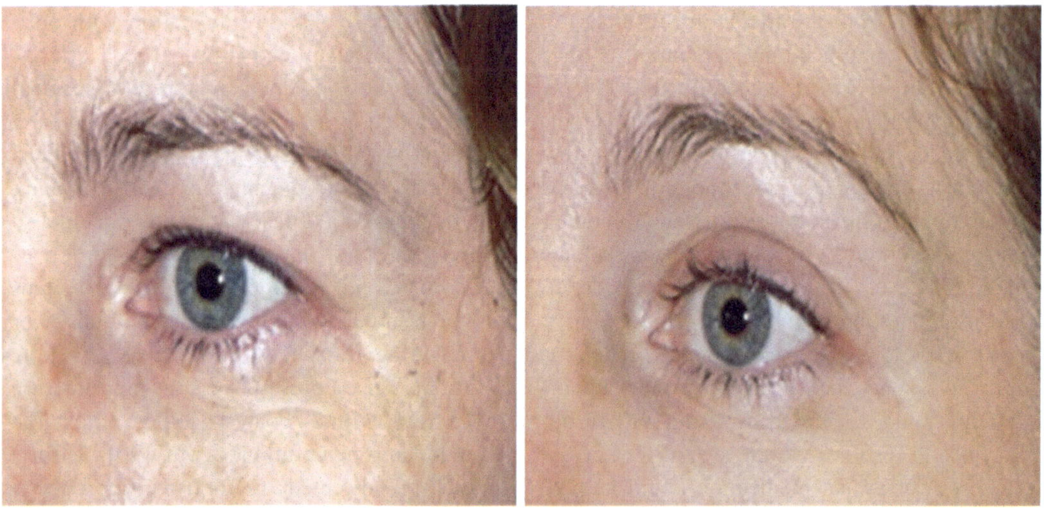

Before Thermage 2 Months Post Treatment

Fig. 7.8 Treatment of upper eyelids and forehead with Thermage, with small eyelid tip treating upper lids and lateral forehead, 400 pulses, Level 3. Left pre-treatment; Right 2 months post-treatment

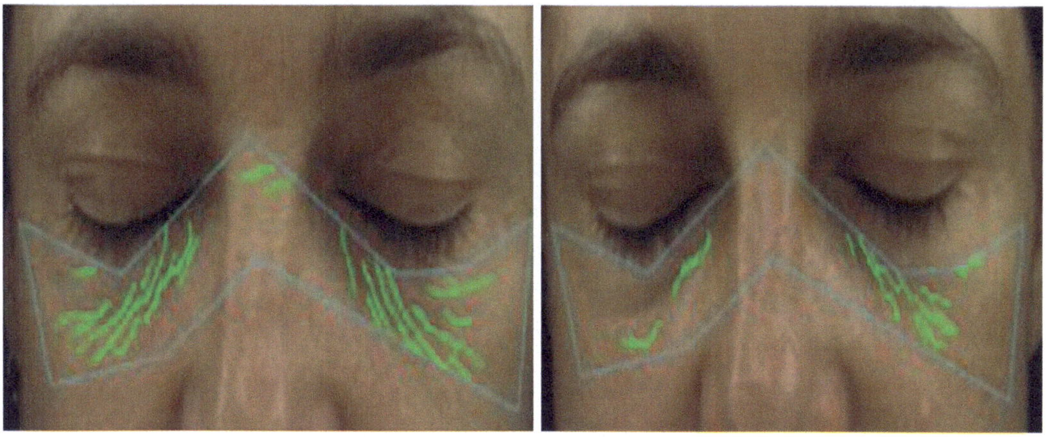

Fig. 7.9 Treatment of lower eyelids with Thermage. Small treatment tip lower lip and upper cheek periorbital area, 200 pulses, level 3. Laxity score measured by VISIA skin analysis system. Left pre-treatment laxity score 7.358; Right post-treatment laxity score 2.317

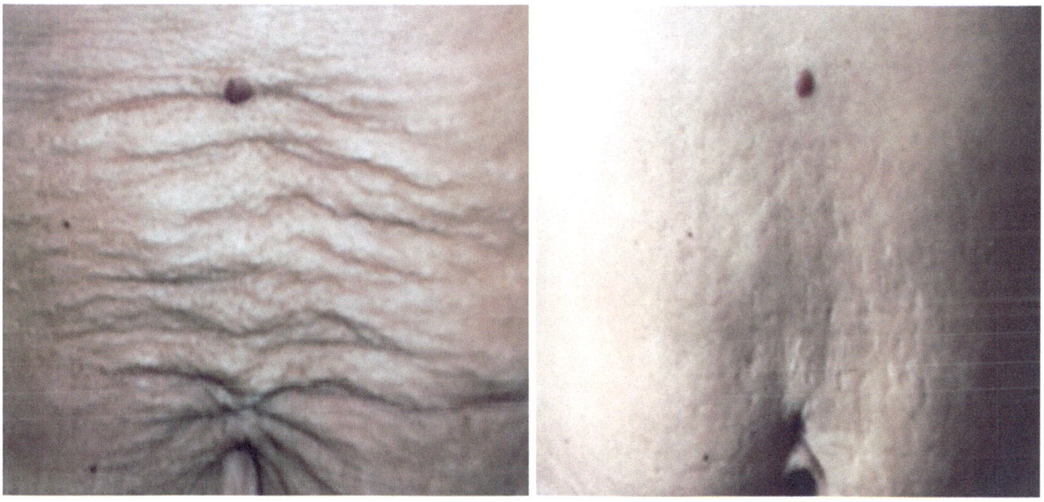

Fig. 7.10 Treatment of abdominal skin laxity using Thermage system, Level 4, 600 pulses, two sessions

Teleangiectatic Haemangioma An example of laser resistant telangiectatic haemangioma successfully treated with microneedle RF is showed in Fig. 7.17.

Acne Scars Improvement of icepick acne scars and overall skin tone was achieved by NJ Lowe following three treatments with insulated microneedle radiofrequency (Fig. 7.18).

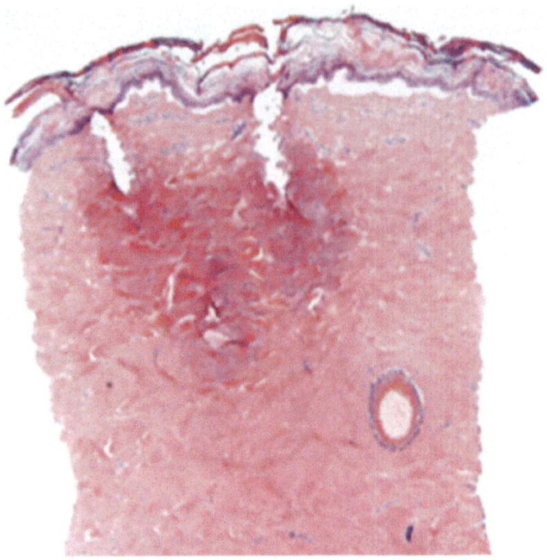

Fig. 7.11 Histology of skin treated with insulated needle radiofrequency. Intracel Fractional RF Microneedling (https://intraceluk.com)

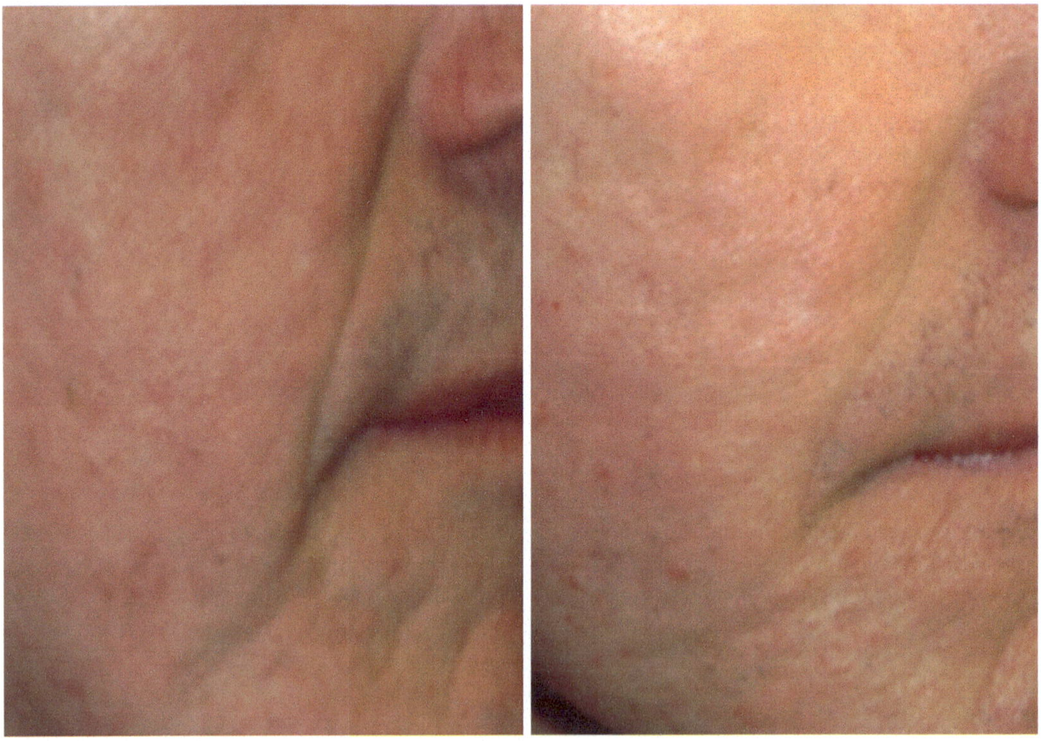

Fig. 7.12 Facial rejuvenation with 5 treatments of microneedle radiofrequency. Power setting 6, Depth 0.8 mm, 1.5 mm and 2 mm. Top: clinical photography; Bottom: VISIA scores

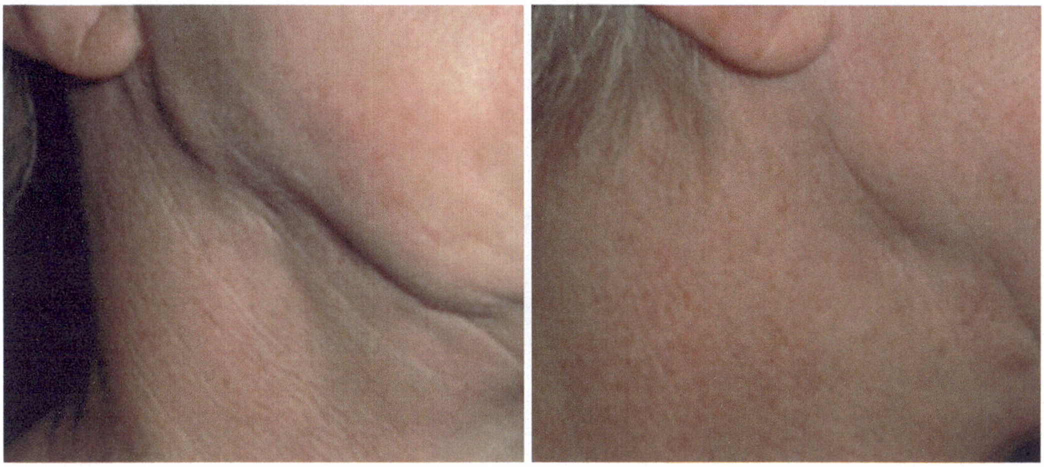

Fig. 7.13 Microneedle radiofrequency treatment of scars and photodamage in the lower face and neck. Power setting 6, Depth 0.5 mm, 1.5 mm and 2 mm. Left pre-treatment; Right post-treatment

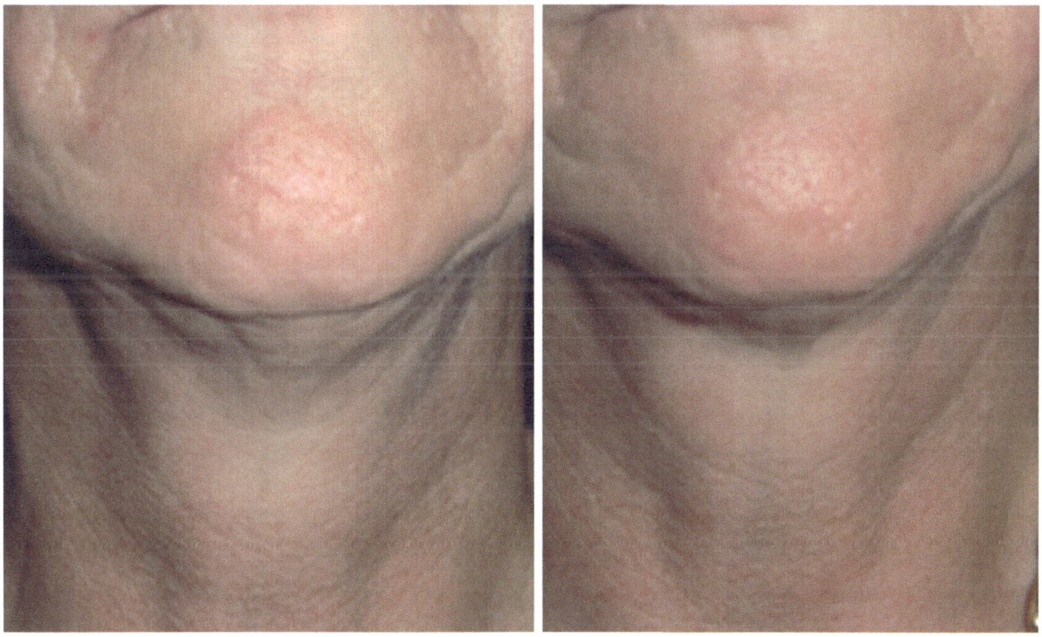

Fig. 7.14 Microneedle radiofrequency treatment of lower face and neck. Power setting 6, Depth 0.5 mm, 1.5 mm and 2 mm. Left before treatment; Right after 4 treatments

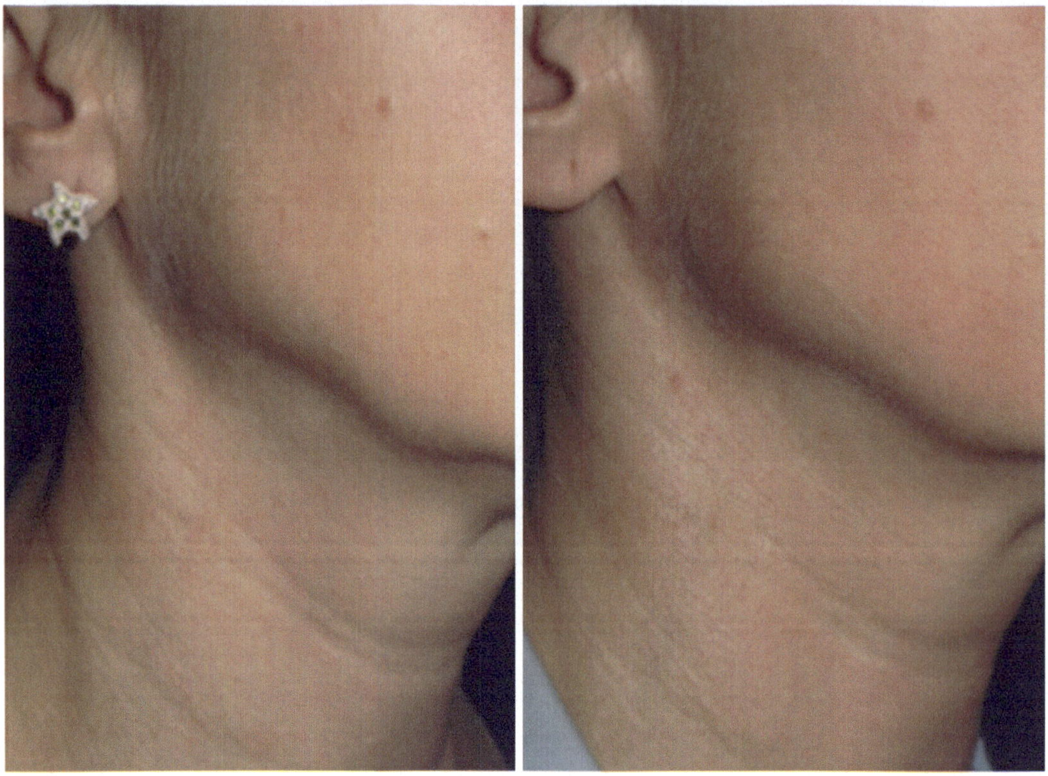

Fig. 7.15 Microneedle radiofrequency treatment for lower face and neck rejuvenation. Power setting 6, Depth 0.5 mm, 1.5 mm and 2 mm. Left before treatment; Right after 4 treatments

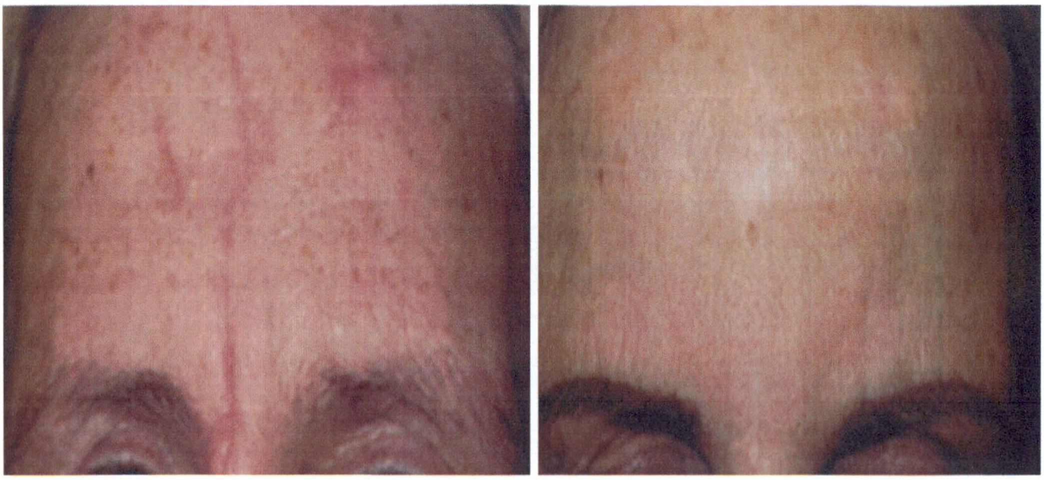

Fig. 7.16 Treatment of post-traumatic scars and photodamage. Left before treatment; Right after treatment with botox, 4 sessions of microneedle RF, level 6, depth 0.8 mm and 1.5 mm, and 4 sessions of IPL

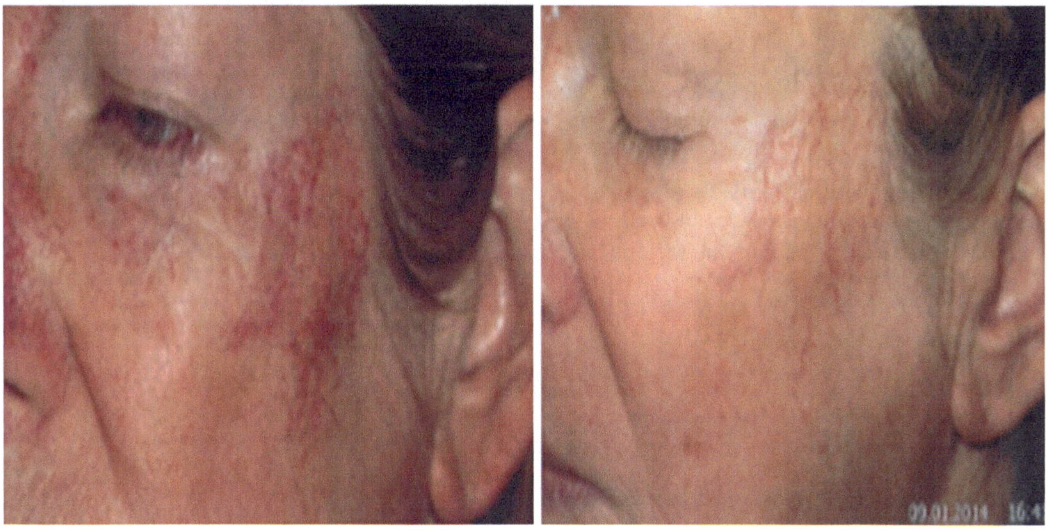

Fig. 7.17 Treatment of laser resistant telangiectatic haemangioma with microneedle RF, Power setting 4, Depth 0.5 mm and 0.8 mm. Left pre-treatment; Right post-treatment

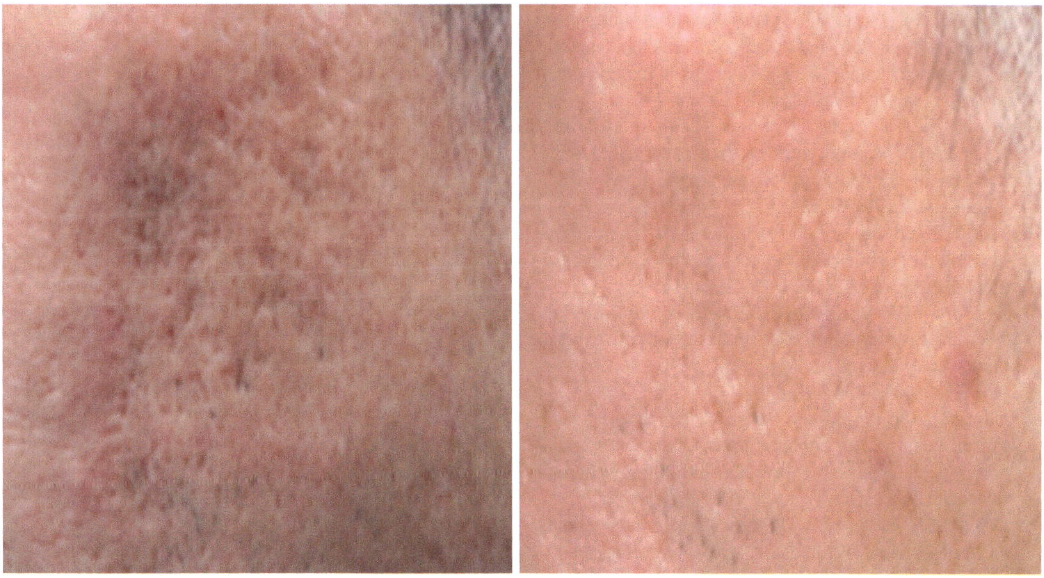

Fig. 7.18 Icepick scars treated with insulated microneedle radiofrequency, Power settings 6, Depth 0.8 mm, 1.5 mm, 2 mm. Left before treatment; Right after 3 treatments

Conclusion

New sophisticated radiofrequency devices have become increasingly popular aiming to meet requirements for optimal efficacy, reduced downtime and minimal side-effects. Studies are encouraging in various aesthetic indications but continued research is paramount to guide new technology development.

References

1. Diffey BL. Sources and measurement of ultraviolet radiation. Methods. 2002;28:4–13.
2. Jauchem JR. Effects of low-level radio-frequency (3kHz to 300GHz) energy on human cardiovascular, reproductive, immune, and other systems: a review of the recent literature. Int J Hyg Environ Health. 2008;211:1–29.
3. Massarweh NN, Cosgriff N, Slakey DP. Electrosurgery: history, principles, and current and future uses. J Am Coll Surg. 2006;202:520–30.
4. Henriques FC, Moritz AR. Studies of thermal injury: I. the conduction of heat to and through skin and the temperatures attained therein. A Theoretical and an Experimental Investigation. Am J Pathol. 1947;23:530–49.
5. Moritz AR, Henriques FC. Studies of thermal injury: II. The relative importance of time and surface temperature in the causation of cutaneous Burns. Am J Pathol. 1947;23:695–720.
6. Moritz AR. Studies of thermal injury: III. The pathology and pathogenesis of cutaneous Burns. An experimental study. Am J Pathol. 1947;23:915–41.
7. Dewhirst MW, Viglianti BL, Lora-Michiels M, et al. Thermal dose requirement for tissue effect: experimental and clinical findings. Proc SPIE--the Int Soc Opt Eng. 2003;4954:37.
8. Dams SD, de Liefde-van Beest M, Nuijs AM, et al. Pulsed heat shocks enhance procollagen type I and procollagen type III expression in human dermal fibroblasts. Skin Res Technol. 2010;16:354–64.
9. Mayes AE, Holyoak CD. Repeat mild heat shock increases dermal fibroblast activity and collagen production. Rejuvenation Res. 2008;11:461–5.
10. Arnoczky SP, Aksan A. Thermal modification of connective tissues: basic science considerations and clinical implications. J Am Acad Orthop Surg. 2000;8:305–13.
11. Lee SJ, Kim J-I, Yang YJ, et al. Treatment of periorbital wrinkles with a novel fractional radiofrequency microneedle system in dark-skinned patients. Dermatol Surg [Internet]. 2015;41:615–622. Available from: http://ovidsp.ovid.com/ovidweb.cgi?T=JS&PAGE=reference&D=med8&NEWS=N&AN=25899885.
12. Alvarez N, Ortiz L, Vicente V, et al. The effects of radiofrequency on skin: experimental study. Lasers Surg Med. 2008;40:76–82.
13. Ruiz-Esparza J, Gomez JB. The medical face lift: a noninvasive, nonsurgical approach to tissue tightening in facial skin using nonablative radiofrequency. Dermatol Surg 2003;29:325–332; discussion 332.
14. Kennedy J, Verne S, Griffith R, et al. Non-invasive subcutaneous fat reduction: a review. J Eur Acad Dermatol Venereol. 2015;29:1679–88.
15. Alster TS, Lupton JR. Nonablative cutaneous remodeling using radiofrequency devices. Clin Dermatol. 2007;25:487–91.
16. Lolis MS, Goldberg DJ. Radiofrequency in cosmetic dermatology: a review. Dermatol Surg. 2012;38:1765–76.
17. Weiss RA. Noninvasive radio frequency for skin tightening and body contouring. Semin Cutan Med Surg. 2013;32:9–17. Available from: http://ovidsp.ovid.com/ovidweb.cgi?T=JS&PAGE=reference&D=med7&NEWS=N&AN=24049924
18. Sadick NS, Nassar AH, Dorizas AS, et al. Bipolar and multipolar radiofrequency. Dermatol Surg. 2014;40(Suppl 1):S174–9.
19. Manstein D, Herron GS, Sink RK, et al. Fractional photothermolysis: a new concept for cutaneous remodeling using microscopic patterns of thermal injury. Lasers Surg Med. 2004;34:426–38.
20. 20171121_INFINI1.2_quickguide_rev3.0.pdf - Google Drive [Internet]. [cited 2018 Jul 25]. Available from: https://drive.google.com/file/d/1DXiwsdI6lM9Rx4m9AWAwLwFntt_ecuis/view.
21. Hantash BM, Renton B, Berkowitz RL, et al. Pilot clinical study of a novel minimally invasive bipolar microneedle radiofrequency device. Lasers Surg Med. 2009;41:87–95.
22. Alexiades-Armenakas M, Newman J, Willey A, et al. Prospective multicenter clinical trial of a minimally invasive temperature-controlled bipolar fractional radiofrequency system for rhytid and laxity treatment. Dermatol Surg. 2013;39:263–73. Available from: http://cochranelibrary-wiley.com/o/cochrane/clcentral/articles/068/CN-00912068/frame.html
23. Ramaut L, Hoeksema H, Pirayesh A, et al. Microneedling: where do we stand now? A systematic review of the literature. J Plast Reconstr Aesthet Surg [Internet]. 2018;71:1–14. Available from: http://ovidsp.ovid.com/ovidweb.cgi?T=JS&PAGE=reference&D=prem&NEWS=N&AN=28690124.
24. Brightman L, Goldman MP, Taub AF. Sublative rejuvenation: experience with a new fractional radiofrequency system for skin rejuvenation and repair. J. Drugs Dermatol [Internet]. 2009;8:s9–13. Available from: http://ovidsp.ovid.com/ovidweb.cgi?T=JS&PAGE=reference&D=med6&NEWS=N&AN=19916261.
25. Gold MH. Update on tissue tightening. J Clin Aesthet Dermatol. 2010;3:36–41.

26. Lolis MS, Goldberg DJ. Assessment of safety and efficacy of a bipolar fractionated radiofrequency device in the treatment of periorbital rhytides. J Cosmet Laser Ther [Internet]. 2014;16:161–164. Available from: http://ovidsp.ovid.com/ovidweb.cgi?T=JS&PAGE=reference&D=med8&NEWS=N&AN=25003480.
27. Fitzpatrick R, Geronemus R, Goldberg D, et al. Multicenter study of noninvasive radiofrequency for periorbital tissue tightening. Lasers Surg Med. 2003;33:232–42.
28. Nahm WK, Su TT, Rotunda AM, et al. Objective changes in brow position, superior palpebral crease, peak angle of the eyebrow, and jowl surface area after volumetric radiofrequency treatments to half of the face. Dermatol Surg 2004;30:922–928; discussion 928.
29. Han SH, Yoon YM, Lee YW, et al. Usefulness of monopolar thermal radiofrequency treatment for periorbital wrinkles. Ann Dermatol. 2018;30: 296–303.
30. Bassichis BA, Dayan S, Thomas JR. Use of a nonablative radiofrequency device to rejuvenate the upper one-third of the face. Otolaryngol Head Neck Surg. 2004;130:397–406.
31. Jacobson LGS, Alexiades-Armenakas M, Bernstein L, et al. Treatment of nasolabial folds and jowls with a noninvasive radiofrequency device. Arch. Dermatol. 2003:1371–2.
32. Alster TS, Tanzi E. Improvement of neck and cheek laxity with a nonablative radiofrequency device: a lifting experience. Dermatol Surg 2004;30:503–507; discussion 507.
33. Alhaddad M, Wu DC, Bolton J, et al. A randomized, Split-face, evaluator-blind clinical trial comparing monopolar radiofrequency versus microfocused ultrasound with visualization for lifting and tightening of the face and upper neck. Dermatol Surg. 2019;45:131–9.
34. Chipps LK, Bentow J, Prather HB, et al. Novel nonablative radio-frequency rejuvenation device applied to the neck and jowls: clinical evaluation and 3-dimensional image analysis. J Drugs Dermatol. 2013;12:1215–8.
35. Weiss RA, Weiss MA, Munavalli G, et al. Monopolar radiofrequency facial tightening: a retrospective analysis of efficacy and safety in over 600 treatments. J Drugs Dermatol. 2006;5:707–12.
36. de Felipe I, Del Cueto SR, Perez E, et al. Adverse reactions after nonablative radiofrequency: follow-up of 290 patients. J Cosmet Dermatol. 2007;6: 163–6.
37. Vega JM, Bucay VW, Mayoral FA. Prospective, multicenter study to determine the safety and efficacy of a unique radiofrequency device for moderate to severe hand wrinkles. J Drugs Dermatol. 2013;12:24–6.
38. Zelickson BD, Kist D, Bernstein E, et al. Histological and ultrastructural evaluation of the effects of a radiofrequency-based nonablative dermal remodeling device: a pilot study. Arch Dermatol. 2004;140: 204–9.
39. Anolik R, Chapas AM, Brightman LA, et al. Radiofrequency devices for body shaping: a review and study of 12 patients. Semin Cutan Med Surg. 2009;28:236–43.
40. Ruiz-Esparza J, Gomez JB. Nonablative radiofrequency for active acne vulgaris: the use of deep dermal heat in the treatment of moderate to severe active acne vulgaris (thermotherapy): a report of 22 patients. Dermatol Surg 2003;29:333–339; discussion 339.
41. Emilia del Pino M, Rosado RH, Azuela A, et al. Effect of controlled volumetric tissue heating with radiofrequency on cellulite and the subcutaneous tissue of the buttocks and thighs. J Drugs Dermatol. 2006;(5):714–22.
42. Goldberg DJ, Fazeli A, Berlin AL. Clinical, laboratory, and MRI analysis of cellulite treatment with a unipolar radiofrequency device. Dermatol Surg 2008;34:204–209; discussion 209.
43. Alexiades-Armenakas M, Dover JS, Arndt KA. Unipolar radiofrequency treatment to improve the appearance of cellulite. J Cosmet Laser Ther. 2008;10:148–53.
44. Alexiades-Armenakas M, Dover JS, Arndt KA. Unipolar versus bipolar radiofrequency treatment of rhytides and laxity using a mobile painless delivery method. Lasers Surg Med. 2008;40:446–53.
45. Sadick NS, Alexiades-Armenakas M, Bitter PJ, et al. Enhanced full-face skin rejuvenation using synchronous intense pulsed optical and conducted bipolar radiofrequency energy (ELOS): introducing selective radiophotothermolysis. J Drugs Dermatol. 2005;4:181–6.
46. Yu CS, Yeung CK, Shek SY, et al. Combined infrared light and bipolar radiofrequency for skin tightening in Asians. Lasers Surg Med. 2007;39:471–5.
47. Choi YJ, Lee JY, Ahn JY, et al. The safety and efficacy of a combined diode laser and bipolar radiofrequency compared with combined infrared light and bipolar radiofrequency for skin rejuvenation. Indian J Dermatol Venereol Leprol. 2012;78: 146–52.
48. Gold AH, Pozner J, Weiss R, et al. A fractional bipolar radiofrequency device combined with a bipolar radiofrequency and infrared light treatment for improvement in facial wrinkles and overall skin tone and texture. Aesthetic Surg J [Internet]. 2016;36:1058–1067. Available from: http://cochranelibrary-wiley.com/o/cochrane/clcentral/articles/619/CN-01246619/frame.html.
49. Verner I, Kutscher TD. Clinical evaluation of the efficacy and safety of combined bipolar radiofrequency and optical energies vs optical energy alone for the treatment of aging hands. Lasers Med Sci. 2017;32:1387–92.
50. El-Domyati M, El-Ammawi TS, Medhat W, et al. Electro-optical synergy technique: A new and effective nonablative approach to skin aging. J Clin Aesthet Dermatol. 2010;3:22–30.
51. Gold MH, Goldman MP, Rao J, et al. Treatment of wrinkles and elastosis using vacuum-assisted bipolar

radiofrequency heating of the dermis. Dermatol Surg. 2007;33:300–9.
52. Prieto VG, Zhang PS, Sadick NS. Evaluation of pulsed light and radiofrequency combined for the treatment of acne vulgaris with histologic analysis of facial skin biopsies. J Cosmet Laser Ther. 2005;7:63–8.
53. Cameli N, Mariano M, Serio M, et al. Preliminary comparison of fractional laser with fractional laser plus radiofrequency for the treatment of acne scars and photoaging. Dermatol Surg [Internet]. 2014;40:553–561. Available from: http://cochranelibrary-wiley.com/o/cochrane/clcentral/articles/384/CN-01117384/frame.html.
54. Min S, Park SY, Moon J, et al. Comparison between Er:YAG laser and bipolar radiofrequency combined with infrared diode laser for the treatment of acne scars: differential expression of fibrogenetic biomolecules may be associated with differences in efficacy between ablative and non-abl. Lasers Surg Med. 2017;49:341–7.
55. van der Lugt C, Romero C, Ancona D, et al. A multicenter study of cellulite treatment with a variable emission radio frequency system. Dermatol Ther. 2009;22:74–84.
56. Nootheti PK, Magpantay A, Yosowitz G, et al. A single center, randomized, comparative, prospective clinical study to determine the efficacy of the VelaSmooth system versus the Triactive system for the treatment of cellulite. Lasers Surg Med. 2006;38:908–12.
57. Sadick NS, Mulholland RS. A prospective clinical study to evaluate the efficacy and safety of cellulite treatment using the combination of optical and RF energies for subcutaneous tissue heating. J Cosmet Laser Ther. 2004;6:187–90.
58. Romero C, Caballero N, Herrero M, et al. Effects of cellulite treatment with RF, IR light, mechanical massage and suction treating one buttock with the contralateral as a control. J Cosmet Laser Ther. 2008;10:193–201.
59. Hexsel DM, Siega C, Schilling-Souza J, et al. A bipolar radiofrequency, infrared, vacuum and mechanical massage device for treatment of cellulite: a pilot study. J Cosmet Laser Ther. 2011;13:297–302.
60. Sadick NS, Shaoul J. Hair removal using a combination of conducted radiofrequency and optical energies--an 18-month follow-up. J Cosmet Laser Ther. 2004;6:21–6.
61. Sadick NS, Laughlin SA. Effective epilation of white and blond hair using combined radiofrequency and optical energy. J Cosmet Laser Ther. 2004;6:27–31.
62. Goldberg DJ, Marmur ES, Hussain M. Treatment of terminal and vellus non-pigmented hairs with an optical/bipolar radiofrequency energy source-with and without pre-treatment using topical aminolevulinic acid. J Cosmet Laser Ther. 2005;7:25–8.
63. Jeon IK, Chang SE, Park G-H, et al. Comparison of microneedle fractional radiofrequency therapy with intradermal botulinum toxin a injection for periorbital rejuvenation. Dermatology [Internet]. 2013;227:367–372. Available from: http://cochranelibrary-wiley.com/o/cochrane/clcentral/articles/238/CN-01070238/frame.html.
64. Kim JK, Roh MR, Park G, et al. Fractionated microneedle radiofrequency for the treatment of periorbital wrinkles. J Dermatol [Internet]. 2013;40:172–176. Available from: http://ovidsp.ovid.com/ovidweb.cgi?T=JS&PAGE=reference&D=med7&NEWS=N&AN=23252484.
65. Shin J-W, Park J-T, Chae J-B, et al. The efficacy of micro-insulated needle radiofrequency system for the treatment of lower eyelid fat bulging. J Dtsch Dermatol Ges. 2019;17:149–56.
66. Roh NK, Yoon YM, Lee YW, et al. Treatment of periorbital wrinkles using multipolar fractional radiofrequency in Korean patients. Lasers Med Sci [Internet]. 2017;32:61–66. Available from: http://ovidsp.ovid.com/ovidweb.cgi?T=JS&PAGE=reference&D=med8&NEWS=N&AN=27686890.
67. Calderhead RG, Goo BL, Lauro F, et al. The clinical efficacy and safety of microneedling fractional radiofrequency in the treatment of facial wrinkles: a multicenter study with The Infini System in 499 patients. 2013 [cited 2018 Jun 8]; Available from: https://int.aesthetic.lutronic.com/assets/PDFs/INFINI-WP-multicenter-Dr.Glen-2013.pdf.
68. Alexiades-Armenakas M, Rosenberg D, Renton B, et al. Blinded, randomized, quantitative grading comparison of minimally invasive, fractional radiofrequency and surgical face-lift to treat skin laxity. Arch Dermatol. 2010;146:396–405. Available from: http://cochranelibrary-wiley.com/o/cochrane/clcentral/articles/672/CN-00743672/frame.html
69. Lu W, Wu P, Zhang Z, et al. Curative effects of microneedle fractional radiofrequency system on skin laxity in Asian patients: a prospective, double-blind, randomized, controlled face-split study. J Cosmet Laser Ther. 2017;19:83–8.
70. Seo KY, Yoon MS, Kim DH, et al. Skin rejuvenation by microneedle fractional radiofrequency treatment in Asian skin; clinical and histological analysis. Lasers Surg Med [Internet]. 2012;44:631–636. Available from: http://ovidsp.ovid.com/ovidweb.cgi?T=JS&PAGE=reference&D=med7&NEWS=N&AN=22936274.
71. Park HJ, Kim HM, Oh MJ. Clinical study of facial wrinkle treatment with fractional microneedle radio frequency system. Med Lasers [Internet]. 2014 [cited 2018 Jun 8];3:59–64. https://doi.org/10.25289/ML.2014.3.2.59. Available from: http://www.jkslms.or.kr/journal/view.html?.
72. Gold M, Taylor M, Rothaus K, et al. Non-insulated smooth motion, micro-needles RF fractional treatment for wrinkle reduction and lifting of the lower face: International study. Lasers Surg Med [Internet]. 2016;48:727–733. Available from: http://ovidsp.ovid.com/ovidweb.cgi?T=JS&PAGE=reference&D=medl&NEWS=N&AN=27490716.
73. Hruza G, Taub AF, Collier SL, et al. Skin rejuvenation and wrinkle reduction using a fractional radiofrequency system. J Drugs Dermatol [Internet].

2009;8:259–265. Available from: http://ovidsp.ovid.com/ovidweb.cgi?T=JS&PAGE=reference&D=med6&NEWS=N&AN=19271373.
74. Akita H, Sasaki R, Yokoyama Y, et al. The clinical experience and efficacy of bipolar radiofrequency with fractional photothermolysis for aged Asian skin. Exp Dermatol [Internet]. 2014;23 Suppl 1:37–42. Available from: http://ovidsp.ovid.com/ovidweb.cgi?T=JS&PAGE=reference&D=med8&NEWS=N&AN=25234835.
75. Jiang Y, Zhang X, Lu Z, et al. Assessment of efficacy and safety of a fractionated bipolar radiofrequency device for the treatment of lower face wrinkles and laxity. J Cosmet Laser Ther. 2018:1–6.
76. Lyons A, Roy J, Herrmann J, et al. Treatment of Decolletage Photoaging with fractional microneedling radiofrequency. J Drugs Dermatol. 2018;17:74–6. Available from: http://ovidsp.ovid.com/ovidweb.cgi?T=JS&PAGE=reference&D=prem&NEWS=N&AN=29320590
77. Cho SI, Chung BY, Choi MG, et al. Evaluation of the clinical efficacy of fractional radiofrequency microneedle treatment in acne scars and large facial pores. Dermatol Surg. 2012;38:1017–24.
78. Gold MH, Biron JA. Treatment of acne scars by fractional bipolar radiofrequency energy. J Cosmet Laser Ther [Internet]. 2012;14:172–178. Available from: http://ovidsp.ovid.com/ovidweb.cgi?T=JS&PAGE=reference&D=med7&NEWS=N&AN=22548644.
79. Dai R, Xie H, Hua W, et al. The efficacy and safety of the fractional radiofrequency technique for the treatment of atrophic acne scar in Asians: A meta-analysis. J Cosmet Laser Ther. 2017;19:337–44.
80. Kaminaka C, Uede M, Matsunaka H, et al. Clinical studies of the treatment of facial atrophic acne scars and acne with a bipolar fractional radiofrequency system. J Dermatol. 2015;42:580–7.
81. Phothong W, Wanitphakdeedecha R, Sathaworawong A, et al. High versus moderate energy use of bipolar fractional radiofrequency in the treatment of acne scars: a split-face double-blinded randomized control trial pilot study. Lasers Med Sci. 2016;31:229–34. Available from: http://cochranelibrary-wiley.com/o/cochrane/clcentral/articles/263/CN-01139263/frame.html
82. Kravvas G, Al-Niaimi F. A systematic review of treatments for acne scarring. Part 2: Energy-based techniques. Scars, Burn Heal. 2018;4:2059513118793420.
83. Abtahi-Naeini B, FF N, Saffaei A, et al. Treatment of primary axillary hyperhidrosis by fractional microneedle radiofrequency: is it still effective after long-term follow-up? Indian J Dermatol 2016;61:234. Available from: http://cochranelibrary-wiley.com/o/cochrane/clcentral/articles/763/CN-01141763/frame.html.
84. Schick CH, Grallath T, Schick KS, et al. Radiofrequency thermotherapy for treating axillary hyperhidrosis. Dermatol Surg. 2016;42:624–30.
85. Kim M, Shin JY, Lee J, et al. Efficacy of fractional microneedle radiofrequency device in the treatment of primary axillary hyperhidrosis: a pilot study. Dermatology [Internet]. 2013;227:243–249. Available from: http://ovidsp.ovid.com/ovidweb.cgi?T=JS&PAGE=reference&D=med7&NEWS=N&AN=24107595.
86. Alexiades M, Munavalli G, Goldberg D, et al. Prospective multicenter clinical trial of a temperature-controlled subcutaneous microneedle fractional bipolar radiofrequency system for the treatment of cellulite. Dermatol Surg. 2018;44:1262–71.
87. Harmelin Y, Boineau D, Cardot-Leccia N, et al. Fractionated bipolar radiofrequency and bipolar radiofrequency potentiated by infrared light for treating striae: A prospective randomized, comparative trial with objective evaluation. Lasers Surg Med. 2016;48:245–53.
88. Di Stefano N. The idea of beauty and its biases: critical notes on the aesthetics of Plastic surgery. Plast Reconstr surgery Glob Open. 2017;5:e1523.
89. www.PlasticSurgery.org. PLASTIC SURGERY STATISTICS REPORT 2017 Plastic Surgery Statistics Report. [cited 2018 Jul 15]; Available from: www.plasticsurgery.org.
90. Dayan E, Chia C, Burns AJ, et al. Adjustable depth fractional radiofrequency combined with bipolar radiofrequency: A minimally invasive combination treatment for skin laxity. Aesthetic Surg J. 2019;39:S112–9.
91. Kleidona IA, Karypidis D, Lowe N, et al. Fractional radiofrequency in the treatment of skin aging: an evidence-based treatment protocol. J Cosmet Laser Ther [Internet]. 2019. https://doi.org/10.1080/14764172.2019.1674448, 9, 25, 22.

Light Emitting Diodes and Low Level Laser Light Therapy

8

Caiwei Zheng, Ali Rajabi-Estarabadi,
Melanie M. Hirsch, and Keyvan Nouri

Mechanism of Action

Low Level Laser Therapy

The terms low level laser therapy (LLLT), phototherapy, and photobiomodulation are sometimes used interchangeably to refer to the use of photons at non-thermal irradiance to alter the biological activity of cells [1]. LLLT typically uses light with wavelengths between 390 nm to 1100 nm (Fig. 8.1a.). It is referred to as "low level" because it uses light at lower power densities (<100 mW/cm^2) and fluences (0.04–50 J/cm^2), unlike that of lasers use for ablation, cutting, or thermal coagulation of tissue [1, 2]. LLLT can use a coherent light source (e.g. lasers), a non-coherent light source (e.g. filtered lamps or light-emitting diodes-LEDs), or a combination of both [1]. Photobiomodulation by LLLT has wide-ranging effects and the specific mechanisms of action are not yet well understood. Generally, photobiomodulation at lower power are associated with stimulation and higher doses are associated with inhibition of cell metabolism.

Lasers with red and near-infrared light emission have wavelengths that correspond to the absorption spectra of key mitochondrial chromophores, particularly the cytochrome c oxidase of the respiratory chain [3]. Absorbed light energy can excite electrons in the chromophore to jump from a low-energy orbit to a higher-energy orbit, which then leads to a cascade of downstream effects at the molecular, cellular, and tissue levels [1, 2]. This downstream effect is hypothesized to be achieved through photodissociation of inhibitory nitric oxide from cytochrome c oxidase, leading to enhancement of enzyme activity in electron transport, mitochondrial respiration and ATP production [1, 4]. LLLT also alters the cellular redox state which induces the activation of numerous intracellular signaling pathways through activation of transcription factors such as: Nuclear factor kappa B (NFkB), Hypoxia inducible factor (HIF-1α), and ERK/FOXM1 (Fig. 8.1b.) [2, 4].

LEDs

Laser emitting diode phototherapy is a more recently introduced modality falling under the broader category of LLLT. In LED technology, high efficiency semiconductor chips are situated on a reflective surface to produce non-coherent, non-collimated light when electricity passes through [5, 6]. Electrons recombine with

C. Zheng · A. Rajabi-Estarabadi (✉) · M. M. Hirsch
K. Nouri
Department of Dermatology and Cutaneous Surgery, University of Miami Miller School of Medicine, Miami, USA
e-mail: c.zheng@med.miami.edu; arajabi@med.miami.edu; melaniehirsch@ufl.edu; knouri@med.miami.edu

V. Madan (ed.), *Practical Introduction to Laser Dermatology*,
https://doi.org/10.1007/978-3-030-46451-6_8

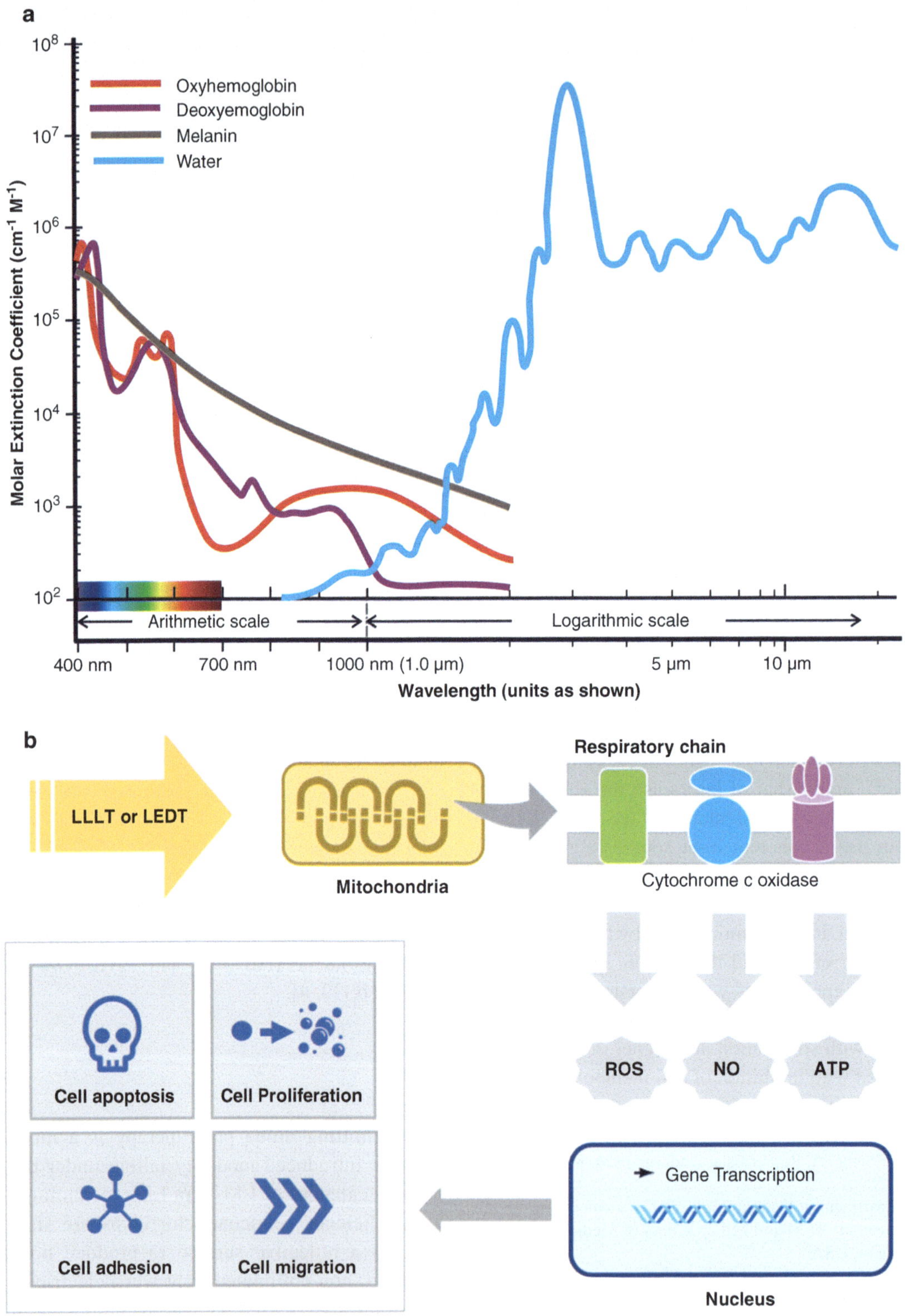

Fig. 8.1 (**a**) Absorption spectra for the biological chromophores of blood (oxyhemoglobin and deoxyhemoglobin) [26] (**b**) Mechanism of action of Low level laser (LLLT) and light emitting diode (LLED) therapies. *LLLT* Low level laser therapy, *LLED* light emitting diode therapy, *ROS* reactive oxygen species, *NO* Nitric oxide, *ATP* Adenosine triphosphate

electron holes within the device to release energy in the form of photons [1]. Depending on the energy gap of the semiconductors, different wavelengths of light are produced in the range of approximately 255–1300 nm, corresponding to the ultra violet, visible, and near-infrared ranges of the electromagnetic spectrum [5, 6]. LED emitted light also affect cellular metabolism by acting on the mitochondria to stimulate intracellular photochemical reactions [5, 6]. Properties of the light emitted and pattern of delivery dictates the effect on cells. Commercially available LEDs can be set to deliver continuously or in photomodulated fashion, with specific sequences of pulse and durations [6]. Wavelengths can also be set to produce light in the red, yellow, blue and near-infrared spectrum [6].

Light emitting diode red light (LED-RL) stimulates the copper/heme iron centers of cytochrome C oxidase in the electron transport chain, which increases reactive oxygen species (ROS) and ATP production [7]. Alterations in ROS levels have effects on the release of TGF-beta 1 and TGF-beta 3, which further acts on the pro-fibrotic cascade, decreasing fibroblast proliferation and collagen biosynthesis [7]. ROS levels also act on redox-sensitive transcription factors (ie. AP-1, NF-kB, p53 etc.) which have downstream effects on transcription, cellular proliferation and migration speed, as well as the production of extracellular matrix [7].

Photomodulated light emitting diode yellow light (LED-YL) has been found to upregulate the collagen type 1(COL-I) gene leading to increases in collagen production and ATP production through increase of cytochromes [8]. Yellow light is also known to reduce MMP-1 level, an important target in skin rejuvenation [8].

The mechanism of light emitting diode blue light is not yet well defined, but it is hypothesized to exert its effect either by directly generating ROS or by photostimulating the flavin group on complex I of the mitochondrial electron transport chain [9]. Downstream, blue light results in alterations in fibroblast proliferation and antioxidant capacity, TGF-beta signaling and myofibroblast differentiation. Blue light is also known for its effects on cytokine levels and inflammatory mediators (Fig. 8.1) [9].

Near-infrared light, also known as monochromatic infrared energy (MIRE), is currently known to induce the release of guanylate cyclase and nitrous oxide, which stimulates circulation. This in turn promotes vasodilation and growth factor production which ultimately encourages angiogenesis, a helpful factor in wound healing [6].

Indications in Dermatology

LLLT has been actively studied for use across a multitude of conditions in dermatology for decades, but still faces skepticism due to the remaining uncertainties in its mechanism of action and limited standardization of dosimetry parameters [1]. Currently, LLLT is known for its application in a number of conditions including wound healing, hair growth, skin rejuvenation, acne, psoriasis, vitiligo, hypertrophic scars, and photoprotection, giving it great potential to grow as a versatile modality in dermatology in the near future.

LLLT for Wound Healing

Wound healing is one of LLLT's earliest applications. Currently, LLLT has been recognized to promote tissue repair via release of substances such as histamine, serotonin, and bradykinin, which stimulate the production of ATP and inhibit the production of prostaglandins that induce inflammation and pain [10]. These effects are further enhanced by the bioelectric effects of laser light leading to improved functioning of the sodium–potassium pump (Na^+/K^+-ATPase), and thus improved maintenance of cell membrane potential [10]. Resulting ATPs can then be used to normalize cellular and tissue functions, thus promoting more consistent tissue repair [11, 12]. Clinically, these changes yield promising effects on healing skin, including: acceleration of tissue repair, increased formation of granulation tissue, wound contraction, inflammation modulation, and pain reduction [11, 12].

Trelles et al. assessed LED phototherapy's effect on wound healing in a study of female patients undergoing laser ablative resurfacing. Twenty-eight female patients underwent ablative Er:YAG/CO_2 laser resurfacing were treated with LLLT immediately after the resurfacing and then again after 72 h—on both occasions with infrared 830 nm light (55 J/cm^2) for 20 min, followed by red 633 nm light (98 J/cm^2) for 20 min [13]. All patients were treated only on one side of the face (the other side was covered with an opaque mask), and the untreated side was and assessed as the control. Three additional treatments were administered within the next three weeks after the resurfacing procedure: two of which were performed 3 days apart in the first week, and the last during the third week [13]. The study reported that the LED-treated facial halves showed 50% faster resolution of exudation, crusting, pain, and edema [13]. Also, although there was no significant difference in wrinkle appearance, the treated skin looked younger when assessed after 6 months [13]. Several subsequent studies have also reported consistent results.

Chaves et al. tested the use of LED-nIR phototherapy on the healing of nipple trauma in breastfeeding women. In this randomized, placebo-controlled pilot study (N = 16), the experimental group (N = 8) was given a training session on nipple care and adequate breastfeeding techniques in addition to active LED phototherapy [14]. For comparison, the control group (N = 8) was given the same training session but with placebo phototherapy. The active LED phototherapy had the following parameters: wavelength of 860 nm, frequency of 100 Hz, average power of 50 mW, power density of 50 mW/cm^2, total emission area of 1 cm^2, pulsed emission mode with 50% duty cycle, and dose of 4 J/cm^2 [14]. Treatment application time was 79 s. The phototherapy was delivered twice a week for a period of 4 weeks, resulting in 8 total sessions. Lesion area was then assessed via digital photography and the images were analyzed by the software Quantikov, which calculated lesion area based on the user's definition of the lesion boundaries [14]. The study reported that the experimental group showed significantly faster healing than the control group, with complete healing of the lesion achieved by the fourth session compared to the eighth session for the control group. The experimental group also showed a statistically significant reduction of pain vs. control, as measured by an 11-point pain intensity numerical rating scale (PI-NRS).

LED's effect on healing of burns was also recently investigated in a double blinded study. A series of cases of second and third degree burns in 5 patients were treated with low intensity LED therapy in the red light spectrum of 658 nm at 7 J/cm^2, power 40 mW, power density 0.31 W/cm^2 [15]. Treated areas were evaluated both clinically and via histopathologic analysis before and after treatment. Histopathologic results revealed that irradiated areas presented greater epithelialization, with greater keratinocytes and fibroblasts proliferation as well as increasing collagen synthesis (Fig. 8.2) [15].

LLLT's effect on chronic wounds, such as venous ulcers have also been investigated. Of the studies available, a study treated a total of 68 patients with chronic (more than 4 weeks) Meggitt-Wagner Grade I foot ulcers from Type 2 DM. Participants were randomized into two groups of 34 [16]. The treatment group was treated with LLLT of 660 and 850 nm at 2–4 J/cm^2 (depending on ulcer size) daily for 15 days, while the control was treated with conventional therapy. The study reported significant reduction of ulcer area after the 15-day treatment regimen [16]. It is worth noting that this study, along with others presenting similar positive results, were limited in its small sample size and the lack of screening to exclude rapid healers [11]. Thus, larger clinical trials with appropriate screening are needed to further investigate efficacy. So far, no significant adverse events had been reported for any of the LLLT treatments of wounds.

LLLT for Hair Growth

LLLT's use to stimulate hair regrowth is more robustly supported, particularly in the treatment of androgenic alopecia (AGA) and alopecia areata (AA). Hair growth is divided into three

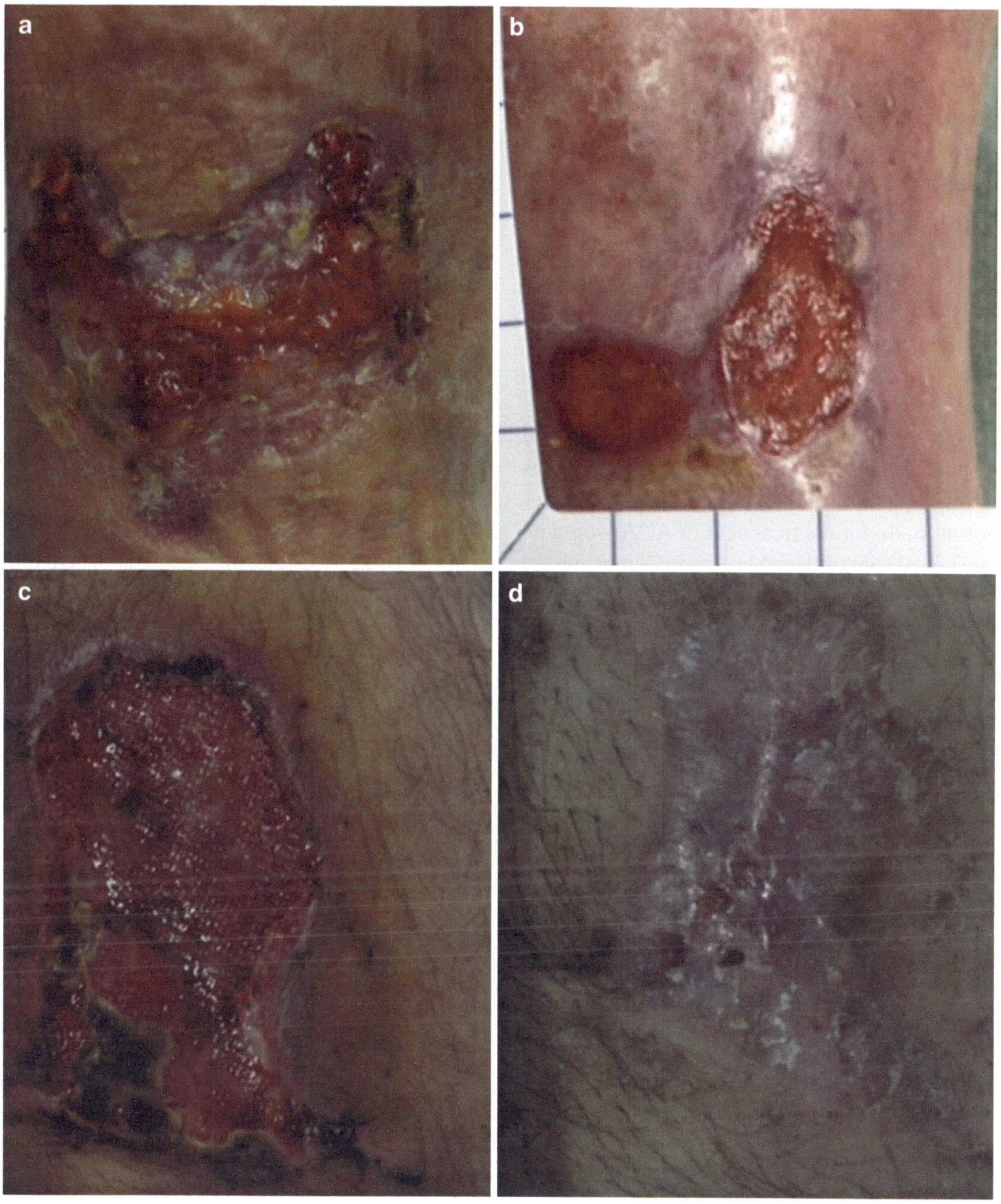

Fig. 8.2 Chronic wound in a 70-year-old female without diabetes (**a**), partially healed after 8 weeks of LED therapy (**b**). Chronic wound in a 58-yearold male with diabetes (**c**). the wound was completely healed 5 weeks after LED therapy (**d**)

phases: anagen, the active growth phase; catagen, the transitional phase; and telogen, the resting phase. It has been found that photobiomodulation applied to the scalp may be able to encourage hair follicles to move from the telogen phase into the anagen phase and increase the duration of the anagen phase itself to augment hair growth, yielding thicker and more pigmented hair [2, 4]. The exact mechanism is not yet fully established, but recently, new mechanisms has been proposed.

Studies reported that the activation of the Wnt10b/β-catenin signaling pathway may be responsible for inducing the anagen phase of hair follicles, as significantly higher expression of Wnt10b and β-catenin was observed with LLLT treatment in mouse models [17, 18]. Wnt10b and β-catenin pathway and ERK pathway activation may be responsible for irradiation induced human outer root sheath cell proliferation and inhibition of its apoptosis, which provides a likely mechanism for LLLT's effects on hair growth [18].

A systematic review and meta-analysis was done on randomized clinical trials studying LLLT's stimulating effect on hair growth and concluded that LLLT is an effective treatments for male-pattern hair loss [19]. The most noteworthy study for the treatment of AGA would be the clinical trial for HairMax LaserComb®, tested by Leavitt et al. in a double-blind, sham device-controlled randomized trial involving 110 male AGA patients [20]. The device is a hand-held LLLT device that that administers 9 beams at a wavelength of 655 nm (+/−5%) to the user's scalp while parting their hair with an attached comb [20]. Patients were instructed to use the device three times per week in 15-min sessions for 26 weeks [20]. Results showed that subjects in the HairMax LaserComb® group exhibited a statistically significant increase in mean terminal hair density compared to the control group, proving the device to be effective and well tolerated [20]. The effect of HairMax LaserComb® on hair growth and tensile strength was further tested in a study by Satino et al. on 28 male and 7 female AGA patients. Patients were instructed to use the LLLT at home for 6 months in 5–10 min sessions every other day. Results were assessed by an experienced hair transplant surgeon and using a computer-assisted hair counting software. Although the study found the device to work yield better results in males, both male and females experience significant improvement in both hair count and tensile strength [21]. HairMax LaserComb is now approved by the FDA as a safe treatment for male and female AGA (Fig. 8.3b) [1].

To investigate treatment of alopecia areata, a study was conducted with 15 patients (6 men, 9 women) using Super Lizer™, which emits polarized pulsed linear light (600–1600 nm) at 1.8 W [22]. Patients received irradiation treatment on their scalps for 3 min either once a week or once every other week until vellus hair regrowth was observed in at least half of the irradiated area and carpronium chloride 5% was applied topically twice daily to all the lesions [22]. As a result, the study observed induced hair growth in irradiated areas 1.6 months earlier than in non-irradiated areas in 47% of the patients [22].

No serious side effects were reported in any of the studies [19]. In short, for the subset of patients who are unwilling or unable to undergo surgical treatment and medical treatment for hair loss, LLLT serves as a notable alternative.

Suchonwanit et al. evaluated the efficacy and safety of LLLT device in the treatment of AGA in a 24-week, prospective, randomized, double-blind, sham device-controlled clinical trial. Twenty men and twenty women with AGA were randomized into two groups to be treated with a laser helmet (RAMACAP) or a sham helmet in the home-based setting for 24 weeks. Hair density, hair diameter, and adverse events were evaluated at baseline and at weeks 8, 16, and 24. Nineteen in the laser group and 17 in the sham group completed the study. At week 24, the laser helmet was significantly superior to the sham device for increasing hair density and hair diameter ($p = 0.002$ and $p = 0.009$, respectively) and showed a significantly greater improvement in global photographic assessment by investigators and subjects (Fig. 8.3a). Temporary hair shedding and scalp pruritus was reported as side effects [23].

LLLT for Skin Rejuvenation

LEDs also have aesthetic applications, primarily in non-thermal, non-ablative skin rejuvenation. Yellow (570–590 nm), red (630–700 nm), and near-infrared (800–1200 nm) wavelengths have been used for their photobiomodulation effects on mitochondria, which stimulates fibroblast proliferation, collagen synthesis, growth factors, and extracellular matrix production [24].

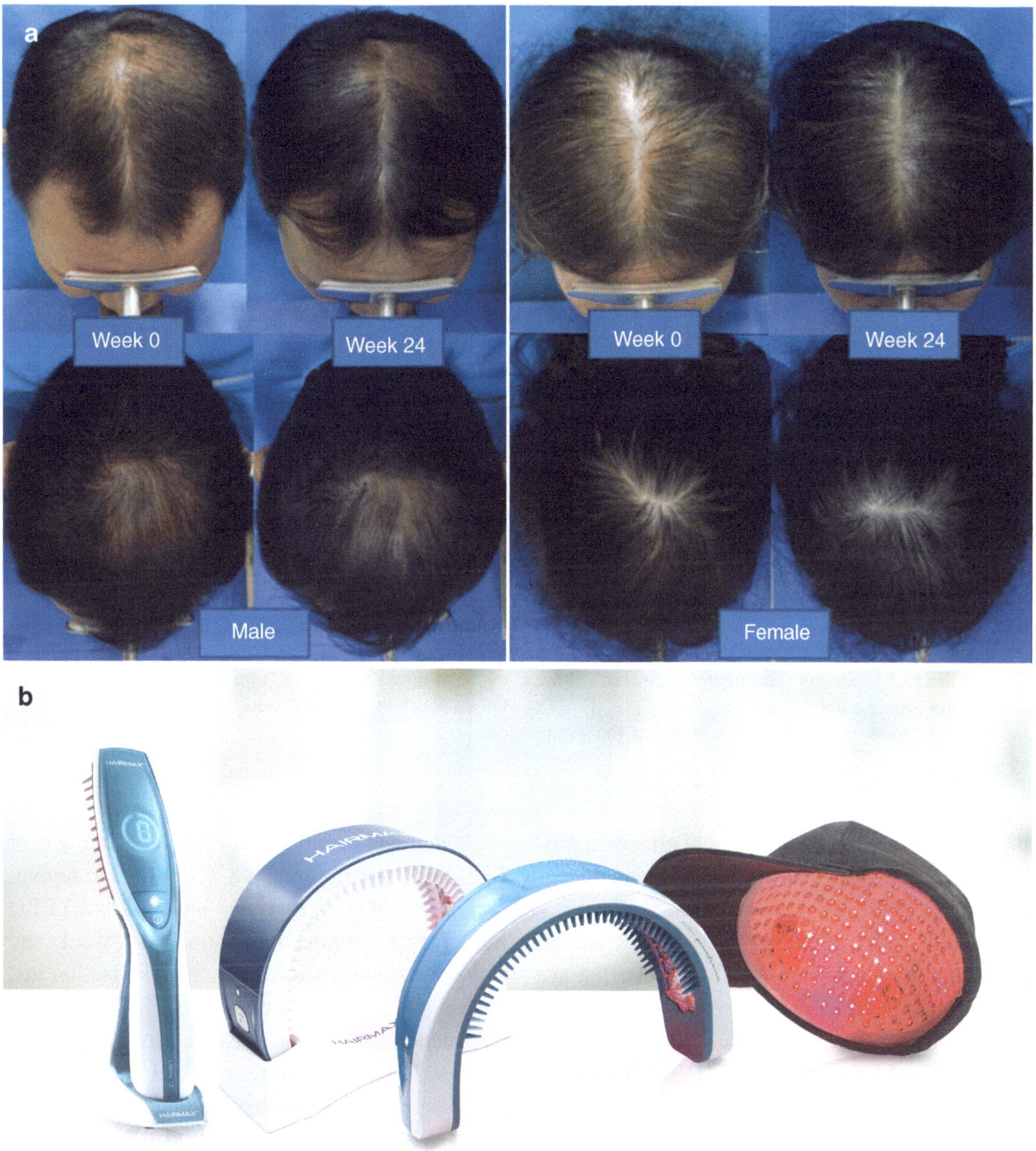

Fig. 8.3 (**a**) Moderate improvement of hair growth in patients treated with laser helmet at baseline and at 24 weeks [23]. (**b**) Commonly used light devices for hair loss

Specifically, increased mRNA levels of interleukin-1 beta (IL-1ß), tumor necrosis factor alpha (TNF-α), intercellular adhesion molecule 1 (ICAM-1), and connexin 43 (Cx43) along with decreased IL-6 have been reported after LED phototherapy treatment with red and infrared laser light [25]. IL-1ß and TNF-α are thought to be responsible for downstream stimulation of MMP activity, which contributes to the removal of photodamaged collagen fragments and, in turn, new collagen biosynthesis (Fig. 8.4) [25]. Augmented expression of Cx43 may contribute to enhanced cell-to-cell communication between fibroblasts, resulting in greater synchrony between cellular responses [25]. Collectively, these changes are thought to result in lifting and tightening of lax skin and the reduction of rhytids [24]. Red and near-infrared lights in particular,

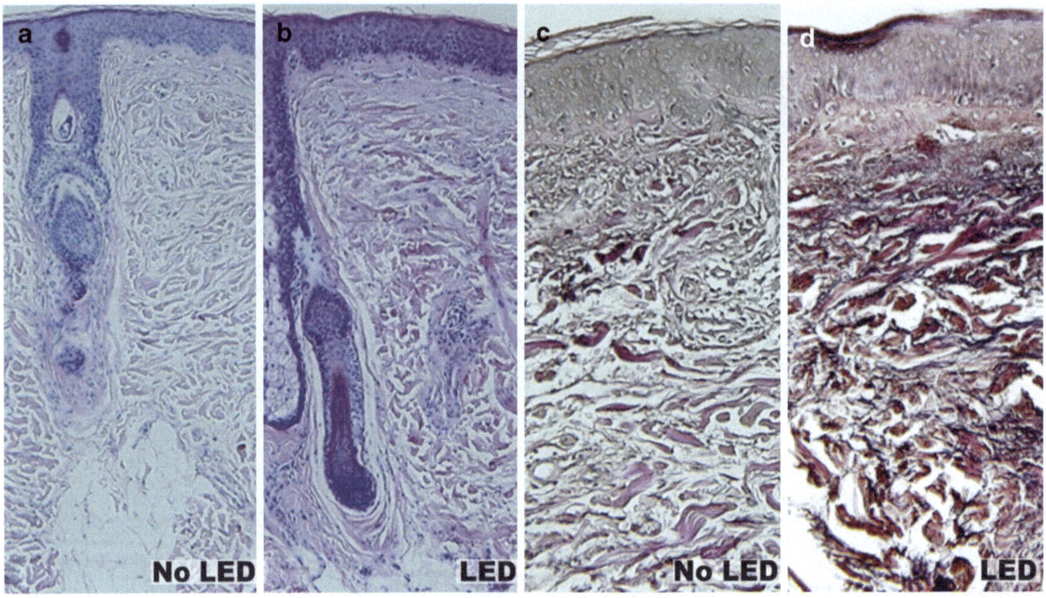

Fig. 8.4 Biopsy specimens of not treated site (**a**, **c**) and the treated side with with 830-nm LED (**b**, **d**) at 2 weeks after the final LED session. The treated sides both show significantly higher collagen (**a**, **b**) and elastin (**c**, **d**) fiber density with good alignment, particularly at the grenz zone, a thicker and more cellular epidermis, and a better organized stratum corneum. ([**a**, **b**]: hematoxylin and eosin, original magnifica- tion 100; [**c**, **d**]: elastica van Giessen, original magnification 200) [25]

are also reported to have additional effects in promoting dermal restructuring due to their deeper penetration [1, 26].

Clinical trials demonstrating LED's use in skin rejuvenation have reported results that are largely in consensus. A multicenter clinical trial treated 90 patients with a full panel 590 nm non-thermal LED array at 0.1 J/cm^2 for 8 sessions over 4 weeks and found significant improvement in the appearance of photoaged skin [27]. It was reported that 90% of patients improved by at least one Fitzpatrick photoaging category, with 65% of patients noting global improvement in facial texture, fine lines, background erythema, and pigmentation [27] This was bolstered by a larger clinical trial by Weiss et al., in which 900 patients were treated with LED therapy: 300 of which using 590 nm LED at 0.10 J/cm^2 alone, and 600 of which were treated with both LED therapy and a thermal-based photorejuvenation procedure [28]. Those treated with LED alone reported similar favorable results.

A number of studies investigated the use of LED light of 633 nm and 830 nm in skin rejuvenation. Bahat et al. used 633 nm (96 J/cm^2) LED light for 20-minute, three times per week and found the same positive aesthetic results after just 3 weeks [29]. Russell et al. (N = 31) employed treatments combining wavelengths of 633 nm and 830 nm (with fluences of 126 J/cm^2 and 66 J/cm^2 respectively) to treat patients with facial rhytids [24, 30]. Subjects were evaluated at after 9 weeks and 12 weeks using profilometry performed on periorbital casts [30]. The study reported that 52% of patients had reported 25–50% improvement in photoaging scores by week 12 [30].

These promising results were further supported by a larger, randomized, double-blind, controlled study designed to further validate the efficacy of 830 nm and 633 nm LEDs. Seventy-six subjects with facial wrinkles were randomized to one of 3 groups that received treatment on one side of the face, or to a fourth group that received sham treatment on the same side of the face [25]. Of the first three groups, subjects were treated using 830 nm (126 J/cm^2) LED alone, 633 nm (66 J/cm^2) LED alone, or 830 nm, 633 nm LEDs sequentially respectively [25]. A significant difference was reported between the experimental groups versus control: 95.2%, 72.3%, and 95.5% of subjects showed improvement versus 13.3% of subjects in the control group (Fig. 8.4) [25]

The Barolet et al. assessed the effects of light treatment on aged/photoaged skin. The study followed 12 patients treated with 660 nm LED light. And similarly, favorable outcomes were reported with 90% of individuals showing a reduction in rhytid depth and surface roughness (based on profilometry quantification), and 87% of the individuals reporting a reduction in the Fitzpatrick wrinkling severity score [31].

LLLT for Acne

Acne vulgaris is an inflammatory condition of the pilosebaceous units associated with increased sebum production, hyperkeratinization, discharge of inflammatory mediators, and the overgrowth of the bacteria Propionibacterium acnes (*P. acnes*) [32]. LLLT at 415 nm (blue) and 630 nm (red) wavelengths match the absorption peaks of porphyrins produced by *P. acnes* and is used for acne vulgaris treatment due to its ability to induce ROS formation as well as its anti-inflammatory properties [6, 33].

Blue light irradiation has been demonstrated to be particularly effective in killing *P. acnes* by photoactivation of endogenous porphyrins, which leads to formation of free radicals that destruct bacterial cell membrane [34]. Thirty patients, with mild-to-moderate acne, were treated with 415 nm blue light LED in a study by Morton et al. Treatments were delivered as 8-min, 10-min, or 20-min sessions over a period of four weeks, which resulted in a decrease of inflammatory lesion counts by 25%, 53%, and 60%, at 5, 8, and 12 weeks respectively [35]. Effect on non-inflammatory lesions were minimal. Another clinical trial conducted by Tremblay et al. investigated the use of blue LED (415 nm) for 20-min, twice per week for 4–8 weeks and reported a 50% reduction in lesion counts with nine patients' lesions completely cleared.

Red light therapy at low doses has also been investigated for acne treatment in different studies. An in-vitro model study used oleic acid (OA) to induce inflammatory response in human epidermal equivalent tissue, which mimics acne lesions in vivo [32]. Results showed that red light at 0.2–1.2 J/cm^2 showed inhibitory effects on OA-induced IL-1α release, and mitigated unsaturated fatty acid induced stratum corneum thickening and hyperkeratinization [32]. Red light therapy was also shown to reduce barrier defects induced by OA, another helpful factor suggesting a potential application of red light in the treatment of Acne vulgaris.

Photodynamic Therapy Using Blue and Red Light

Different types of photosensitizers, such as 5-aminolevulinic acid (ALA) and methyl ester aminolevulinate (MAL), are available for LED therapy and the use of these photosensitizers in conjunction with light therapy is known as photodynamic therapy (PDT) [36]. Blue light 's use in aminolevulinic acid photodynamic therapy (ALA-PDT) and red light's use in methyl aminolevulinate photodynamic therapy (MAL-PDT) for treatment of acne has also been explored. Its results were compared with that of LED therapy alone. In a study comparing blue light therapy alone and with ALA-PDT, difference in results were not found to be statistically significant [37]. No significant changes in sebum excretion, erythema or the melanin index were noted in the group treated with both ALA-PDT and blue light. However, side effects of pain, stinging, peeling, pruritus, oozing and pustules were more severe in the ALA-PDT group than that of blue light therapy alone [37]. Similar results were reported in a review of a series of studies comparing MAL-PDT with red light and red light LED therapy alone.

Metanalysis of the studies showed that four sessions of MAL ranging from 400-mg/g to 160-mg/g plus red light, had little effect on investigator-assessed change in the number of inflamed lesions compared with placebo cream plus red light when evaluated at 6 weeks [38]. Red-light MAL-PDT was not associated with higher rates of severe adverse effect than placebo or no treatment [38].

One of commonly used device for blue and red light therapies (Fig. 8.5).

LLLT for Psoriasis

The pathogenesis of psoriasis is known to be associated with abnormal interactions among innate immunity, such as T cells and keratinocytes [39]. In psoriasis, these immune cells release excess pro-inflammatory factors, which results in uncontrolled activation of immune response, including the nuclear factor-κB (NF-kB) signaling pathway and the differentiation of T helper (Th) cells toward Th1 and/or Th17 cells

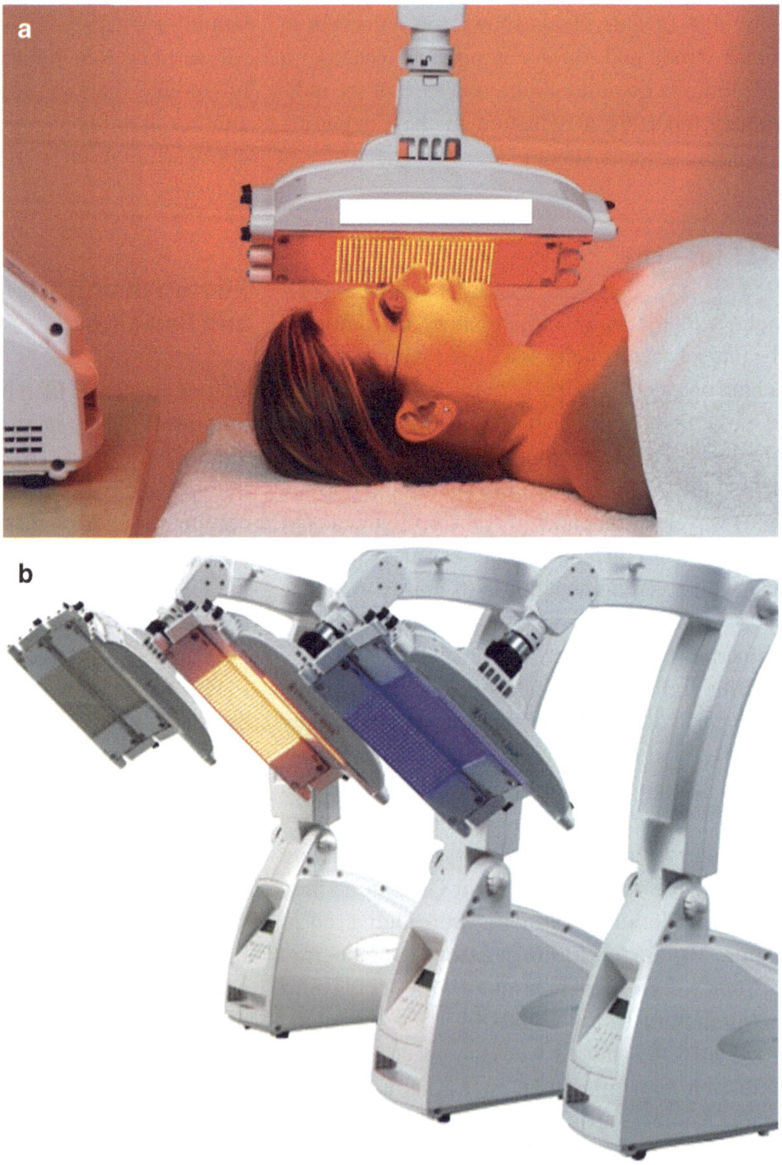

Fig. 8.5 Skin rejuvenation: Commonly used light device (**a**), (**b**)

[39]. LLLT of several wavelengths has been shown to have beneficial effects in modulating this process.

Blue light at 400–480 nm has been shown to reduce the proliferative activity of keratinocytes, lower T cell immune responses, and hence improve mild plaque psoriasis [40]. In a study by Weinstabl et al., 37 patients with mild to moderate psoriasis vulgaris (PV) were treated with blue light LED at 420 nm or at 453 nm once daily for 4 weeks [41]. Plaques were assessed using the Local Psoriasis Severity Index (LPSI) and both groups showed significant improvement [41].

Pfaff et al. also conducted a randomized long-term study on blue light treatment for mild PV with 47 patients using both high intensity treatment (453 nm LED 200 mW/cm^2) and low-intensity treatment (453 nm LED 100 mW/cm^2) [40]. The study showed statistically significant improvement in both LED settings compared to the control plaques, demonstrating the treatment safety and patient satisfaction achieved by blue light therapy [40].

Red light (620–770 nm) and near infrared light (800–1200 nm) at higher wavelengths, are known to be able to deeply penetrate the skin, allowing it to stimulate mitochondrial activity, and to modulate cytokine release to reduce inflammation [42]. A pilot study tested the efficacy of LED therapy in the treatment of recalcitrant psoriasis using a combination of 830 nm (near infrared) and 630 nm (visible red light) irradiation. Patients with chronic plaque psoriasis ($n = 8$) and guttate psoriasis ($n = 1$) of up to 35 years duration were enrolled, most of whom had psoriasis that are resistant to conventional therapy. Participants were sequentially treated with near infrared and red light in two 20-min sessions 48 h apart for 4–5 weeks [43]. The results showed psoriasis clearance ranging from 60 to 100% with high patient satisfaction and no adverse side effects [43]. In conclusion, these positive reports show great promise in the application of LLLT in psoriasis treatment. Its advantages of being non-invasive with few side effects merit to be explored further in the treatment of psoriasis.

LLLT for Vitiligo

Vitiligo is an acquired pigmentary disorder for which the underlying mechanism of the lack of functional melanocytes is still under investigation. Some progress has been made that suggests the involvement of keratinocytes, fibroblasts, melanoblasts and melanocytes, and thus stimulation of these epidermal and dermal cells, are thought to present a possible treatment option [1].

LLLT's use as alternative therapy for vitiligo goes back to 1997, when Mandel et al. reported noteworthy re-pigmentation after having treated 18 vitiligo patients with low-energy Helium-Neon (He-Ne) laser (632 nm, 25 mW/cm^2) therapy [44]. He-Ne laser use was then proposed for segmental-type vitiligo, a variant known to be more resistant to conventional therapies [45]. In the Yu et al. study, cultured keratinocytes and fibroblasts were treated with He-Ne laser at 0.5–1.5 J per cm^2 [45]. The irradiation lead to a significant increase in bFGF release in both keratinocytes and fibroblasts as well as an increase in NGF release from keratinocytes [45]. Applied clinically, the results sustained: 30 patients were treated with HeNe laser light (632.8 nm) administered locally at 3 J/cm^2, 1.0 mW with point stimulation 1–2 times weekly, and marked perilesional and perifollicular re-pigmentation (>50%) was observed in 60% of patients [45]. Lan et al.'s study helped clarify the theoretic basis for the positive results in vitiligo treatment. The study showed that the He-Ne laser (632.8 nm, 1 J/cm^2 and 10 mW) stimulates melanocyte proliferation through enhanced $\alpha 2\beta 1$ integrin expression and cyclic-AMP response element binding protein (CREB) expression, a key regulator of melanocyte growth [46].

Recently, the effects of LLLT on the ultrastructure and number of melanosomes in normal cultured human melanocytes was investigated. In a study by Khalid et al., melanocytes were irradiated by light therapy at an energy level of 2.0 J/cm^2, using a blue (457 nm), red (635 nm), or ultraviolet (UV) (355 nm) laser and compared to a control group that received sham treatment [47]. Developmental stages of melanosomes were observed and their numbers were counted. A significantly higher amount of Stage I melanosomes was reported in the LLLT treated cells compared to the control [47]. Red laser light treatment yielded a larger amount than that of others, indicating more effective stimulation of melanogenesis [47]. The same research team also tested different LLLT's effect on human melanocyte migration in vitro. The study reported that LLLT at low energy densities has promising effects on increasing melanocyte viability, proliferation, and migration, while LLLT at higher energy densities yielded non-stimulatory results [48]. Despite these advances, LLLT's clinical application in vitiligo would benefit from larger clinical trials.

LLLT for Scars: Hypertrophic and Keloid

Hypertrophic scars and keloids that arise from surgery, trauma, or acne have long been a challenge in dermatology despite a wide range of treatment options. The pathogenesis of these conditions is thought to involve an imbalance between the rate of collagen biosynthesis and degradation leading to fibroblastic proliferation and excess collagen deposits [1]. Recent studies have proposed that inadequate regulation of interleukin (IL)-6 signaling pathways and transforming growth factor beta-I (TGF-βI) expression have a significant role in this process, making inhibition of the IL-6 pathway and/or TGF-βI a potential therapeutic target [49–53]. Since some wavelengths in the LED-RL (633 nm) spectrum and infrared spectrum (830 nm) have been shown to lead to a decrease in IL-6 (despite the increase of IL-1ß and TNF-a), LLLT has been suggested as a prophylactic to avoid or attenuate the formation of hypertrophic scars or keloids [25].

In a case report study, the efficacy of LLLT is investigated on three patients with different type of scars. In each, a single scar of bilateral scars was treated daily at home with NIR—LED 805 nm at 30 mW/cm^2 and 27 J/cm^2 [54]. In the first case, the LED treatment was applied to pre-auricular linear keloids resulting from a face lift procedure, which had been treated surgically for scar revision [54]. A second case was performed on a patient with hypertrophic scars on the chest resulting from acne, where CO_2 laser was used for resurfacing [54]. A third case treated a patient with hypertrophic scars on the back post-excision, which was also treated with CO_2 laser for resurfacing [54]. Results show significant improvements on the nIR-LED treated scar compared to the control scar [54]. No significant treatment-related adverse effects were reported [54].

LLLT's efficacy in the treatment of post-burn hypertrophic scars in children was recently explored. In a randomized controlled trial consisting of 15 children ranging from 2 to 10 years of age was conducted and results were assessed using the *Vancouver Scar Scale* (VSS). Each scar in this study was divided in half. One side of each scar was treated with a Helium -Neon laser (wave length 632.8 nm, power density of 119 mW/cm^2, and energy density of 16 J/cm^2) for 25 min. Significant improvement after treatment was reported, with a pre-treatment median VSS score of 9 (whole scar) vs 6 (whole scar) after treatment (Fig. 8.6) [55].

LLLT for Photoprotection

The application of LLLT's application in photoprotection is still in its early stages and is still being contested. Recent studies have proposed that infrared light exposure delivered at certain parameters may have protective effects on the skin by triggering protective/repair responses to UV irradiation (Table 8.1) [1]. However, the effect is highly parameter specific and conflicting views also exist [2]. This discrepancy may be explained by the fact that only a specific range of optimal combination of irradiance and time for stimulation yields desired results: suboptimal doses lead to lack of response, higher-than-optimal doses lead inhibition of response—a phenomenon known as the biphasic dose response [2]. Despite some disagreements on the skin's natural mechanism to prepare for UV damage, some studies showed that non-coherent near

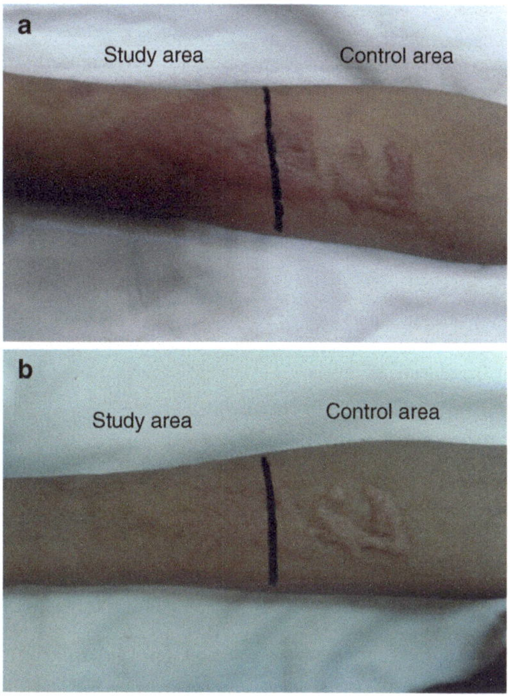

Fig. 8.6 The study and control halves of post-burn hypertrophic scars before treatment (**a**) and after 12 weeks of treatment with HE-Ne laser (**b**)

infrared radiation (NIR) (700–2000 nm) prepares cells to resist UVB-induced damage by inhibiting UVB-induced apoptosis [56–58]. In preventing activation of caspase-9 and -3, decreasing pro-apoptotic proteins (ie, Bax) and increasing anti-apoptotic proteins (ie, Bcl-2 or Bcl-xL), IR was reported to have modulating effects on the Bcl2/Bax balance that is assumed to be lasting and cumulative [56–58].

A series of studies by Barolet and Boucher investigated the clinical effects of such findings. Thirteen healthy subjects and two subjects with polymorphous light eruption (PLE) were treated with LED to investigate the protective effect of LED treatment (660 nm) when administered prior to UV exposure [59]. Results showed that dose-dependent LED irradiation of 660 nm was effective in achieving a >50% reduction UVB induced erythema in at least one occasion in 85% of subjects, including those with PLE [59]. An in-vitro study was then done in 2009, which reported that non-thermal non-coherent deep red visible LED exposure (660 nm, sequential pulsing mode) lead to an increase of dermal fibroblast

Table 8.1 Indications of LLLT

Indications	Laser specification	Mechanism	Referenced trial
Wound healing	Infrared 830 nm light (55 J/cm^2) followed by red 633 nm light	Stimulate production of ATP and inhibit the production of prostaglandins via release of histamine, serotonin, and bradykinin.	Trelles et al
	LED-nIR phototherapy 860 nm		Chaves et al.
Hair growth	HairMax LaserComb® 655 nm	Wnt10b and β-catenin pathway and ERK pathway activation	Leavitt et al.
Skin rejuvenation	590 nm non-thermal LED array	Increased mRNA levels of interleukin 1 beta (IL-1ß), tumor necrosis factor alpha (TNF-α), intercellular adhesion molecule 1 (ICAM-1), and connexin 43 (Cx43) along with decreased IL-6	McDaniel et al. Weiss et al
	LED light of 633 nm and 830 nm		Bahat et al. Lee et al.
Acne	Blue light 415 nm	Formation of free radicals that destruct P. acnes bacterial cell membrane	Morton et al.
	Red light 630 nm	Inhibitory effects on OA-induced IL-1α release, and stratum corneum thickening and hyperkeratinization	Li et al.
Psoriasis	Blue light (400–480 nm)	Modulate the nuclear factor-κB (NF-kB) signaling pathway and the differentiation of T helper (Th) cells	Weinstabl et al.
	Red light (620–770 nm) and near infrared light (800–1200 nm)	Stimulate mitochondrial activity, and to modulate cytokine release to reduce inflammation	Ablon et al.

continued

Table 8.1 (continued)

Indications	Laser specification	Mechanism	Referenced trial
Vitiligo	Helium-neon (he-ne) laser 632 nm	Stimulation of melanocytes and karatinocytes	Mandel et al. Yu et al.
	Blue (457 nm), red (635 nm), or ultraviolet (UV 355 nm) laser		Khalid et al.
Hypertrophic/keloid scars	NIR—LED 805 nm	Decrease IL-6	Barolet et al.
	Helium-neon laser 632.8 nm		Alsharnoubi et al.
Photoprotection	NIR 700–2000 nm	Inhibition of UVB-induced apoptosis	Menezes et al. Frank et al. Applegate et al.
	LED exposure (660 nm	Increase dermal fibroblast procollagen secretion and reduction of metalloproteinases (MMP) or collagenase production	Barolet et al.

procollagen secretion, which reduced metalloproteinases (MMP) or collagenase production [54]. These findings were correlated with significant clinical improvement of rhytids in vivo [54].

Pre-Treatment Preparation and Precautions

LLLT's application in dermatology is still in its early stages and thus it is mostly used as adjunct therapy to established therapeutic options. Among the concerns for its use, the most notable are those regarding its safety and efficacy. The relatively more well-established indications of use include hair loss, and as prophylaxis against scar formation [60]. Other indications include wound healing, photodamaged skin rejuvenation, acne vulgaris and fibrosis. Dosimetry is an important factor that largely dictates efficacy. Choosing amongst a large number of illumination parameters such as wavelength, fluence, power density, pulse structure, and treatment timing is a complex task and is a potential explanatory factor for the wide range of different outcomes that have been reported [2]. LLLT is generally a safe, well tolerated treatment option, but some contraindications have been proposed (Table 8.2). Due to the laser's biostimulating effects, malignancy and direct irradiation over the thyroid gland are well-recognized contraindications [61–65]. Direct irradiation over the fetus during pregnancy is also generally recognized as a contraindication out of precaution, though animal models have reported no teratogenic effects [65]. LLLT is inherently an eye irritant, therefore direct irradiation of the retina should be avoided as well as use in those with photophobia or photosensitive dermatoses [65]. Other contraindications that are still under consideration include: infectious disease and fever due to the biostimulating effect of the laser on infectious agents, and the potential bacteriostatic effect of the laser on microflora [65]. Regarding LLLT use in children, so far, no literature has reported any adverse effects from the use

Table 8.2 Contraindications of Low level laser therapy (LLLT)

Contraindications of LLLT
– Malignancy – Pregnancy – Irradiation of retina – Photophobia – Photosensitive dermatoses
Under consideration:
– Infectious disease – Fever – Irradiation of growth plates (children) – Tattooed skin

of LLLT on open growth plates. However, because it is sometimes listed as a contraindication in equipment operation manuals as well as textbooks, it may be best to avoid irradiation directly over growth plates as a precautionary measure. LLLT is not otherwise contraindicated in children. Tattooed skin and skin with darker pigmentation may absorb light energy more efficiently and predict an increased risk for adverse effects; it is recommended that a patch test be done prior to treatment. Lower dosage—decreased to 50–75% of the recommended dosage is also recommended.

Treatment Technique

Prior to treatment, the targeted area of skin should be cleaned with alcohol and excess body hair should be removed. It is important to note that no coupling media, such as lotions, gels, or ointments should be between the applicator and the patient's skin during the delivery of LLLT. A stationary technique should be used to allow for the most efficient transfer of energy. To ensure depth of penetration, the clinician should maintain firm, direct contact with the patient's intact skin throughout the procedure. Both the recipient and the administrator of the low-level laser treatment should be wearing manufacturer-provided protective eyewear before beginning light administration.

Post Treatment Care Advice and Plan

There are no established guidelines specifically for treatment follow-up for LLLT. As with many other laser therapies, patients should be closely examined and monitored for any side effects after treatment and be instructed for proper skin care. Adherence to general suggestions for skin care after laser surgery is advised. Note that the treated area may be pink or red for the first 4–8 h after treatment with possible stinging/tingling sensation. Patient should be instructed not to rub, scratch, or put pressure on the treated area until erythema or crusting clears. Make-up or lotion should be avoided until signs of redness and stinging have dissipated. An appropriate moisturizing lotion is encouraged for the duration of the treatment and for at least three months after the final treatment. Washing of the treated area is allowed if done gently with water, but swimming is generally not suggested until after 2–4 weeks depending on the procedure done. Ice packs or cold compress can be applied to alleviate erythema, edema and tingling. Irritation to the treated area should be avoided in general by using milder cleaning agents. Direct sun exposure should be avoided, and appropriate sunscreen should be applied if needed.

Complications

LLLT is generally a safe, low-risk, well-tolerated therapeutic modality with minimal side effects and complications. Currently, side effects reliably reported by studies include: post-treatment erythema, hyperpigmentation, edema, dry skin, and burning sensation of treated areas [5]. However, when used by clinicians who are properly trained in the indications, contraindications, dosing and administration of LLLT, there should be very little downtime and scarce adverse events. In literature, very few side effects were reported, even when tested at higher than optimal doses. Even in the event of adverse side effects, symptoms are often transient. In fact, in a 2018 systematic review of 31 controlled trials of LED treatment across all aforementioned indications (i.e. acne vulgaris, skin rejuvenation, wound healing etc.), only 8 reported any side effects at all.

References

1. Avci P, Sadasivam AGM, Vecchio D, Pam Z, Pam N, Hamblin MR. Low-level laser (light) therapy (LLLT) in skin: stimulating, healing, restoring. Semin Cutan Med Surg. 2013;32(1):41–52.
2. Chung H, et al. The nuts and bolts of low-level laser (light) therapy. Ann Biomed Eng. 2012;40(2): 516–33.
3. Ketty Peris TM, Piccolo D, Concetta M. Dermoscopic features of actinic keratosis. J German Soc Dermatol. 2007;5(11):970–5.

4. de Freitas LF, Hamblin MR. Proposed mechanisms of photobiomodulation or low-level light therapy. IEEE J Selected Top Quantum Electron. 2016;22(3):7000417.
5. Jagdeo J, et al. Light-emitting diodes in dermatology: a systematic review of randomized controlled trials. Lasers Surg Med. 2018;50(6):613–8.
6. Opel DR, Hagstrom E, Pace AK, Sisto K, Hirano-Ali SA, Desai S, Swan J. Light-emitting diodes: a brief review and clinical experience. J Clin Aesthet Dermatol. 2015;8(6):36–44.
7. Andrew Mamalis DS, Jagdeo J. Visible red light emitting diode photobiomodulation for skin fibrosis: key molecular pathways. Curr Dermatol Rep. 2016;5(1):121–8.
8. Kim SK, You HR, Kim SH, Yun SJ, Lee SC, Lee JB. Skin photorejuvenation effects of light-emitting diodes (LEDs): acomparative study of yellow and red LEDs in vitro and in vivo. Clin Exp Dermatol. 2016;41(7):798–805.
9. Andrew Mamalis MG, Jagdeo J. Light emitting diode-generated blue light modulates fibrosis characteristics: fibroblast proliferation, migration speed, and reactive oxygen species generation. Lasers Surg Med. 2015;47(2):210–5.
10. Taline Bavaresc AP, Moraes VM, Osmarin VM, Silveira DT, de Fátima Lucena A. Low-level laser therapy for treatment of venous ulcers evaluated with the nursing outcome classification: study protocol for a randomized controlled trial. Trials. 2018;19:372.
11. Tchanque-Fossuo CN, Ho D, Dahle SE, Koo E, Li CS, Isseroff RR, Jagdeo JA. A systematic review of low-level light therapy for treatment of diabetic foot ulcer. Wound Repair Regen. 2016;24(2):418–26.
12. Andrade F, de Oliveira Clark RM, Ferreira ML. Effects of low-level laser therapy on wound healing. Rev Col Bras Cir. 2014;41(2):129–33.
13. Trelles MA, Allones I, Mayo E. Combined visible light and infrared light-emitting diode (LED) therapy enhances wound healing after laser ablative resurfacing of photodamaged facial skin. Med Laser Appl. 2006;21:165–75.
14. Emı'lia de Abreu Chaves M, Araujo AR, Santos SF, Pinotti M, Oliveira LS. LED phototherapy improves healing of nipple trauma: a pilot study. Photomed Laser Surg. 2012;30(3):172–8.
15. de Oliveira RA, et al. Low-intensity LED therapy (658 nm) on burn healing: a series of cases. Lasers Med Sci. 2018;33(4):729–35.
16. Kajagar BM, Godhi AS, Pandit A, Khatri S. Efficacy of low level laser therapy on wound healing in patients with chronic diabetic foot ulcers—a randomised control trial. Indian J Surg. 2012;74(5):359–63.
17. Tiran Zhang LL, Fan J, Tian J, Gan C, Yang Z, Jiao H, Han B, Liu Z. Low-level laser treatment stimulates hair growth via upregulating Wnt10b and β-catenin expression in C3H/HeJ mice. Lasers Med Sci. 2017;32(5):1189–95.
18. Kim JE, Woo YJ, Sohn KM, Jeong KH, Kang H. Wnt/β-catenin and ERK pathway activation: a possible mechanism of photobiomodulation therapy with light-emitting diodes that regulate the proliferation of human outer root sheath cells. Laser Surg Med. 2017;49(10):940–7.
19. Adil A, Godwin M. The effectiveness of treatments for androgenetic alopecia: a systematic review and meta-analysis. J Am Acad Dermatol. 2017;77(1):136–41.
20. Leavitt M, Charles G, Heyman E, Michaels D. HairMax LaserComb laser phototherapy device in the treatment of male androgenetic alopecia: a randomized, double-blind, sham device-controlled, multicentre trial. Clin Drug Investig. 2009;29(5):283–92.
21. Satino JL, Markou M. Hair regrowth and increased hair tensile strength using the HairMax LaserComb for low-level laser therapy. Int J Cosmet Surg Aesthet Dermatol. 2003;5:113–7.
22. Yamazaki M, Miura Y, Tsuboi R, Ogawa H. Linear polarized infrared irradiation using super Lizer is an effective treatment for multiple-type alopecia areata. Int J Dermatol. 2003;42(9):738–40.
23. Suchonwanit P, Chalermroj N, Khunkhet S. Low-level laser therapy for the treatment of androgenetic alopecia in Thai men and women: a 24-week, randomized, double-blind, sham device-controlled trial. Lasers Med Sci. 2019;34(6):1107–14.
24. Ablon G. Phototherapy with light emitting diodes: treating a broad range of medical and aesthetic conditions in dermatology the journal of clinical and aesthetic. Dermatology. 2018;11(2):21–7.
25. Lee SY, Ki-Ho P, Jung-Woo C, Jung-Kyun K, Rak LD, Sun SM, Sung LJ, Eui YC, Youn PM. A prospective, randomized, placebo-controlled, double-blinded, and split-face clinical study on LED phototherapy for skin rejuvenation: clinical, profilometric, histologic, ultrastructural, and biochemical evaluations and comparison of three different treatment settings. J Photochem Photobiol: Biol. 2007;88(1):51–67.
26. Glen Calderhead R, Vasily DB. Low level light therapy with light-emitting diodes for the aging face. Clin Plast Surg. 2016;43(3):541–50.
27. McDaniel DH, Newman J, Geronemus RG, Weiss MA. Non-ablative non-thermal LED photomodulation—a multicenter clinical photoaging trial. Laser Surg Med. 2003;25:22.
28. Weiss RA, McDaniel D, Geronemus RG, et al. Clinical experience with light-emitting diode (LED) photomodulation. Dermatol Surg. 2005;31(9 Pt 2):1199–205.
29. Bhat J, Birch J, Whitehurst C. A single-blinded randomised controlled study to determine the efficacy of Omnilux revive facial treatment in skin rejuvenation. Lasers Med Sci. 2005;20(6):6–10.
30. Russell BA, Kellett N, Reilly LR. A study to determine the efficacy of combination LED light therapy (633nm and 830nm) in facial skin rejuvenation. J Cosmet Laser Therap. 2005;7:196–200.
31. Barolet D, Roberge C, Auger FA, Boucher A, Germain L. Regulation of skin collagen metabolism in vitro using a pulsed 660 nm LED light source: clin-

ical correlation with a single-blinded study. J Investig Dermatol. 2009;12:2751–9.
32. Li W-H, Fassih A, Binner C, Parsa R, Southall MD. Low-level red LED light inhibits hyperkeratinization and inflammation induced by unsaturated fatty acid in an in vitro model mimicking acne. Laser Surg Med. 2018;50(2):158–65.
33. Gold MH, Goldberg DJ, Nestor MS. Current treatments of acne: medications, lights, lasers, and a novel 650-μs 1064-nm Nd: YAG laser. J Cosmet Dermatol. 2017;16(3):303–18.
34. Ashkenazi H, Malik Z, Harth Y. Eradication of Propionibacterium acnes by its endogenic porphyrins after illumination with high intensity blue light. FEMS Immunol Med Microbiol. 2003;35(1):17–24.
35. Morton CA, Scholefield R, Whitehurst C, Birch J. An open study to determine the efficacy of blue light in the treatment of mild to moderate acne. J Dermatol Treat. 2005;16:219–23.
36. Sorbellini E, Rucco M, Rinaldi F. Photodynamic and photobiological effects of light-emitting diode (LED) therapy in dermatological disease: an update. Lasers Med Sci. 2018;33(7):1431–9.
37. Akaraphanth R, Kanjanawanitchkul W, Gritiyarangsan P. Efficacy of ALA-PDT vs blue light in the treatment of acne. Photodermatol Photoimmunol Photomed. 2007;23:186–90.
38. Pawel Posadzki JC. Light therapies for acne. JAMA Dermatol. 2018;154(5):597–8.
39. Greb JE, Golminz AM, Elder JT, Lebwohl MG, Gladman DD, Wu JJ, Mehta NN, Finlay AY, Gottlieb AB. Psoriasis. Nat Rev Dis Primers. 2016; 24:2.
40. Pfaff S, Liebmann J, Born M, Merk HF, von Felbert V. Prospective randomized long-term study on the efficacy and safety of UV-free blue light for treating mild psoriasis vulgaris. Dermatology. 2015;231(1):24–34.
41. Weinstabl A, Hoff-Lesch S, Merk HF, von Felbert V. Prospective randomized study on the efficacy of blue light in the treatment of psoriasis vulgaris. Dermatology. 2011;223(3):251–9.
42. Niu T, Tian Y, Ren Q, Wei L, Li X, Cai Q. Red light interferes in UVA-induced photoaging of human skin fibroblast cells. Photochem Photobiol. 2014;90(6):1349–58.
43. Ablon G. Combination 830-nm and 633-nm light-emitting diode phototherapy shows promise in the treatment of recalcitrant psoriasis: preliminary findings. Photomed Laser Surg. 2010;28(1):141–6.
44. Mandel AS, Haberman HF, Pawlowski D, Goldstein E. Non PUVA nonsurgical therapies for vitiligo. Clin Dermatol. 1997;15(6):907–19.
45. Yu HS, Wu C, Yu CL, Kao YH, Chiou MH. Helium-neon laser irradiation stimulates migration and proliferation in melanocytes and induces repigmentation in segmental-type vitiligo. J Investig Dermatol. 2003;120(1):56–64.
46. Lan CC, Wu C, Chiou MH, Chiang TY, Yu HS. Low-energy helium-neon laser induces melanocyte proliferation via interaction with type IV collagen: visible light as a therapeutic option for vitiligo. Br J Dermatol. 2009;161(2):273–80.
47. Alghamdi KM, Kumar A, Al-ghamdi A, Al-rikabi AC, Mubarek M. Ultra-structural effects of different low-level lasers on normal cultured human melanocytes: an in vitro comparative study. Lasers Med Sci. 2016;31(9):1819–25.
48. AlGhamdi KM, Kumar A, Ashour AE, AlGhamdi AA. A comparative study of the effects of different low-level lasers on the proliferation, viability, and migration of human melanocytes in vitro. Lasers Med Sci. 2015;30(5):1541–51.
49. Wolfram D, Tzankov A, Pulzl P, Piza-Katzer H. Hypertrophic scars and keloids—a review of their pathophysiology, risk factors, and therapeutic management. Dermatol Surg. 2009;35(2):171–81.
50. Bouzari N, Davis S, Nouri K. Laser treatment of keloids and hypertrophic scars. Int J Dermatol. 2007;46(1):80–8.
51. Uitto J. IL-6 signaling pathway in keloids: a target for pharmacologic intervention? J Investig Dermatol. 2007;127(1):6–8.
52. Ghazizadeh M, Tosa M, Shimizu H, Hyakusoku H, Kawanami O. Functional implications of the IL-6 signaling pathway in keloid pathogenesis. J Investig Dermatol. 2007;127(1):98–105.
53. Liu W, Wang D, Cao YL. TGF-beta: a fibrotic factor in wound scarring and a potential target for anti-scarring gene therapy. Curr Gene Ther. 2004;4(1): 123–6.
54. Barolet D, Boucher A. Prophylactic low-level light therapy for the treatment of hypertrophic scars and keloids: a case series. Laser Surg Med. 2010;42(6):597–601.
55. Alsharnoubi J, Shoukry KE-S, Fawzy MW, Mohamed O. Evaluation of scars in children after treatment with low-level laser. Lasers Med Sci. 2018;33:1991.
56. Menezes S, Coulomb B, Lebreton C, Dubertret L. Non-coherent near infrared radiation protects normal human dermal fibroblasts from solar ultraviolet toxicity. J Investig Dermatol. 1998;111(4): 629–33.
57. Frank S, Oliver L, Coster CL-D. Infrared radiation affects the mitochondrial pathway of apoptosis in human fibroblasts. J Investig Dermatol. 2004;123(5):823–31.
58. Applegate LA, Scaletta C, Panizzon R, Frenk E, Hohlfeld P, Schwarzkopf S. Induction of the putative protective protein ferritin by infrared radiation: implications in skin repair. Int J Mol Med. 2000;5(3):247–51.
59. Barolet D, Boucher A. LED photoprevention: reduced MED response following multiple LED exposures. Laser Surg Med. 2008;40(2):106–12.

60. Won-Serk Kim RGC. Is light-emitting diode phototherapy (LED-LLLT) really effective? Laser Therapy. 2011;20(3):205–15.
61. Baxter D. Electrotherapy: evidence-based practice. 11th ed. London: WB Saunders; 2003.
62. Belanger AY. Evidence-based guide to therapeutic physical agents. Philadelphia, PA: Lippincott Williams & Wilkins; 2002.
63. Ann Reed JL. Electrotherapy explained: principles and practice. 3rd ed. London: Elsevier Health Sciences; 1999.
64. Jan Tuner LH. Laser therapy clinical practice & scientific background. Grangesberg: Prima Books; 2014.
65. Leos Navratil JK. Contraindications in noninvasive laser therapy: truth and fiction. J Clin Laser Med Surg. 2002;20(6):341–3.

9 Intense Pulsed Light in Dermatology

Sam Hills and Miguel Montero

Introduction

Lasers have found use in dermatological applications since shortly after the first laser was demonstrated in 1960, however, it wasn't until the late 1990s that the first polychromatic light sources entered the aesthetics market. These Intense Pulsed Light (IPL) systems, also known as Intense Light Sources (ILS) are based upon flash-lamp technology and deliver non-coherent, polychromatic light.

Typically an IPL consists of the main unit, which houses the power supply and user interface, and a handpiece, in which the light is produced (Fig. 9.1). The light source within the handpiece is usually a Xenon arc lamp. When an electric current is passed through the pressurised gas, light is generated over a broad spectral range from UV to infrared (approximately 350–1200 nm). The IPL handpiece will generally have an internal parabolic reflector which collects and directs the light out of the handpiece, to be applied to the skin via a quartz treatment applicator, which may be fixed or interchangeable (Fig. 9.1).

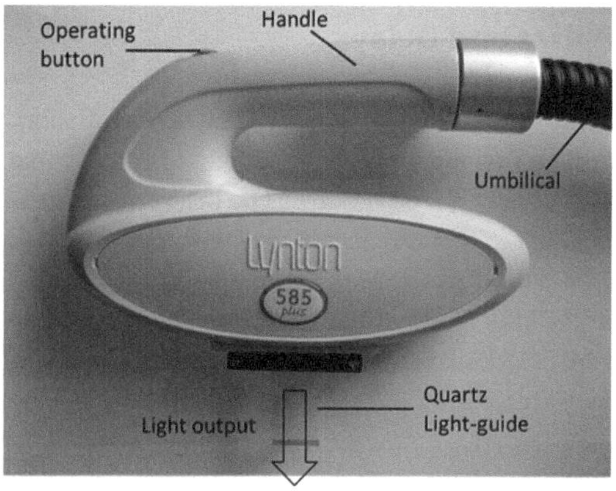

Fig. 9.1 An example of an IPL handpiece

The lamp and reflector are water-cooled, and the water and the power are delivered to the handpiece from the main unit, via a flexible conduit or umbilical. Many of the longer IR wavelengths are filtered out before reaching the skin via the water, but dichroic filters are also utilised to narrow down the spectral output and to target specific skin chromophores; namely melanin for hair removal and pigmentation treatments, and haemoglobin for the treatment of superficial vascular lesions. These filters generally remove any light below a given wavelength, for example a 650 nm filter means that the handpiece will typically emit light of a wavelength range of 650 to approximately 1200 nm. This wavelength range will target melanin in preference to haemoglobin or water, and is therefore a useful tool for hair

S. Hills
Lynton Lasers Ltd, Holmes Chapel, UK
e-mail: shills@lynton.co.uk

M. Montero (✉)
Discover Laser Clinic,
Crow Wood Leisure, Burnley, UK
e-mail: miguel@discoverlaser.co.uk

V. Madan (ed.), *Practical Introduction to Laser Dermatology*,
https://doi.org/10.1007/978-3-030-46451-6_9

removal. In contrast, using a cut-off filter of approximately 550 nm will allow targeting of haemoglobin absorption peaks, and the treatment of a variety of vascular conditions, such as rosacea or telangiectasia.

Eliminating the shorter wavelengths means there is no unnecessary absorption by the superficially penetrating shorter wavelengths, that can cause unwanted epidermal heating. This ability to deliver different wavelengths to the skin means that IPLs are versatile systems that can be used to treat a wide range of skin conditions.

Pulses and Delays

Most IPL systems emit light via a series of short, millisecond pulses separated by a pulse delay that may or may not be variable. The benefit of delivering light in this way is that the epidermis is able to cool during the short delay. Because the Thermal Relaxation Time of the epidermis is shorter than that of a hair follicle or blood vessel, the delay time (typically of the order of 5–50 ms) is long enough to allow the epidermis to cool but it is short enough to have little cooling effect on the target skin structure. Thus over the entire pulse sequence (typically 2–5 pulses) the target temperature rises yet the epidermis is able to remain cooler and a temperature differential is established which will damage the target without damaging the epidermis.

The number of pulses can often be altered, as can the delay, and in some cases, the individual pulse on-time. Adjusting any of these variables will have the end result of changing the overall pulse train duration. In general, delivering the light to the skin in the shortest possible time will give the most effective results, while extending the pulse train duration will make treatments more gentle and suitable for the treatment of darker skin types.

Comparison with Laser

Laser light is monochromatic, coherent and non-divergent, whereas IPL light is polychromatic, non-coherent and divergent. The property of coherence offers no advantage for skin treatments, in fact, due to the scattering nature of the skin tissue, any coherent incident light source may be considered diffuse on entering the tissue.

As dermatological lasers generally have fixed wavelength outputs, there are few laser options available that can effectively treat both hair and vascular lesions, however, by the use of variable cut off filters, IPL sources can be used to effectively target both chromophores, and can treat a variety of skin conditions.

The large, rectangular treatment heads also mean that treatments can be carried out quickly, and, the avoidance of the typical laser round spot (which can't be tessellated, and can sometimes leave a 'dotty' appearance on the skin), can sometimes be beneficial.

IPLs tend to be more compact and robust than traditional solid state lasers, which means they can be a cost-effective solution for a clinic looking to offer light-based treatments. However, it is worth noting that there is more discrepancy with power outputs than is typically seen with laser system, and low power models will give inadequate outcomes.

IPL Indications and Techniques

Common indications for IPL devices are shown in Table 9.1.

Rosacea

Introduction

Rosacea is a chronic inflammatory condition, which affects an estimated 5.46% of the adult population, but the true figure will vary depending on the diagnostic criteria used [1]. It has an unknown aetiology, but both genetic and environmental factors have been implicated. Recent advances in molecular biology and immunology have improved our understanding of the pathophysiology of this condition. The consen-

Table 9.1 Common indications for IPL

Vascular:
• Facial
– Telangiectasia: arborizing, linear – Port Wine Stains – Rosacea
• Truncal and limbs:
– Telangiectasia – Poikiloderma of Civatte
Sun damage: Photo-rejuvenation
Pigmentation
• Lentigos/ lentigines • Ephelides • Melasma (caution) • Post inflammatory hyperpigmentation (caution)
Hair removal: Photoepilation
Other
• Acne • Activation of PDT

sus in recent years seems to be that there is a persistently anomalous innate immune response that results in the appearance of the typical inflammatory and vascular features [2]. The interaction of known triggers like UV light, spicy food, alcohol, bacteria like *H. Pylori* [3] or skin parasites like Demodex, with the toll-like receptors (TLR) present in keratinocytes, will have in normal circumstances a mild or no effect. The TLR activation (signalling) triggers the production of reactive oxygen species (ROS) [4], neuropeptides (substance P, serotonin) [5] and antimicrobial peptides (cathelicidins) [6]. These will, in turn, activate cascades of other mediators which will eventually activate cytokines and chemokines, that will recruit and activate different types of leucocytes as they promote inflammation [7, 8]. The different leucocytes will be ultimately responsible for the different histopathological features of the rosacea [2, 6]. There is another interesting hypothesis which relates rosacea to neurogenic inflammation, a condition caused by damaged sensory nerves which release neuromediators [8]. There is also a broad consensus that there is an impairment of the epidermal barrier function [2, 7] which may be responsible for some of the above problems, and needs to be addressed as part of the treatment plan.

Classification and Clinical Presentation

Primary symptoms of rosacea include flushing (transient erythema), persistent erythema, telangiectasia, papules and pustules. Secondary features include as burning or stinging, plaques, dry appearance, oedema or development of phymatous rosacea and ocular involvement [9]

Treatment Protocol

Due to the less selective nature of IPL's compared to lasers, their safe use is limited to the lighter skin types which are also the most commonly affected with rosacea. The optimum wavelengths and settings to achieve treatment of facial telangiectasias have been subject of a multitude of publications [10, 11]. There cannot be any standard recommendations as the settings for one machine cannot be safely exchanged to another [12]. Papageorgiou et al. [11] treated successfully patients with a 560 nm filter single pass, 3–5 ms double pulses, at a relatively high fluence of 23–27 J/cm [2]. The American Acne and Rosacea Society includes IPL amongst the physical treatments and devices recommended for rosacea [13], and a Cochrane review [14] in 2011 concluded that IPL and lasers are likely to be effective for rosacea but the evidence to support their use is not robust enough. A more recent systematic review found only level 2 evidence to support the use of IPL in rosacea [15]. The best evidence is for a small RCT ($n = 29$) by Neuhaus et al., comparing PDL and IPL [16]. They found no difference in outcomes in the laser and IPL groups, and both were superior to the control group.

The author (MM) uses a triple pass approach in treating rosacea with IPL. The starting fluence for a Fitzpatrick skin type III patient would be 19–20 J/cm^2 with 1 J/cm^2 increments with every pass as tolerated. The treatment is delivered using the largest spot size (15x 35 mm) in three pulses with a duration of 3.5–5 ms, and pulse delays of 30 ms.

The first pass targets the more superficial capillaries and telangiectasia (up to 1 mm depth) with a wavelength of 560–590 nm. The second pulse targets the blood vessels between the papillary and reticular dermis (1–2 mm) with a wavelength of 650 nm, and the third one targets the deep dermal/ subdermal plexus (2–3 mm) with the wavelength of 695 nm.

Most patients receive 4 IPL treatments 1 month apart, with maintenance treatments once or twice every year,

IPL treatments are delivered at 90° of each other to reduce the possibility of creating a 'zebra effect' on the skin (560/590, 650 and 695 nm filters, triple pulses of 4–5 ms, with 30 ms delays, and fluence starting at 19–20 J/cm [2] as described above). Although not routinely practiced, in the authors' own experience combining low fluence long pulsed Nd:YAG laser and subpurpuric PDL treatments to IPL treatments can improve outcomes in patients with severe flushing and telangiectatic rosacea.

Treatment end-point is generally erythema which will take up to 2–3 days to resolve.

Strict sun protection measures and, sun avoidance are essential to the success of the treatment. Generally, most patients will require one to two IPL/laser treatments per year for maintenance.

Photorejuvenation

Signs and symptoms of photoageing include:

- Fine and coarse wrinkles
- Epidermal and dermal atrophy
- Dyspigmentation, causing some areas of irregular, mottled hyperpigmentation, lentigines and other patches of hypopigmentation
- Sallow colour
- Rough, coarse skin leading to solar elastosis
- Loss of elasticity and sagging
- Telangiectasias on cheeks and nose
- Blemishes: benign seborrhoeic keratosis, premalignant actinic keratosis, and malignant pigmented and non-pigmented skin cancers

Not all of these signs of photoageing can be treated with non-ablative options such as IPLs.

IPL are useful in treatment of:

- Telangiectases
- Pigmentation, e.g. lentigenes and ephelides
- Fine wrinkles
- Dull skin
- Uneven complexion
- Combinations of the above

For superficial pigmented and vascular lesions in skin Fitzpatrick type III the authors use 560 nm filter, double 3.5–4 ms pulses with a pulse delay of 15–20 ms. Fluence starts at 14 J/cm^2 up to 20 J/cm^2 for the larger spot size 15 × 35 mm. Deeper lesions will benefit from using the 590 nm filter, also using double pulses of 3.5–4 ms with a pulse delay of 15–20 ms with fluence range of 18 J/cm [2] to 22 J/cm [2]. Stacking up two passes, one with each filter, using lower fluence and increasing patient comfort is beneficial as there is some evidence that using different filters helps to reduce fluence, need for cooling and number of treatments [17]. For treating difficult to reach areas such as the sides of the nose, smaller spot sizes like the 8 × 15 or the round 6 mm may be more appropriate, and those settings will need adjusting accordingly.

Very superficial lesions not responding to the above settings can be treated with the 515 nm filter, single 3–4 ms single or double pulses, 15–25 ms delay and fluence of 14–20 J/cm [2] for the 8 × 15 or 28–30 J/cm [2] for the round 6 mm spot size.

There is some evidence of morphological changes of the skin treated with IPL: in one study [18], histological analysis showed that both type 1 and type 3 collagens increased whereas the elastin content decreased but elastin fibres were more neatly arranged after IPL treatments. This explains the clinical improvement in skin texture which varies from subtle to more marked.

Treatment endpoints vary depending on the target lesions. Vascular lesions may blanch, darken, become redder or even bruise. Pigmented lesions may darken if they are very superficial, or develop a red hue if they are deeper. Around the eyelids, one can expect more bruising and swelling, and patients need to be warned when treating lesions close to that area. At these settings, very little downtime is expected and most patients should be able to return to work within 24 h. Most people will need four treatments 1 month apart.

Photofractional treatment for photoageing is the term for combined, same day sequential use of IPL and non-ablative fractional laser resurfacing to reduce the signs of ageing.

IPL can be combined with non-ablative fractional 1565 nm fibre laser using a protocol recently described by Knight and Kautz [19]. For skin type III, a single pass with the 560 nm filter, 16–18 J/cm^2, double pulse 3–5 ms, with 15–20 ms delay [19]. This will be followed by quickly removing the gel and drying the skin before proceeding to perform the non- ablative fractional laser, at parameters appropriate for the condition to treated.

Other Options: Notch Filters

Notch filters, band-stop or band-rejection filters, are designed to transmit most wavelengths with little intensity loss while attenuating light within a specific wavelength range (the stop band) to a very low level.

Notch filters are useful in applications where one needs to block light from a broadband light source. The rationale in the case of vascular filters is to target the areas of the spectrum where the absorption of those wavelengths by the target chromophore, HbO_2, is maximum, minimising the waste of energy to target those regions of the spectrum where we know that the absorption is minimal. It transforms the broadband IPL into a concentrated or narrowband, dual band IPL: 530–650 nm and 900–1200, targeting the main 2 peaks of absorption. The energy is delivered over 2 pulses. A recent retrospective review by Gao et al., found the result of the treatments comparable to PDL and superior to other IPL cut off filters [20].

Treatment of Leg Veins

Attempting the treatment of any superficial leg veins without dealing first with any underlying varicosities is one of the most common causes of treatment failure. Treatment of symptomatic chronic venous insufficiency, from heaviness, aching, and other symptoms to skin ulceration, should only be carried out by vascular experts.

The layered nature of the target veins makes essential the development of a combined treatment protocol, which will vary depending on local availability of equipment and expertise, but at the least should include IPL, long pulse Nd: YAG and microsclerotherapy.

Lasers and IPLs are useful in the treatment of:

- Red/blue spider veins.
- Reticular veins—easily visible small blue veins (less than 3 mm diameter), not associated with valvular incompetence of superficial venous trunks (e.g. long or short saphenous veins).

Treatment options for the superficial veins include: Laser/IPL, and Microsclerotherapy/ Sclerotherapy. Microsclerotherapy is the treatment of choice for reticular feeder veins.

Smaller veins can then be targeted with the long pulsed Nd: YAG [21]. The settings used vary depending on the individual targets,

The most superficial veins can be targeted with different lasers, including PDL, LP Nd: YAG, KTP, or IPL. In the author's experience, IPL is less selective but more comfortable than the LP Nd: YAG, safer than KTP and as effective as the PDL. IPL is very effective in clearing vessels less than 1 mm in diameter [22]. IPL can also be used to deal with some of the complications of microsclerotherapy like matting and hyperpigmentation [22].

Following treatment, patients are advised to wear support tights. We recommend walking for 10–30 min a day but to avoid strenuous exercise, hot baths, saunas and any other activities that produce vasodilation for 2 weeks. Patients should continue to wear tights during the day for the same duration. Regular exercise, a high-fibre diet, and maintaining a healthy weight are recommended long term to help discourage new visible vein formation.

Photoepilation

Laser photoepilation has been discussed in detail in Chap. 4. IPL has a role to play as it is based on the same principle of selective photothermolysis to damage the tissue in the hair follicle, the bulge or both, whilst protecting the surrounding tissue. There are a small number of quality papers documenting the efficacy of the treatment compared to lasers. Some like Cameron et al. used a split face study to compare a 755 nm Alexandrite with a 625–1100 nm IPL [23]. There was no statistically significant difference in the hair number reduction but patient preference was for the laser based on the experience. McGill et al. found significant differences in patients with PCOS in favour of an Alexandrite laser but the settings used for the IPL were too conservative in this author's opinion [24]. A systematic review in 2006 found that there was not enough evidence of long term effect of hair removal with IPL, but this is only related to the very low number of quality papers analysed, compared to the larger number for ruby, alexandrite, diode and Nd:YAG lasers [25]. Safety data has always matched the clinical outcomes in most studies, but there has been always the concern of using broadband light in skin of colour, as experience tells us that there is a higher risk of side effects. A recent systematic review by Dorgham and Dorgham found that the safety profile of IPL, diode and alexandrite lasers is very similar for skin types III–VI [26].

We have an alternative to the in-office systems, as some patients prefer the convenience and reduced cost of using home devices. Alster and Karzi performed a study of one of the home systems, and found satisfactory hair count reduction at 6 months in some body areas, but longer term safety and efficacy studies are needed about these devices [27].

Difficult to Treat Conditions

Melasma

Melasma is an acquired hypermelanosis affecting the epidermis and/or dermis in sun-exposed areas, particularly the face. The areas of pigmentation are asymmetric, irregular and on dermoscopy, look reticulated. The pathogenesis of melasma has not been fully elucidated; however, there are some factors which have been proposed to play a role in the development of melasma: chronic ultraviolet (UV) exposure causing solar elastosis, female hormone stimulation and predisposed genetic background [28]. It has been demonstrated that as well as the melanocytic component, there is a dermal component with fibroblasts and endothelial cells which is also part of the pathophysiology of the disease [29]. Melasma is probably the most complex hyperpigmentary disorder, and its management requires particular expertise and a multifaceted approach, especially because it is prone to frequent relapse despite successful clearance.

The gold standard treatment for melasma is topical bleaching agents, in particular Kligman's solution [30]. High relapse rates and darkening of melasma with laser/IPL devices is not uncommon, therefore, these devices should only be considered after topical depigmenting agents and peelings have failed [30]. IPLs, laser toning using long pulse Nd:YAG laser are used by some in refractory melasma.

Post-Inflammatory Hyperpigmentation (PIH)

PIH is a reactive acquired hypermelanosis resulting from cutaneous inflammation or injury. Depending on the cause and the duration of progression, the proportion of epidermal and dermal melanin changes and significantly influences the response to the treatment. Although many treatment modalities have been tried for PIH, its management remains a challenge due to its recurrent and refractory nature [30].

Early treatment of the dermatosis or insult causing PIH is important for resolution and to stop further accumulation of pigment in the tissue. The treatment of choice should cause no irritation to the skin to avoid exacerbation of the pigmentation. Topical treatments such as those for melasma are the first-line. IPL and laser can eventually improve some PIH but they still carry the risk of inducing or exacerbating PIH [31]. Test patch in a small area before further application of IPL on the whole lesion is recommended.

Pre-Treatment Preparation and Precautions: Post-Treatment Care Advice and Plan

The preparation of the skin and advice to the patients before any IPL treatment is very similar to that prior to any other laser treatment (Including LP- Nd: YAG):

Contraindications for Treatment

- Sun exposure one month before treatment.
- Recent intake of oral retinoids e.g. isotretinoin—advice to wait 6 months post treatment or as long as the local policy advices.
- Acute skin infection.
- Recent self-tanning, spray tanning products or chemical peels on the area to be treated.
- Fitzpatrick skin type VI. Types IV and V need caution.

The **preparation prior to treatment** involves the following procedures:

- Diagnosis of condition. Do not proceed without a clear indication to treatment.
- Informed consent involving explanation of procedure, alternatives, benefits and risks.
- Removal of all makeup, perfume and sun cream from the area to be treated.
- Pre-procedure photography should be carried out in all cases.
- Adequate eye protection
- Use of chilled IPL coupling gel.
- Carry out a patch test for every set of parameters used and if the same settings will be used in different areas, test them in every area. This should be done at least a week before the treatment, for certain indications even longer intervals are recommended.

During the Treatment

- Apply a thick layer (1–2 mm) of IPL coupling gel, avoid the use of ultrasound gel as this has a much lighter formulation which doesn't disperse the heat produced as easily.
- Make sure that the IPL tip is in contact with the skin to benefit from the cooling effect that very often is built-in the handpiece. The pressure has to be minimal for treatment of vascular conditions, but can be firmer when dealing with pigmentation as this displaces haemoglobin, the competing chromophore.
- Use chilled air cooling throughout the procedure as it provides a more comfortable experience for the patients. This should be used in addition to contact cooling [32].
- Intermittent visual inspection of the treated area and patient feedback are important to ensure safe end points and adequate tissue response from treatment.

Following the Treatment

- Continue cooling the skin for as long as needed.
- Extra comfort can be obtained by applying soothing lotions. As they are water-based, there is a degree of evaporation that will enhance the cooling effect.
- Once a patient is comfortable, apply sun cream to facial or exposed areas before they go.
- When treating body areas, and especially when treating leg veins it is a very important to request that patients bring lose clothes and light footwear.
- Chilled *Aloe vera* gel applied in the first 24–48 h can be very soothing for the treated skin. *Aloe vera* can also be used for the duration of the treatment as the moisturiser.
- Patients should avoid:
  - Sun or sunbed exposure to the treated area for at a minimum of 4 weeks after treatment.

- Self-tanning products throughout the entire course of treatment.
- Chemical peels on the area to be treated for 30 days prior to treatment and throughout the entire course of treatment.
- Application of gels, oils, deodorants or perfumes to the area for at least 48 h after to treatment.
- Saunas, steam rooms, Jacuzzis, hot baths/showers or take excessive exercise or swimming for 48 h after treatment.
- Make-up (except mineral powder) for 48 h after treatment.
- Touch, pick or scratch the area

• Sun protection of at least SPF30 must be worn daily on the treated, exposed area for a minimum of 4 weeks after treatment.

Complications of IPL

As IPL emits a range of wavelengths it often induces undesired absorption by haemoglobin and melanin despite the appropriate filter. The nonspecific heating of epidermal melanin is the reason for most side effects [33], which fortunately are very rare. The best way to prevent side effects is to carry out patch tests. Most common undesirable effects post IPL treatment include:

- Hypo- or depigmentation
- Burns, erosions, crusts
- Infections
- Post-inflammatory hyperpigmentation
- Scarring—both hypertrophic and keloid scars

Case Studies

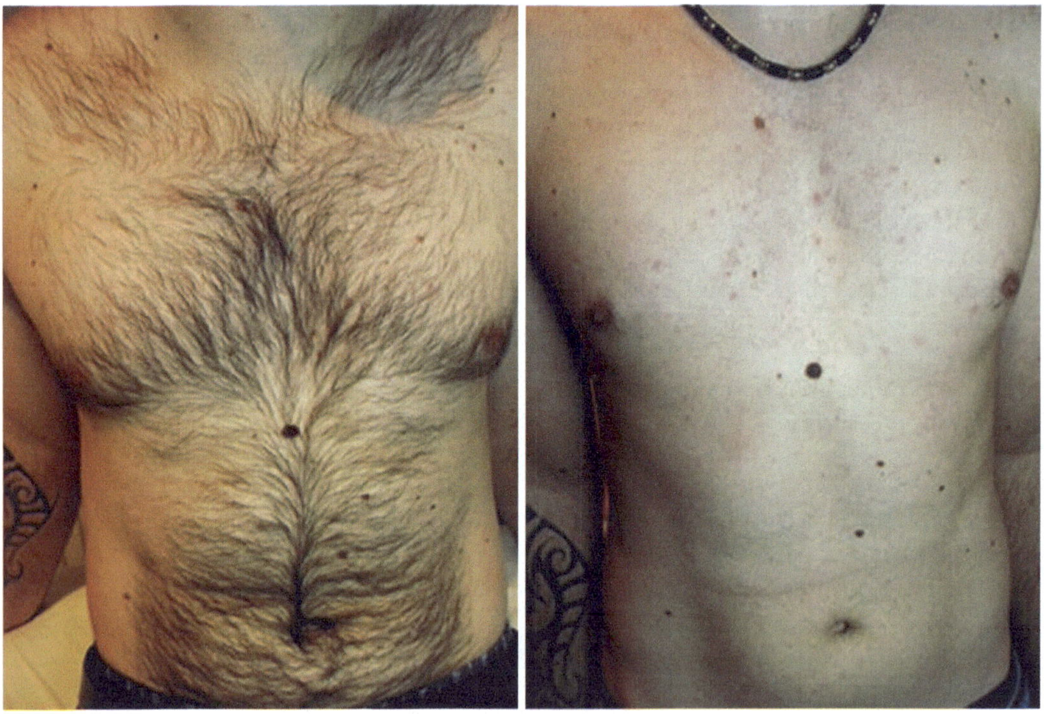

A 25 year old male before and after six hair removal treatments with an IPL system. Courtesy of Laser Skin Solutions, Bournemouth.

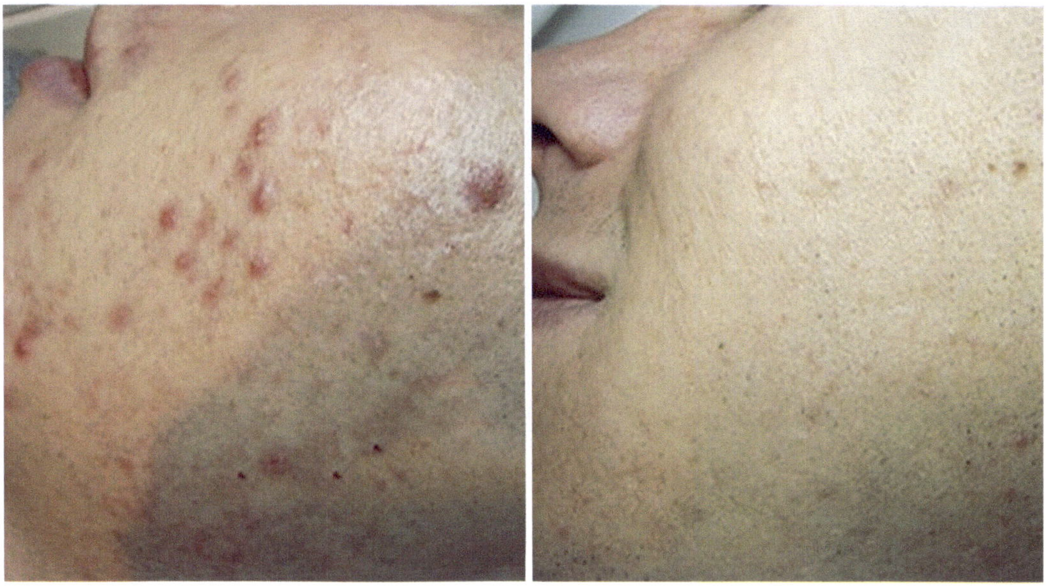

Improvement in inflammatory lesions in acne 22 year old male before and after four treatments with an IPL system. (Courtesy of Laser Skin Solutions, Bournemouth).

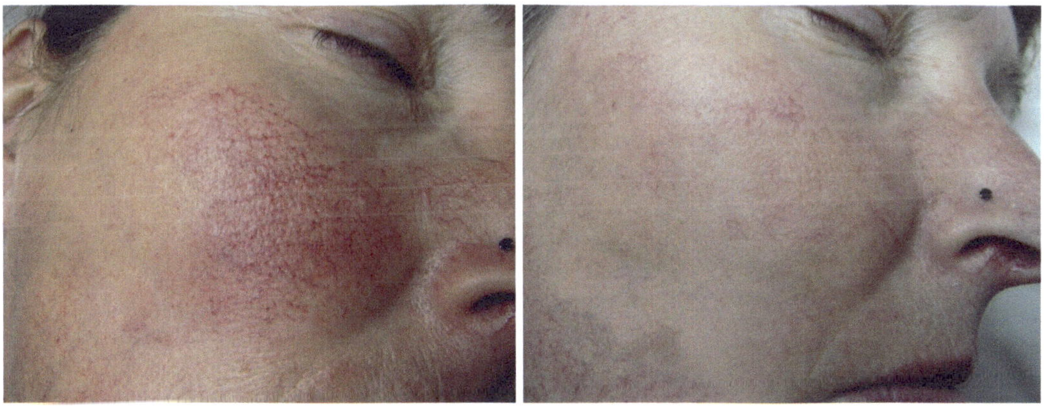

A 40 year old woman presented with facial telangiectasia that she was finding increasingly difficult to cover with make-up. She had four IPL treatments at 6–8 week intervals. (Courtesy of Laser Skin Solutions, Bournemouth).

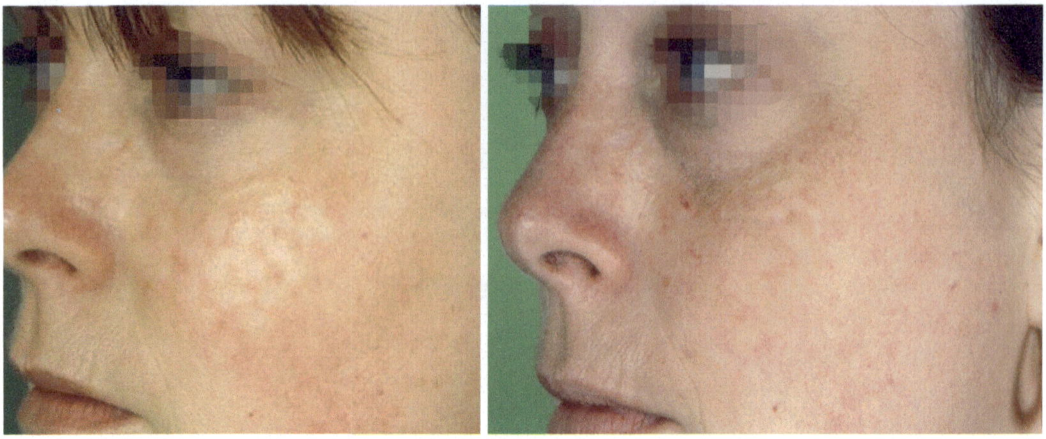

Spotted effect apparent on cheeks after one treatment with pulsed dye laser. Good improvement seen following one IPL treatment.

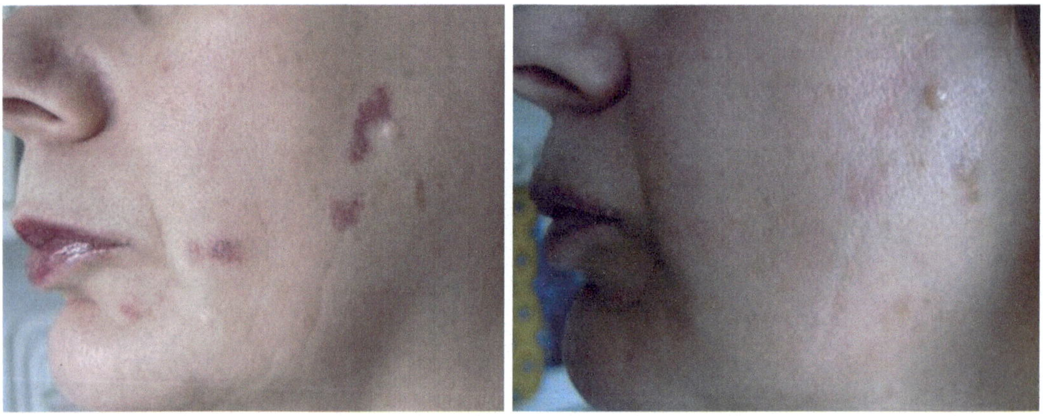

Facial port wine stain treated with IPL. Before and after four treatments. Results were obtained without the purpura typical of pulse dye laser treatment.

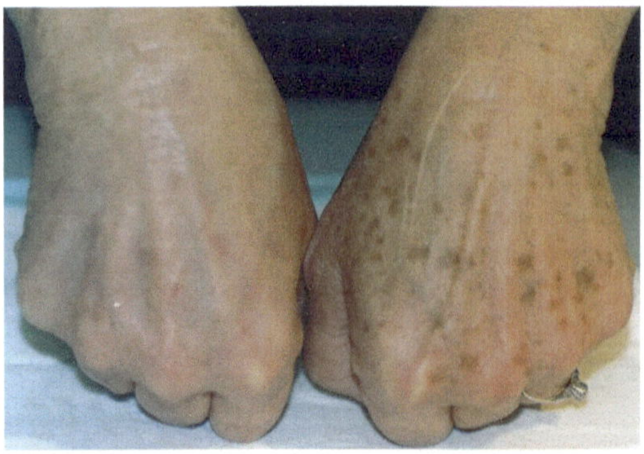

Lentigines on right hand treated with one session of IPL. Left hand subsequently treated with the same results.

References

1. Gether L, Overgaard LK, Egeberg A, Thyssen JP. Incidence and prevalence of rosacea: a systematic review and meta-analysis. Br J Dermatol. 2018;179(2):282–9.
2. Yamasaki K, Gallo RL. Rosacea as a disease of cathelicidins and skin innate immunity. J Investig Dermatol Symp Proc. 2011;15(1):12–5.
3. Gravina AG, Federico A, Ruocco E, Lo Schiavo A, Masarone M, Tuccillo C, Peccerillo F, Miranda A, Romano L, de Sio C, de Sio I. *Helicobacter pylori* infection but not small intestinal bacterial overgrowth may play a pathogenic role in rosacea. United Eur Gastroenterol J. 2015;3(1):17–24.
4. Baz K, Cimen MB, Kokturk A, Aslan G, Ikizoglu G, Demirseren DD, Kanik A, Atik U. Plasma reactive oxygen species activity and antioxidant potential levels in rosacea patients: correlation with seropositivity to *Helicobacter pylori*. Int J Dermatol. 2004;43(7):494–7.
5. Powell FC, Corbally N, Powell D. Substance P and rosacea. J Am Acad Dermatol. 1993;28(1):132–3.
6. Schauber J, Gallo RL. Antimicrobial peptides and the skin immune defense system. J Allergy Clin Immunol. 2008;122(2):261–6.
7. Aroni K, Tsagroni E, Lazaris AC, Patsouris E, Agapitos E. Rosacea: a clinicopathological approach. Dermatology. 2004;209(3):177–82.
8. Schwab VD, Sulk M, Seeliger S, Nowak P, Aubert J, Mess C, Rivier M, Carlavan I, Rossio P, Metze D, Buddenkotte J. Neurovascular and neuroimmune aspects in the pathophysiology of rosacea. J Investig Dermatol Symp Proc. 2011;15(1):53–62.
9. Wilkin J, Dahl M, Detmar M, Drake L, Liang MH, Odom R, Powell F. Standard grading system for rosacea: report of the National Rosacea Society Expert Committee on the classification and staging of rosacea. J Am Acad Dermatol. 2004;50(6):907–12.
10. Schroeter CA, Haaf-von Below S, Neumann HA. Effective treatment of rosacea using intense pulsed light systems. Dermatol Surg. 2005;31(10):1285–9.
11. Papageorgiou P, Clayton W, Norwood S, Chopra S, Rustin M. Treatment of rosacea with intense pulsed light: significant improvement and long-lasting results. Br J Dermatol. 2008;159(3):628–32.
12. Hare McCoppin HH, Goldberg DJ. Laser treatment of facial telangiectases: an update. Dermatol Surg. 2010;36(8):1221–30.
13. Tanghetti E, Del Rosso JQ, Thiboutot D, Gallo R, Webster G, Eichenfield LF, Stein-Gold L, Berson D, Zaenglein A. American Acne & Rosacea Society. Consensus recommendations from the American Acne & Rosacea Society on the Management of Rosacea, part 4: A status report on physical modalities and devices. Cutis. 2014;93(2):71–6.
14. Van Zuuren EJ, Kramer SF, Carter BR, Graber MA, Fedorowicz Z. Effective and evidence-based management strategies for rosacea: summary of a Cochrane systematic review. Br J Dermatol. 2011;165(4):760–81.
15. Wat H, Wu DC, Rao J, Goldman MP. Application of intense pulsed light in the treatment of dermatologic disease: a systematic review. Dermatol Surg. 2014;40(4):359–77.
16. Neuhaus IM, Zane LT, Tope WD. Comparative efficacy of nonpurpuragenic pulsed dye laser and intense pulsed light for erythematotelangiectatic rosacea. Dermatol Surg. 2009;35(6):920–8.
17. Bjerring P, Christiansen K, Troilius A, Dierickx C. Facial photo rejuvenation using two different intense pulsed light (IPL) wavelength bands. Lasers Surg Med. 2004;34(2):120–6.
18. Feng Y, Zhao J, Gold MH. Skin rejuvenation in Asian skin: the analysis of clinical effects and basic mechanisms of intense pulsed light. J Drugs Dermatol. 2008;7(3):273–9.
19. Knight JM, Kautz G. Sequential facial skin rejuvenation with intense pulsed light and non-ablative fractionated laser resurfacing in Fitzpatrick skin type II–IV patients: a prospective multicenter analysis. Lasers Surg Med. 2019;51(2):141–9.
20. Gao L, Qu H, Gao N, Li K, Dang E, Tan W, Wang G. A retrospective analysis for facial telangiectasia treatment using pulsed dye laser and intense pulsed light configured with different wavelength bands. J Cosmet Dermatol. 2020;19(1):88–92.
21. Lumenis® Wittig C. Leg veins – Long-pulsed (LP) Nd:YAG Guidelines/CD-1008960 Rev A. 2017.
22. Kunishige JH, Goldberg LH, Friedman PM. Laser therapy for leg veins. Clin Dermatol. 2007;25(5):454–61.
23. Cameron H, Ibbotson SH, Dawe RS, Ferguson J, Moseley H. Within-patient right-left blinded comparison of diode (810 nm) laser therapy and intense pulsed light therapy for hair removal. Lasers Med Sci. 2008;23(4):393–7.
24. McGill DJ, Hutchison C, McKenzie E, McSherry E, Mackay IR. A randomised, split-face comparison of facial hair removal with the alexandrite laser and intense pulsed light system. Lasers Surg Med. 2007;39(10):767 72.
25. Haedersdal M, Wulf HC. Evidence-based review of hair removal using lasers and light sources. J Eur Acad Dermatol Venereol. 2006;20(1):9–20.
26. Dorgham NA, Dorgham DA. Lasers for reduction of unwanted hair in skin of colour: a systematic review and meta-analysis. J Eur Acad Dermatol Venereol. 2020; https://doi.org/10.1111/jdv.15995.
27. Alster TS, Tanzi EL. Effect of a novel low-energy pulsed-light device for home-use hair removal. Dermatol Surg. 2009;35(3):483–9.
28. Kwon SH, Na JI, Choi JY, Park KC. Melasma: updates and perspectives. Exp Dermatol. 2018;28:704–8.
29. Passeron T, Picardo M. Melasma, a photoaging disorder. Pigment Cell Melanoma Res. 2018;31:461–5.

30. Passeron T, Genedy R, Salah L, Fusade T, Kositratna G, Laubach HJ, Marini L, Badawi A. Laser treatment of hyperpigmented lesions: position statement of the European Society of Laser in dermatology. J Eur Acad Dermatol Venereol. 2019;33:987–1005.
31. Agbai O, Hamzavi I, Jagdeo J. Laser treatments for postinflammatory hyperpigmentation: a systematic review. JAMA Dermatol. 2017;153:199–206.
32. Chang CD, Reinisch L, Biesman BS. Analysis of epidermal protection using cold air versus chilled sapphire window with water or gel during 810 nm diode laser application. Laser Surg Med. 2003;32(2):129–36.
33. Stangl S, Hadshiew I, Kimmig W. Side effects and complications using intense pulsed light (IPL) sources. Med Laser Appl. 2008;23(1):15–20.

Cosmeceuticals 10

Rhonda Meys

Abbreviations

AHAs	Alpha-hydroxy acids
BHAs	Beta-hydroxy acids
FDA	Food and Drug Administration
HA	Hyaluronic acid
IPD	Immediate pigment darkening
IR	Infrared radiation
MMP	Metalloproteinases
NAG	*N*-acetyl glucosamine
NCAP	*N*-acetyl-4-*S*-cysteaminylphenol
NMSC	Non-melanoma skin cancer
PIH	Post inflammatory hyperpigmentation
PPD	Persistent pigment darkening
ROS	Reactive oxygen species
SA	Salicylic acid
SPF	Sun protection factor
TC	Triple combination
UV	Ultraviolent-A and -B
VL	Visible light

Introduction

Laser procedures are becoming increasingly common in dermatological practice. The beauty and cosmeceutical industries are worth around £400 billion globally, and around 10% of this is purely cosmeceutical products [1]. The vast majority of individuals globally, including men, purchase skin creams with the aim of improving the appearance their skin. Combining the two together, there is a huge potential emerging role for 'active' cosmeceutical formulations to be used in conjunction with dermatological procedures, including lasers. Dermatologists are frequently asked to advise on skincare products, and it is important we are able to direct patients to effective products with an evidence base for their use.

It is essential to discuss topical products pre-laser with patients. Optimising topical regimes before treatment can be useful "practice" to reduce post-laser complications and maintain the skin after a procedure. The application of ablative lasers such as carbon dioxide, Erbuim:YAG lasers and non-ablative fractional laser in many situations can induce open "channels" in the skin thereby presenting an opportunity of laser-assisted drug delivery of pharmacologically active compounds into the skin. There is 'no' evidence for the use of cosmeceutical agents in this manner [2], but this is nonetheless widespread in dermatological laser practice worldwide.

This chapter will consider cosmeceutical compounds that might be helpful in laser practice: pre-treatment, immediately after laser, as skin maintenance post-treatment laser procedures and as useful post-laser anti-ageing products. The available evidence on sun protection with a particular

R. Meys (✉)
Royal Free London NHS Foundation Trust, Pond Street, London, UK

Dermamed Clinic, Wafi Mall, Dubai, UAE

V. Madan (ed.), *Practical Introduction to Laser Dermatology*,
https://doi.org/10.1007/978-3-030-46451-6_10

reference to commercially available sunscreens will be presented. We will consider some cosmeceutical definitions and the foundation of recommending a skin care regime that is appropriate for each patient, including moisturisers and cleansers. The cosmeceutical ingredients have been classified on composition and mode of action: retinoids, peeling agents, depigmenting agents, anti-oxidants, nanoparticles and newer cosmeceutical peptides. These will be reviewed with their evidence base.

Part 1

Sun Protection: The Evidence

Sun protection is an undeniably vital part of pre- and post-laser care for our patients. Most importantly, laser procedures may heat or damage the epidermis with a consequent risk of dyspigmentation. Post inflammatory hyper-pigmentation (PIH) can be heightened by sunlight exposure. Therefore, it is essential that sun protection is always discussed pre-procedure. Pre-existing pigmentary conditions may be exacerbated or precipitated by laser procedures—for example melasma (that may be very subtle), PIH or lichen planus. Such conditions, undiagnosed, carry a high risk of a poor outcome and should be identified to avoid patient dissatisfaction and medico-legal pitfalls. Additionally, sunscreens reduce UV penetration into the skin and retard ageing. Therefore, this is an important motivating factor to highlight to patients who undergo laser procedures to improve age-related deterioration of their skin texture and colour.

In Europe sunscreens are classed as cosmetics, which means that a wide range of UV filters are on the market and there is a relatively short lead time to market for new agents. In the USA they, have until recently, been treated as over the counter drugs by the Food and Drug Administration (FDA), meaning approvals are more vigorous, take longer and are more expensive to obtain.

Sun exposure is correlated to the risk of non-melanoma skin cancer (NMSC) and melanoma [3, 4]. Dogma dictates that dermatologists advise patients to wear sunscreen, despite limited robust scientific evidence that its application directly reduces the incidence of cancer. The primary hurdle is that it takes several decades to generate tumours and prospective studies require significant numbers of subjects and extended follow-up. However, there is good evidence that UVB and UVA are carcinogenic [5].

The best evidence that sunscreen reduces skin cancer is found from a series of publications from a study conducted in Nambour, Australia [6–8]. The study was a randomised controlled trial that commenced in 2003 (n = 1621) and compared several skin cancer outcomes in (1) one group of individuals who were instructed to apply sunscreen daily versus (2) a control group who were allowed 'ordinary use' of sunscreen, in a geographic location with high ambient solar irradiation. All other sun avoidance behaviour was allowed in both groups. Over 10 years, a reduction in the melanoma incidence of 50%–75% was observed. A reduction in actinic keratoses were observed in the first 2 years, but not in the subsequent 2 years. There was a 35% reduction in the incidence of squamous cell cancers but there was no reduction in basal cell cancers. In this cohort of lighter skinned individuals there was no reduction in vitamin D levels observed due to sunscreen use (or wearing a hat, using an umbrella), tested in the summer. However, lower vitamin D levels were found in individuals who had naturally lower levels of sun exposure *and* tended to stay in the shade [9].

The same group also quite elegantly demonstrated that the application of sunscreen resulted in a reduction in the visible signs of ageing, as measured by microtopography (silicone imprints of the skin on the dorsal hand) [10]. They documented an objective reduction in skin ageing of 24% over a period of 4.5 years, with a small increase in the frequency of sunscreen application; 2/3 of individuals in the "sunscreen group" applied it >3–4 times/week compared with only 1/3 of individuals in the control ("ordinary use") group applying >3–4 times/week.

Not All SPF 30+ Sunscreens Are Equal

Sunlight consists of four types of potentially damaging irradiation that activate skin pigmentation and induce photo-ageing: Ultraviolent (UV)-A and -B, visible light (VL) and Infrared radiation (IR). After exposure to UVA (400–320 nm), human skin undergoes immediate pigment darkening (IPD) that disappears within 2 h. Afterwards, persistent pigment darkening (PPD) is observed. UVB (280–320 nm) also causes burning, IPD, delayed tanning and thickening of the epidermis and dermis. Both UVA and UVB contribute to photoageing [5]. The pigmentary potential of VL has become apparent more recently, and this has changed how we think about photoprotection. In one study, a single exposure to VL (400–700 nm) caused darker and more sustained pigmentation than a single UVA exposure [11]. This was only the case for individuals of Fitzpatrick skin type 4 and above. However, others have proposed that multiple exposures might be required to prime lighter skin (Fitzpatrick skin types 1–3) to produce excess pigmentation and that this may be partially responsible for blotchy pigmentation observed in sun damaged individuals [12].

In addition to UVA, UVB and VR, IR might also contribute to pigmentation and photodamage. IR consists of near IR or IRA (700–1400 nm), IRB (1400–3000 nm) and IRC (3000 nm–1 mm). Biologically, IRA is the most important as it is abundant (comprising 30% of sunlight) and penetrates below the deep dermis [13]. There is emerging evidence that near IR causes the generation of reactive oxygen species (ROS) and activation of metalloproteinases (MMP), resulting in collagen degradation, that is seen as coarse wrinkling in animal models and human skin [13]. IR *may* also be involved in the generation of pigmentation but definitive evidence is lacking. In animal studies (guinea pigs) it is clear that IR induces pigmentation [14]. Although several studies in human skin have documented pigmentation after IR irradiation, the lamps used in these studies emitted *both* VL and IR [15, 16]. However, several experts have proposed anecdotally that recalcitrant melasma in night workers is likely to be IR related (for example in bakers) [17].

Sun Protection Factor (SPF) is a widely used in vivo testing system that gives a sunscreen rating for UVB. However, many sunscreens that protect against UVA are rated by in vitro scales. Sunscreens labelled as "Broad spectrum" (meaning that they absorb UVB and UVA) or have a high star rating (the Boots method) are protective against UVA. Although this label provides some indication of UVA protection, unfortunately neither of these labels correlate with the efficacy of a product in vivo and do not take into account its photostability. The UVA-PF (scale from 0 to 28, or PA+/++/+++) is significantly more accurate; this is based on in vivo protection against persistent pigment darkening (PPD) [18].

The situation for VL and IR is more complex. There is no standardised rating system for either of these wavelengths. However, products containing the opaque mineral blocks such as titanium dioxide, zinc oxide and iron (ferric) oxides are photostable and reflect and scatter all light; they protect against both UV and visible light. But mineral blocks are less palatable to many patients, being thicker white or brown-orange. With respect to IR there is no rating system despite 'novel' patented compounds promoted by several manufacturers that claim to protect against IR. The addition of antioxidants to sunscreens is a relatively new phenomenon. In combination with a photostable mineral block in a topical sunscreen, antioxidants may be helpful to reduce the formation of ROS and cytokines and MMPs in vitro, as a second defence; this may also be the case for other wavelengths [19].

Practical Sun Protection Advice

Excessive sunlight exposure can therefore reverse the beneficial effects of antiageing laser treatments and result in PIH. Advising patients regarding effective post procedure sun protection is paramount. This should form a two-part explanation in the consultation process. Firstly, sun avoidance advice is essential. It is important to discuss the concept that even "normal" sub-erythemal levels of ill-timed sun exposure may trigger pigmentation (for example in melasma or PIH), lasting several months. *Any* outdoor sunlight exposure should be avoided during peak times of ambient UVB (10–4 pm). UVA avoidance is also important for pigmentation also (exposure through water, in a car or behind glass and early/late in the day). Limiting any exposure through physical barriers such as shade, hats and clothing is also helpful if patients must be outside.

Sunscreen is best considered a secondary defence, to limit skin cellular damage level by the few incident rays that may have escaped primary methods of protection. Sunscreen should be applied fastidiously and daily, first thing in the morning, aiming to use 5 ml for the face and neck and reapplied 2–3 hourly during exposure. Many patients will still tan significantly through sunscreen. The author proposes (from professional experience) that there are several reasons for this: that sunscreen is only partially protective in vivo, that most individuals apply significantly less than the recommended amount, and that sunscreen is not reapplied correctly. Many patients fail to take into consideration the level of UVA exposure through car windows, or on cloudy days. For example "wind burn" on a cloudy day is predominantly UVA related. Clearly the level of diligence required on a daily basis is related to the "sunniness" of the country of residence. Year-round strict adherence is required in (for example) Southern Europe, Australia or New Zealand whilst a more slightly relaxed approach can be taken to countries in Northern Europe in the winter months (November to March), bearing in mind that there will still be significant amounts of ambient UVA in the winter. However, it is advisable for post-procedure patients to wear sunscreen daily in case they are caught out by a sunny day in winter. Ideally application of sunscreen should become a year-round part of the laser patient's daily routine.

Sunscreen Concerns

There are several concerns regarding sunscreens: cosmetic, safety and environmental. Mineral sunscreen ingredients (such as zinc oxide and titanium dioxide) are photostable and last longer but have the disadvantage of being chalky white. Micronised minerals are slightly more palatable and nano-sized particles are not white at all (for example in "invisible zinc" products). There is concern that nano mineral particles might scatter UV light into keratinocytes and dermal tissue rather than reflecting it, or their small size means that they penetrate through the skin barrier. However, coatings on nanoparticles are designed to avoid the scatter of ROS into keratinocytes and absorption of particles into the circulation [13]. Chemical sunscreens degrade on exposure to UV, meaning that they are depleted with time. Sunscreen-related contact hypersensitivity and irritation, are most often associated with oxybenzone and cinnamates (octinoxate, cinoxate) and occur in ~1.5% of regular sunscreen users [20]. After 2021, the sale of sunscreens containing oxybenzone and octinoxate will be prohibited in Hawaii after concerns that these compounds contribute to bleaching of coral reefs. Other chemical filters include avobenzone, mexoryl and a wide variety of 'novel' chemical UV filters are found in sunscreens in the UK and Europe. Additionally, recent studies have raised concerns that chemical sunscreens *can* be systemically absorbed through normal skin when full body applications are used four times daily [21]. Although the authors indicated that the results should not discourage sunscreen use, the effect of this in the short term or long term is not known.

Which Sunscreen?

A good sunscreen has a high SPF (30+) and UVA-PF rating (>8 or +++). Products containing visible light protection, such as those containing mineral iron oxide, are advisable for post-laser patients. The brown-orange colour may be acceptable as a 'tinted' sunscreen for women that can act as a makeup foundation. Men generally prefer lighter, oil free preparations or very lightly tinted liquids. Some other important factors to consider when recommending sunscreens include the vehicle—liquids, gels or creams—often sunscreens are too sticky for acne prone or oily skin and the whiteness of the product may limit patient uptake. There is limited evidence that applying topical antioxidants under sunscreens is useful (see also below); theoretically the presence of an antioxidant on sun exposed skin might 'mop up' free radicals that penetrate despite the presence of sunscreen. Examples of some useful products are found in Fig. 10.1.

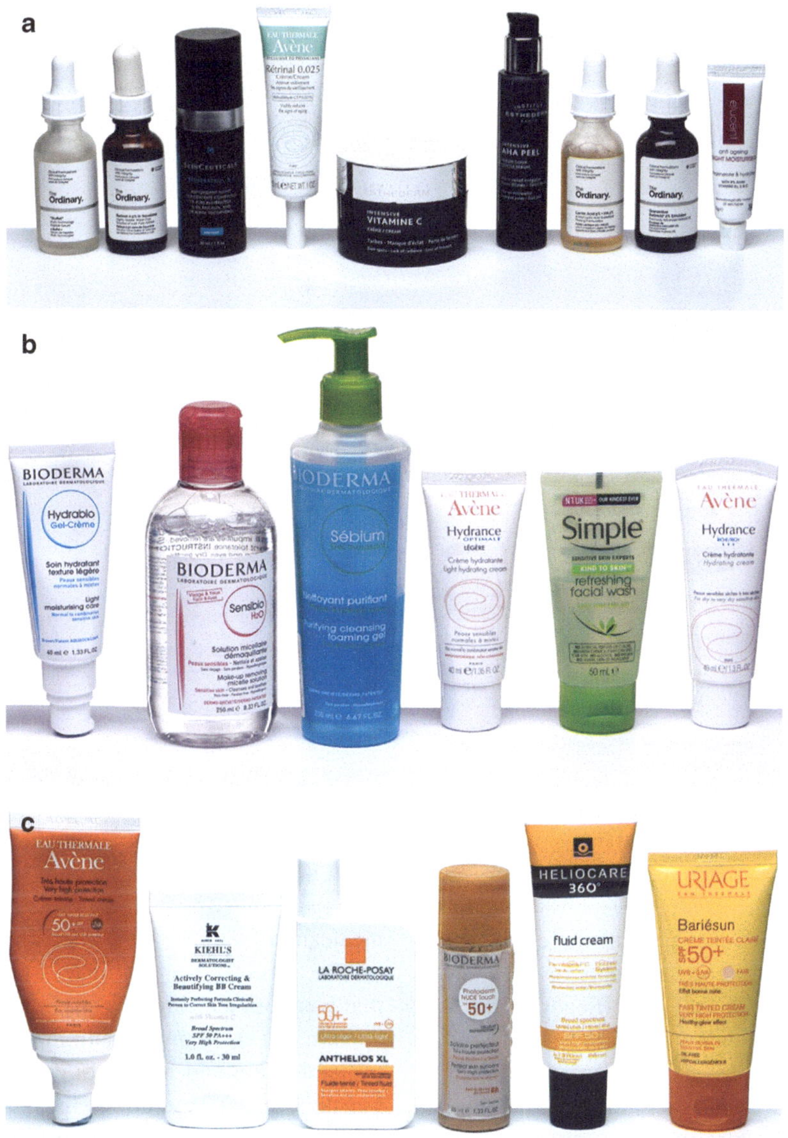

Fig. 10.1 Examples of helpful cosmeceutical products. (**a**) Retinols, alpha-hydroxyacids (AHAs), and anti-oxidants—examples of over the counter products. From left to right: "Buffet" (includes multiple peptides including Matrixyl 3000 and hyaluronic acid); 0.5% retinol in squalene; Resveratrol BE (anti-oxidants, vitamin E); RetrinAL 0.025% (available in several strengths of retinaldehyde 0.1, 0.05 and 0.025—the higher the better); Vitamin C cream (depigmenting, anti-oxidant); AHA peel (containing glycolic acid, citric acid, salicylic acid and used as day or night cream); Lactic acid 5% with hyaluronic acid 2%; Granactive retinoid 2% emulsion (contains retinoic acid ester; minimal side effects with low potency); AHA containing night cream (with vitamins and antioxidants). (**b**) Cleansers and Moisturisers. (i) Examples of acne-friendly 'light' non-comedogenic moisturisers Hydrabio and Hydrance (far left, far right and fourth from left). (ii) Examples of gentle cleansers (second left—micellar water, third from the left—gentle cleanser with some oil removal properties, fifth from the left gentle cleanser). (**c**) A selection of ultra broad spectrum sunscreen products. These are all tinted products that contain iron oxide (that protects against visible light). The only exception is Heliocare products (second from the right) which are not tinted but contains filters protecting against visible and infrared light. (**d**) Anti-pigmentation products. Left to right—CE Ferulic (contains ferulic acid, Vitamin C); Esthe-White (contains Vitamin C and licorice root extract); Pigmentclar (contains niacinamide, resourcinol, ferulic acid); Biluma (contains kojic Acid dipalmitate as an ester, arbutin, and licorice, mulberry, tetrahydrocurcumin and artocarpus extracts). Another very useful product is The Ordinary 2% Arbutin with Hyaluronic acid (not pictured)

d

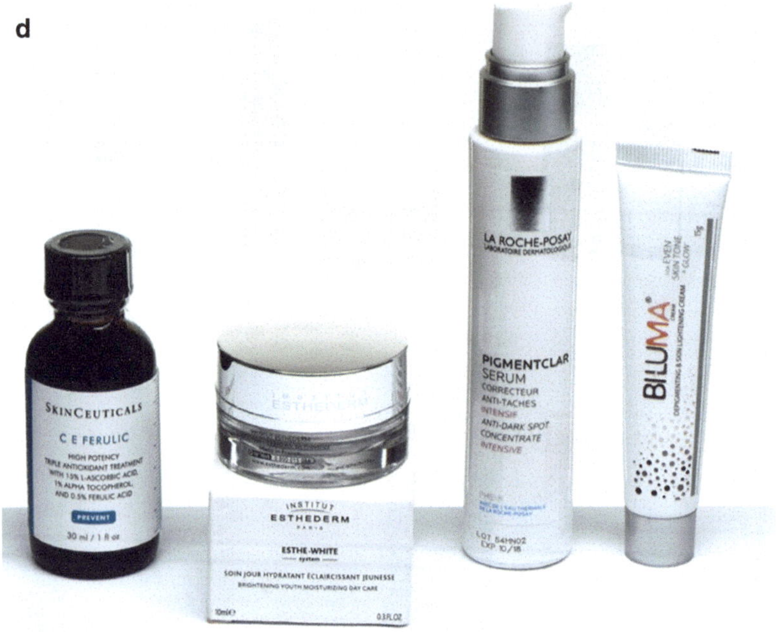

Fig. 10.1 (continued)

Part 2

What Is a Cosmeceutical?

Sun protection is an indispensable topical 'cosmeceutical' cream, but there are many other topicals that are available on the market, with some evidence of efficacy. The vast majority of patients already use them and in some cases the creams they use may even be counterproductive. To commence, it is useful to discuss the definition of cosmetic, pharmaceutical and 'cosmeceutical' agents. Next, we can address the different categories of cosmeceutical agents and their utility before and after laser.

Some Definitions as They Relate to Skincare

A "cosmetic" is a biologically inert agent that is formulated to enhance the skin and should not change the structure or function of the skin, only the appearance.

A "pharmaceutical" agent is a drug, that should have a given clinical effect above that of placebo and rigorous testing and licencing procedures are required. This may be licenced as an over the counter preparation or as a prescription medication.

The term "cosmeceutical" is a substance that has both a cosmetic and, in theory, a therapeutic effect. Many contain ingredients that a probably safe and have a biological effects—but the current regulations means that claims of efficacy do not have to be rigorously substantiated [22].

"Clinically proven" means that there has been a trial of the product in some individuals, and that the outcome is reported back. There is no standard that these "clinical trials" are required to adhere to and are often of low quality, not randomised and conducted on insufficient numbers.

"Dermatologically tested" might mean that the company gave several samples to a dermatologist who tried it themselves or on patients in the clinic and gave some feedback.

Other general points relating to cosmeceutical labelling:

"Fragrance-free" does not necessarily mean there are no fragrances in the product—it can be labelled as parfum, fragrance or cinnamates, limonene, citronellol, benzyl benzoate. Low or fragrance-free products are generally a good idea and are best identified by those that are bland i.e. don't have a strong or pleasant smell.

"Hypoallergenic" means that this product is less likely to cause allergies than similar products or those produced by that manufacturer. If your patient is reactive to products, a good choice might be those that do not contain irritant ingredients (e.g. retinols, retinoids or acids) or are formulated for eczema or 'sensitive' skin.

"Non-comedogenic"—refers to the product not resulting in the formation of comedones (or black heads). In the past comedogenicity was tested on the ears of rabbits, but to avoid animal testing, comedogenicity is now tested on the back skin of human volunteers. In general it relates to the occlusiveness of the product and ability to generate acne pre-cursor lesions.

"Organic"—although there are industry standards that relate to organic certification of food, organic skincare is difficult to endorse as many of the ingredients in skincare are not natural or organic.

"Botanical" or "vegan"—plant derived products can still cause irritation and allergy so are not necessarily any better than chemical products.

"Preservative-free"—most liquid products containing water require preservatives to prevent bacterial growth, so removing these isn't possible and natural alternatives may also cause irritation.

The issue is often with classification. Cosmeceutical actions by definition are limited to improving skin appearance and claims by manufacturers that relate to functional parameters might lead to products being classified as drugs, that is often not desirable by the company. There are several substances that cross the boundaries between cosmetics, supplements and pharmaceuticals— an example is glutathione, that we will touch on briefly later; this is sold as an oral supplement, even though the IV preparation of the same substance is marketed as an antioxidant drug used to reduce the incidence of neurological side effects in patients having platinum-based chemotherapy. The next section details topical agents and cosmeceuticals that are most useful in conjunction with laser therapy as pre- and post-laser anti-ageing treatment and maintenance regimens.

Part 3: Topical Agents

Basic Skincare Products

The patient consultation prior to laser treatment is an excellent time to enquire about and to optimise a patient's topical regime. There is the opportunity to minimise the risk of pigmentary complications through education about sun protection and to introduce an appropriate, evidence-based topical skin care regime. Many patients use inappropriate or ineffective over the counter creams. A pre-treatment "trial" period is also important to identify those patient who are very sensitive, intolerant or non-compliant and who may not be ideal candidates for procedures that are attached to a risk of complications.

Moisturisers

Skin moisturisers are formulated along a spectrum of viscosities and moisturising potentials. Gels are thinner and water based; emulsions are a mix of oils and water and have increasing oil content from lotions (more water) to creams and ointments (mostly oils). Many other ingredients are added including humectants, emollients and occlusives. Humectants applied topically attract and bind water to the skin surface, temporarily increasing the water content and improving the skin appearance, albeit increasing surface evaporation. The down side of using a cream with a high level of humectants is that the deeper skin layers can become dry as a consequence of this water movement. Commonly used humectants include hyaluronic acid (HA), sorbitol, glycerine, glycerol. They are useful in lighter formulations. New formulations of HA (e.g. nano HA) include small HA particles which may produce a longer lasting moisturising effects, particularly when combined with an occlusive agent prevents water loss from the skin (see below). Natural moisturising factor is a concoction of various naturally occurring humectants that simulate the natural milieu in the skin—and include filaggrin breakdown products, humectants such as HA together with amino acids, carbohydrates, minerals, urea, lactate, ammonia.

Emollients include agents such as dimethicone, ceramides, linoleic acid, that replace the natural skin lipids. They are like the cement between the 'building blocks' (or keratinocytes) of the skin barrier. Finally, occlusives are greasy and shiny and form a barrier over the skin surface to prevent water loss. Commonly used occlusive agents are propylene glycol, lecithin, dimethicone, squalene, shea butter, lanolin, petrolatum, paraffin.

Most moisturisers are a concoction of various proportions of these products and it is difficult to ascertain the properties of a topical preparation without being guided by the manufacturers labelling. As a general rule, a low fragrance non-botanical moisturising cream tailored to the patient's skin type is a good start.

Cleansers, Toners and Wash Off-Products

Peri-procedure cleansing regimes should include gentle and non-irritant products. Toners and abrasive cleaning products and equipment (e.g. scrubs and cloths) are best avoided. Cream cleansers can be quite gentle, and can be used as an emollient wash. Micellar water is a relatively recent product to enter the market and is useful as a double cleanser (for oily skin) or a gentle cleanser (for normal-dry skin). It consists of a ready-made solution of micelles of surfactant that, once placed on a pad or cloth attracts dirt without excessive oil removal. Some recommendations based on skin type are made in Table 10.1.

Depigmenting and Pigment Control Agents

The most important topical agents for laser patients (after sunscreens), are creams that can control pigmentation. All laser procedures carry a varying risk of erythema and inflammation and therefore, subsequent PIH, particularly in darker skin types

Table 10.1 Basic guide for skin care products, based on skin type

Type of skin	Cleanser	Moisturiser	Adjucts
Rosacea or red sensitive skin Avoid exfoliants, abrasives	Gentle washes, moisturising washes (e.g. Cetaphil gentle wash, Avene gentle cleanser), cream cleansers or micellar water	Products for atopic or sensitive skin (e.g. Aveeno lotion/cream, or those formulated for skin with acne under treatment e.g. Bioderma Sebium Hydra). Apply topicals at least 10-20 mins after showering or washing to avoid stinging.	Anti-redness creams[a] (e.g. La Roche Posay Rosaliac, Anti-rougeurs), 10% azelaic acid, The Ordinary Prescription Soolantra, Finacea, Rosex cream Use fewer products, moisturising makeup
Dry and sensitive skin e.g. atopic eczema As for rosacea	Wash with water or moisturiser or gentle cleansers (as above)	Heavier moisturisers—containing more occlusive moisturisers and emollients (E.g. emollients, creams, ointments such as La Roche Posay Lipikar Baume, Avene Tolerance).	Moisturising make-up Prescription topicals to treat eczema
Mature skin—often dry	Cleansing oils[b] Gentle washes Micellar water	As for dry skin	Retinol, retinaldehyde and AHA, BHAs Prescription Retinoids

Table 10.1 (continued)

Type of skin	Cleanser	Moisturiser	Adjucts
Oily—prone to acne	Double cleansing (wash with cleanser for oily skin, using micellar water afterwards) Acne cleanser (containing benzoyl peroxide or salicylic acid e.g. Cetaphil, Benzac, Bioderma) ± Toner[c] ? Exfoliant cleansers[d]	Light, non-comedogenic moisturiser formulated for acne prone skin (E.g. Bioderma Sebium Hydra, Avene Hydrance light)	Retinoids and AHA, BHAs Prescription Consider long term prescription topical retinoids
Active acne	Acne wash 2× day Double cleansing (as above) ± Toner[c] ? Exfoliant cleansers[d]	Light, non-comedogenic moisturiser formulated for acne prone skin (as for oily)	Medicated products containing for e.g. Benzoyl peroxide, salicylic acid Prescription Topical retinoids Topical anti-biotics, zinc/niacinamide
Hyperpigmented skin: Melasma, previous PIH of any cause	Cleansing as per skin oil content	Moisturise based on skin oil content	Vitamin C serum/cream Ferulic acid Arbutin Kojic acid Glycolic acid Retinols/retinaldehyde Prescription 'Bleaching' creams e.g. triple combination (Kligmans-type creams), Hydroquinone, topical retinoids
Post-laser regimen for Fitzpatrick skin type 3 and above	Consider as for Hyperpigmented skin	Consider as for Hyperpigmented skin	Consider as for Hyperpigmented skin

AHAs alpha hydroxy acids, *BHAs* beta hydroxy acids

[a]The author does not find anti-redness creams useful (personal view)

[b]Cleansing oils should only be used in dry or mature skin

[c]Toners can be used in addition to cleansers when additional oil control is required e.g. in individuals with acne or very oily skin

[d]Exfoliant cleansers and abrasive skin cleaning equipment can be irritant for many skin types e.g. atopic, dry skin and rosacea. They may be useful in oily, non-sensitive skin types and in individuals who prefer this method of exfoliation. The author prefers chemical exfoliation e.g. retinoids, azelaic acid and AHA/BHAs as these have added anti-ageing benefits. If patients still have oily skin and can tolerate it, the addition of an exfoliating 'scrub' once per week might be appropriate

(Fitzpatrick 3 and above). Avoidance of direct sun (clothes, hats) is the most important preventative element, with sunscreen acting as a 'back stop'. Preparation of the skin with depigmenting agents before laser procedures has three main purposes: reduction in melanocyte activity pre-procedure, reduction of competing chromophores during the procedure and providing the patient with opportunity to 'practice' a topical regimen that minimises side effects post-procedure. Table 10.2 outlines the classification of useful depigmenting cosmeceuticals.

Hydroquinone

Hydroquinone 2–8% without a doubt is the most important depigmenting compound in dermatology. From the year 2000, Hydroquinone has

Table 10.2 Effective depigmenting ingredients found in cosmeceuticals

Class of agent	Agents
Hydroquinone related compounds	Arbutin and deoxyarbutin Rucinol/resorcinol
Acids	Kojic acid AHAs—glycolic acid BHAs—salicylic acid (see below)
Depigmenting antioxidants	Vitamin C Ferulic acid Resveratrol Niacinamide
Botanicals	Aloesin, flavinoids *p*-coumaric acid (ginseng), mulberry extract polyphenols (grape seeds, strawberries) Soy proteases (Bowman-Birk Inhibitor, Soybean Trypsin Inhibitor)
Other	Niacinamide NAG (N-acetyl glucosamine) NCAP (N-acetyl-4-S-cysteaminylphenol)

been limited to prescription in the EU (including the UK) and since 2006 in the US has only been available up to 2% in over the counter preparations [22]. In the UK it is not licensed, although it can be prescribed and its use is therefore limited. It is toxic to melanocytes, there is a risk of contact hypersensitivity (perhaps in up to 5% of individuals) and occasionally it induces exogenous ochronosis (when used for extended periods, usually at concentrations of 5% and above) [23]. Hydroquinone has been linked to sun induced cancers [24], although to date, this and links to other cancers are largely unproven [23, 25, 26]. Nevertheless, hydroquinone containing products are freely available over the counter in many countries. Usually, hydroquinone is combined with a prescription retinoid to aid penetration and a topical steroid to reduce inflammation. It may be prescribed as a compounded bespoke 'Kligmans' formula or obtained as commercially available triple combination (TC) preparations e.g. Pigmanorm or Triluma. TC cream remains the gold standard topical depigmenting agent; it has the most evidence base for its use and it is more effective compared to other topicals, including hydroquinone alone. This author's personal preference is to use three separate creams as 'bespoke' TC treatment: 2–4% hydroquinone daily, topical retinoid 4–7 times/week and 1% hydrocortisone *only when required* for inflammation—to limit steroid side effects. TC is highly effective as a pre-laser lightening agent and it may limit the risk of PIH used post-laser. This is especially relevant for many cosmetic laser applications such as rejuvenating fractional laser (e.g. fractional non-ablative and CO_2 laser), intense pulsed light or 'pigment' lasers (e.g. q-switched Nd:YAG).

Compounds Related to Hydroquinone (Non-prescription)

Several of the ingredients that are included in commercially available bleaching or whitening creams are related to, or derivatives of, hydroquinone. They are purported to have less toxicity than hydroquinone and include arbutin (glycosylated hydroquinone), deoxyarbutin (with –OH groups removed), bearberry extract and mequinol (4-hydroxyanisole, hydroquinone monoethyl ether). Several inhibit tyrosinase and several small studies show efficacy approaching that of 2–4% hydroquinone [27–29]. Although there are no reported cases to date, each has the *potential* to induce exogenous ochronosis if used in high concentrations for extended periods of time, as they are variably converted to hydroquinone in the skin [27]. Although commercially available cosmeceutical agents may contain these compounds in the list the ingredients, it is often not clear from labelling how much they contain—and there is scanty evidence on the optimal topical concentrations.

Arbutin is a naturally occurring glycoside; it is a glycosylated hydroquinone extracted from the bearberry plant in the genus Arctostaphylos. It is converted to hydroquinone by commensal skin bacteria and both forms inhibit tyrosinase and thus prevent the formation of melanin. There are limited clinical studies but it appears to be efficacious and have fewer side effects than hydroquinone [27]. Arbutin can be found in several products at a concentration of 1–2%. Arbutin is also frequently found in skin lightening cosmeceutical products as **bearberry** extract; but it is difficult to quantify the amount of the active ingredients when included as an "extract".

Deoxyarbutin is a newer agent, derived from arbutin, by removal of the hydroxy groups. Deoxyarbutin is metabolized to arbutin and hydroquinone in the skin and induces reversible skin lightening by inhibiting tyrosinase. There is less evidence for its use but it shows potential as deoxyarbutin and its derivates inhibit tyrosinase with less melanocyte toxicity than hydroquinone [27, 30].

Resorcinol, or Rucinol (4-*n* butyl resorcinol) used as 0.03% or 0.01%, is a phenol derivative also related to hydroquinone. It inhibits tyrosinase and tyrosinase related protein. It probably better than placebo but are less effective than hydroquinone, although side effects are minimal [31].

Mequinol is another compound that is related to hydroquinone and is licensed by the FDA to alleviate solar lentigines (as a combination topical with a topical retinoid). It is probably less effective than hydroquinone but also has fewer side effects [31].

Botanicals

It has been claimed that several botanically derived ingredients have depigmenting effects: however, there is only with a little evidence of in vivo effects but limited efficacy in vitro. The agents that are most likely to helpful are: bearberry extract (which contains arbutin), the polyphenol ellagaic acid (from cranberries, geraniums) and licorice extracts (containing glabridin, liquiritin). The same caveat as before should be heeded: that plant extracts, when included as ingredients in cosmeceuticals are largely of undefined purity and concentration. Other depigmenting botanicals include:

(i) Aloesin (from aloe),
(ii) Flavinoids (flavones and flavonols such as liquiritin and isoliquiritin found in many plants and hesperidin found in citrus fruits),
(iii) P-coumaric acid (ginseng),
(iv) Mulberry extract
(v) Other polyphenols such as procyanidins (found in grape seeds, strawberries)
(vi) Soy proteases Bowman-Birk Inhibitor (BBI) and Soybean Trypsin Inhibitor (STI) reduce melanosome transfer (but not whole soy or isoflavines— these contain oestrogens and might actually potentiate pigmentation) [32, 33].

Other Depigmenting Ingredients

Kojic acid is a fungal metabolite that is a by-product of rice fermentation and has been used in depigmenting agents for some time. It competitively and reversibly inhibits tyrosinase and thereby cellular melanin production. It appears to have limited effect as a single agent and is best used in combination. In some studies, used as 1–4%, it was equivalent to 4% hydroquinone (for example, in combination with emblica extract and glycolic acid or with 2% hydroquinone) [34]. A new over the counter product called Biluma shows some promise: it is presumptively named in likeness to Triluma and contains kojic acid dipalmitate (as an ester), arbutin, and extracts of licorice, mulberry, tetrahydrocurcumin and artocarpus extracts.

N-acetyl-4-S-cysteaminylphenol (NCAP) is a derivative of phenol that competitively inhibits tyrosinase by acting as an alternative substrate. It is less irritant than hydroquinone and, as a 4% formulation, it reduces pigmentation in patients with melasma [35].

N-acetyl glucosamine (NAG) is a combination of glucosamine and acetic acid. It is a precursor building block that makes up hyaluronic acid (an alternating polymer of NAG–glucuronic acid), a vital component of the youthful dermis. NAG is also the monomer component of the polymer chitin, that is derived from mollusc shells and small studies indicate it might facilitate wound healing. NAG inhibits the glycosylation of tyrosinase, an obligatory step in the activation of the human enzyme, which is central to formation of melanin. 2% NAG (in combination with niacinamide 4%) is effective in reducing facial hyperpigmentation [36].

Glutathione is an oral, sublingual, IV or topical "supplement" and antioxidant that has depigmenting effects. It is found naturally in human cells. The mechanism of action is not known but it may bind with and inactivate tyrosinase, or reduce free radicals. Higher levels of glutathione are associated with the shift of eumelanogenesis (brown pigment) to slower pheomelanin (red pigment) synthesis [37]. Orally, it is poorly absorbed and in active (reduced) form is very unstable. Concerns about the toxicity of IV Glutathione means that is now carries a boxed warning from the FDA, nonetheless it is still in widespread use worldwide as a skin lightening agent for darker skin types in black market beauty clinics. Topical glutathione in oxidised (stable) form in a small blinded split face trial showed some lightening on the treated side that did not reach statistical significance [38]. It is a relative new kid on the block for dermatology, and has generated a lot of interest and is sold freely orally and topically.

Tranexamic acid is an oral fibrinolytic drug that is currently undergoing very promising trials as an oral treatment for melasma. It is not known if it will be effective for photoageing. Topical tranexamic acid shows a little promise, as a 2–5% solution or cream or a liposomal formulation and there are multiple preparations on the cosmeceutical market that contain it. To date, four studies comparing topical tranexamic acid and hydroquinone for the treatment of melasma showed either: a reduction in the melasma severity index with topical tranexamic acid or no significant difference between the two [39–42].

Antioxidants as Depigmenting Agents

A number of antioxidants are marketed as depigmenting agents and have been used in studies on pigmentation and anti-ageing. The compounds that are most useful in pigment reduction are Vitamin C, resveratrol, ferulic acid and niacinamide. Further discussion of antioxidants can be found below.

Polypodium leucotomos is a species of South American fern and as a cosmoceutical ingredient is also labelled as calaguala or anapsos extract. It is an antioxidant and has photoprotective agent. Studies in vitro, and in small numbers of human subjects, suggest that it reduces oxidative stress and damage in UV exposed cells and reduces UV induced skin immunosuppression in animal studies. It also appears to increase the minimal erythema dose in humans and protect against polymorphic light eruption [43]. It is available as an oral supplement, not a cosmeceutical cream but worthy of a mention here due to the interest it has generated in the supplement market.

Retinoids and Cosmeceutical Peeling Agents

Retinoids are very useful de-pigmenting agents but are limited by tolerability and the long duration required for effect (for example, 40 weeks). Prior to laser treatments, a period of topical retinoid application may allow better penetration of the laser light, diminish the formation of milia post operatively and possibly reduce hyperpigmentation. Topical retinoids can also aid in re-epithelialisation of the skin post-laser and facilitate healing post procedure [44]. They are optimally applied for 3 months prior to anti-ageing laser procedures; a minimum of 2 weeks can be helpful, discontinuing 1 week prior.

Prescription retinoids, such as Tretinoin 0.05% or 0.1% is frequently used as an antiageing topical agent and there is good evidence for its use. Retinoids act on retinoic acid receptors in the cytoplasm and nucleus to produce three main effects (1) epidermal proliferation leading to epidermal thickening, (2) compaction of the stratum corneum and (3) increase in the production of glycosaminoglycans including hyaluronic acid [45]. Tretinoin also appears to alleviate some of the deleterious effects of UV irradiation such as blocking the action of collagenases and gelatinases, preventing collagen breakdown and reducing UV induced nuclear transcription factors [46]. With longer term use (circa 6 months), tretinoin 0.05% results in a significant improvement in fine wrinkling, and a reduction in mottled hyperpigmentation and skin roughness [47]. Continual improvements in skin quality and regeneration of dermal collagen are seen after 12 months of treatment. Both lower strength 0.02% and higher strength (e.g. 1% twice weekly) have demonstrated positive clinical effects [46]. Adapalene 0.1% was equivalent to 0.05% tretinoin in reducing pigmentation in melasma patients over 3 months, with decreased side effects [48]. The evidence for antiageing is less for adapalene than for tretinoin, but the increased tolerability of adapalene (and therefore perhaps extended compliance as a topical agent) makes it a good alternative. Other topical retinoids can also be used but the evidence is less robust (e.g. topical isotretinoin).

Although prescription retinoids such as tretinoin and adapalene have the best evidence for antiageing effects, they are not tolerated by many patients. Over the counter Vitamin A derivatives such as retinol and retinaldehyde are widely available in cosmeceutical creams. Both are less potent but more tolerable than prescription retinoids. Retinol is converted to retinoic acid in vivo and is effective in reducing the action of collagenases, but is unstable and easily degraded by air and light exposure [46]. Retinol derivates such as retinyl acetate, retinyl palmitate and retinyl propionate are less effective than retinoic acid and firm evidence of efficacy is lacking. However, tolerability is significantly improved upon prescription retinoids. Retinaldehyde is converted to retinoic acid in keratinocytes at a key stage of their differentiation, delivering it direct to the cell without inducing the side effects; it is also converted locally to retinol and retinol esters. It is also highly tolerable [46]. There is a little controversy regarding which is superior, but probably retinaldehyde is a marginally more effective compound [49]. To be effective either compound should be used with a strength of at least 1%.

Tazarotene 0.1% is effective at reducing the signs of photoageing, modifies abnormal keratinocytes and can reduce fine lines, and alleviate lentigines, irregular pigmentation and wrinkles, but has a high incidence of side effects. Studies evaluating 0.1% tazarotene against topical tretinoin 0.05% suggest that it may be equivalent, but there is less evidence for its use [46].

Azelaic acid (AA) as 15% or as 20%, whichever is tolerated, is an alternative prescription topical for pigmentation and a desquamative agent for pregnant patients or those who are not able to tolerate retinoids. It is effective in reducing hyperpigmentation but has no depigmenting effect on normal skin. Studies have shown superiority of AA 20% over 2% hydroquinone and an equivalence with 4% hydroquinone, with fewer side effects [27]. However, many patients also find AA intolerable due to pruritus, burning and stinging.

Alpha-hydroxy acids (AHAs) are derived from plants. The best known is glycolic acid (derived from sugar); other AHAs include citric acid (fruit), lactic acid (milk), malic acid (apples), tartaric acid (wine), mandelic acid (almonds). AHAs are hydrophilic, so do not penetrate beyond the waterproof stratum corneum. Glycolic acid peels, and also daily use creams, have good evidence of pigment reduction in melasma and actinic damage by removal of epidermal pigmentation [50]. They are thought to disrupt cell adhesion molecules (such as cadherins in desmosomes) by chelation of the calcium ions, resulting in desquamation of the superficial layers of the skin. This also leads to irritation—the main side effect of AHAs—and increased sun sensitivity. AHA-mediated reduction of calcium ions in the epidermis also results in a shift in enzymatic processes in the stratum corneum, resulting in increased cell growth and reduced differentiation. They may also modify dermal collagen and elastin, these additive effects resulting in improvement of skin texture and younger appearing skin [51]. They are a good choice for dry skin as they draw moisture into the skin by acting as humectants.

Beta-hydroxy acids (BHAs) usually refers to salicylic acid (SA), a relative of aspirin that is also derived from the bark of the willow tree. However, there is some controversy regarding classification; several AHAs are technically speaking also BHAs, and SA is not a true BHA (although it is usually classified as BHA) [52]. SA is lipophilic and it can penetrate deeper into the skin and sebaceous glands. It removes the lipids between keratinocytes, causing the stratum corneum to swell, soften, macerate, and desquamate. It is a desmolytic; it loosens desmosomal proteins, leading to disruption of keratinocyte cohesion and cell exfoliation. It also reduces sebum production and promotes dermal regeneration without full thickness epidermal disruption. In the longer term, the corneal layer is thinned, with the epidermal thickness remaining constant. SA is very useful for oily and acne-prone skin as it causes selective desquamation around the pores, therefore reducing the formation of comedones. It can be helpful as a topical anti-acne and anti-comedogenic agent at concentrations of 0.5%–3%; it is desmolytic at 3–6%. Above 6% it is destructive and can be used as a chemical peel from 10–30% for superficial peeling and 30–50% to remove pigmented lesions such as solar keratoses [53].

Antioxidants

Traditionally, antioxidants such as Vitamin E (as tocopherol and tocotrienols) and Vitamin A have been formulated into "anti-ageing" night creams, but there is sketchy evidence for their use in this manner [54]. A more intelligent approache to skincare involves the application of antioxidants during the *day*, as an adjunct to sun protection during exposure to solar irradiation. "Antioxidants" by their nature are reactive free radical scavenging molecules, and therefore, are also innately unstable. Although in vitro activity may be documented, degradation may occur before application or on the skin surface. Recent advances in delivery via liposomes or carrier nanoparticles (see below), may mean that stability of these compounds are maintained until they are required.

Vitamin C (L-ascorbic acid) has used as a topical preparation for many years. It is irritant in higher concentrations and many creams contain it in low and probably ineffective concentrations. It is unstable and hydrophilic (so poorly absorbed into the skin) although some derivatives of Vitamin C have improved stability and are lipophilic e.g. magnesium-ascorbyl-phosphate (MAP), ascorbyl-6-palmitate. Vitamin C through its antioxidant effect has been shown to inhibit collagenases such as matrix metalloproteinase (MMP) and increase collagen [44]. It chelates copper, interfering with tyrosinase and acts as a reducing agent at several steps in the production of melanin; its anti-pigmentary effect may also be a consequence of its antioxidant effect. Topically, as 10% it may be equal/inferior to hydroquinone as a depigmenting agent and is able to inhibit UV induced damage due to UV [35, 51]. At 5–10% concentration there were minimal side effects [35].

Niacinamide is a derivative of Vitamin B_3 but unlike nicotinic acid, does not cause facial flushing. Niacinamide inhibits the transfer of melanosomes, thereby reducing pigmentation [51]. Several studies have shown it is effective as a single agent or in combination with other active ingredients in concentrations of 2–5% [49]. It is a precursor to the NADP family of coenzymes; its topical application increases reduced forms (NADPH) that are effective antioxidants [49]. It also improves the skin barrier, reduces transepidermal water loss, minimizes redness and blotchiness and reduces fine lines and wrinkles. Studies have shown it stimulated collagen synthesis and the epidermal proteins keratin, fillagrin, and involucrin [49]. It has also been used as an anti-inflammatory in acne.

Vitamin E (alpha-tocopherol) taken orally has been shown to reduce sunburn cells after UV exposure and that it counteracts free radicals; it also acts as a humectant [51]. It is synergistic with Vitamin C, which regenerates oxidised Vitamin E. Unfortunately, as a topical it has shown limited efficacy. However, when delivered in an optimal formulation and in combination with Vitamin C it may ameliorate UV damage and act as a depigmenting agent [55].

Ubiquinone (coQ10) is a natural fat soluble anti-oxidant that in vitro reduced UVA induces collagen breakdown by fibroblasts and UVB-related oxidative stress in keratinocytes. Therefore, it may reduce skin ageing [51].

Other Botanically derived anti-oxidants such as green tea extracts (containing polyphenols) reduce the deleterious effects of UV irradiation e.g. sunburn, carcinogenic activity and photoageing [51]. Ferulic acid is phenolic phytochemical extracted from plant cell walls. It is a good anti-oxidant and exerts anti-UV protective effect that is independent of sunscreens [51]. Ferulic acid also has a significant effect in the retardation of melanogenesis, possibly by inhibiting tyrosine hydroxylase activity in an indirect manner [27]. Soy protease inhibitors (Bowman-Birk inhibitor and soybean trypsin inhibitor) inhibit pigmentation, but *not* soy isoflavones (that have a phytoestrogen effect, and therefore may potentiate pigmentation). Isoflavines are good anti-oxidants and promote collagen and hyaluronic acid [55].

Other anti-oxidants such as synthetic molecules are of intellectual interest in terms of anti-ageing, although to date, good evidence of efficacy is lacking. One such compound is EUK-134 (ethylbisiminomethylguaiacol manganese chloride). This is a synthetic porphyrin-manganese superoxide dismutase and catalase that prolongs the survival of cells exposed to UVB irradiation and reduces UV-induced mutations in vivo [56]. Copper peptides may inhibit proteases and assist in collagen rebuilding and are also mentioned below. They are also purported to be anti-inflammatory and may also be useful adjuncts to corticosteroids post-laser [44].

Whats New in Cosmeceuticals

Nanoparticles are materials 1–100 nm in size. They may be rigid, for example gold, silver, iron oxide or ceramic particles that deliver medication to the site of action. They can also be malleable; for example liposomes that are composed of hydrophilic and lipophilic micelles, fullerenes that have potential to absorb UV light and free radicals, and solid lipid nanoparticles. In dermatology these have great potential as drug delivery systems and also in protecting formulations from environmental factors, improving shelf life of perishable substances. Chitin nanofibrils (from crustacean shells) might also be of assistance in facilitating wound healing [57]. Other nanoparticles can optimise skin hydration by forming a superficial lipid layer on the skin, preventing evaporation. Hyaluronic acid nanoparticles show great potential in moisturisers. Hyaluronic acid (HA) is usually a very large molecule 3000 nm attracts and binds huge numbers of water molecules. Therefore, it usually cannot penetrate beyond the stratum corneum. Nanosized (5 nm) hyaluronic acid have the potential to penetrate deeply into the epidermis and below. Small studies using of nanosized HA over 2 months show significant wrinkle reduction and enhancement of skin hydration, skin firmness and elasticity [44, 58].

Novel cosmeceutical peptides are emerging as ingredients in cosmeceuticals with many potential benefits in dermatology, including peri-laser. Unfortunately, as is the case for many cosmeceutical creams, robust evidence of in vivo efficacy is largely lacking. Peptides have many other applications in dermatology. One of the first agents to be discovered was the copper tripeptide transport peptide Cu-GHK (Lamin). It stimulates wound healing and synthesis of collagen, elastin, proteoglycan and glycosoaminoglycan and acts as an anti-inflammatory agent, perhaps even with efficacy similar to a weak topical steroid [44]. Various effects have been attributed to Cu-GHK, such as keratinocyte proliferation, stimulating hair growth, improving skin firmness, thickness, elasticity and appearance [59]. Manganese carrier peptides (e.g. Manganese tripeptide-1) also have limited data of efficacy in anti-ageing and anti-pigmentation.

One of the most exciting is "topical Botox" or Argireline (also known as acetyl hexapeptide-3). It is a mimic of the synaptosomal-associated protein 25 and competitively destabilises the SNARE (the soluble *N*-ethylmaleimide-sensitive factor attachment protein receptors) complex, preventing acetyl choline release at the pre-synaptic membrane. As a 5–10% emulsion, it is much less efficacious than botulinum toxin but has been shown to penetrate into the skin and inhibit facial muscle contraction [59]. Its role is probably best considered as a mild wrinkle reductant in those who do not wish to have injections, or as an adjunct to injectable botulinum toxin, reducing the units required and increasing the duration between treatments. There are also other peptides tested for topical use that inhibit actetylcholine and are based on snake venom such as pentapeptide-3 (Vialox) and tripeptide-3 (also called dipeptide diamino butyroyl benzylamide diacetate, or Syn-Ake). Others reduce muscle contraction by mimicking enkephalins, substances that inhibit acteylcholamine release in the synapse, e.g. pentapeptide-18 (Leuphasyl) [59]. Some manufacturers suggest they may be synergistic when used in combination.

Other peptides are reported to act as antioxidants and 'matricins'—compounds that are released by the extracellular matrix and might stimulate collagen neogenesis. A mixture of the water based antioxidant Carnosine (β-Ala-His) and several other stimulatory peptides, in several small randomised studies, improved periorbital skin smoothness and reduced wrinkle depth. Another study examined a formulation including carnosine and SPF 50, photolyase, endonuclease, 8-oxoguanine glycosylase, arazine, and ergothionine—and found that it was able to reduce the formation of pyrimidine photoproducts and inhibit protein degradation [59]. Carnosine has also been formulated in a lipophilic version palmitoyl carnitine (β-Ala-His) that penetrates through the skin to the dermis [59]. Several other peptides are of interest for their abilities to stimulate collagen, elastin and other dermal structural components and improve skin appearance—again with the caveat that the studies are small and of limited quality: palmitoyl tripeptide-1 (pal-GHK), pal-GQPR (as a combination with a tradename of Matrixyl 3000), palmitoyl tripeptide-3/5 (Syn-Coll), palmitoyl pentapeptide-4 (Matrixyl).

Post-treatment Applications

Many companies promote cosmeceutical creams that are specifically aimed at post-treatment application. Patients, too often request a post-treatment 'serum' to apply. After treatment with an ablative laser or another treatment that weakens the epidermal barrier, it is a good opportunity to apply a topical that might have some activity. Examples might include topical tranexamic acid, vitamin C or arbutin for pigmentation or topicals containing anti-ageing or anti-inflammatory peptides (as discussed above). Alternatively, a bland emollient preparation containing hyaluronic acid or dimethicone are also good choices e.g. Epidermal Repair (Skinceuticals), Cicalfate, Crème peaux Intolerantes (Avene), Cicaplast (La Roche Posay) or Hyaluronic acid serum (Esthetaderm). Many clinics apply sunscreen immediately after procedures to treated skin due to concern about sun exposure after patients leave the clinic (and post inflammatory pigmentation). This practice might facilitate the absorption of sunscreen chemicals which seems counter-productive; strict clothing coverage is likely to be a better option if there is a concern about sun exposure on the journey home.

Summary

Cosmeceuticals are now so commonly used by patients, that it is vital to have a basic working knowledge of what is available on the market. It is important to establish what regimen a patient is using prior to embarking on laser treatment and to optimise this prior to treatment. Vigilant sun protection is vital in conjunction with Laser for all skin types especially Fitzpatrick type 3 and above. Ideally, a tinted sunscreen in a vehicle suitable for each patient's skin type should be recommended to provide extra protection against high energy visible light. If a tinted block is not palatable, then a suitable alternative broad spectrum sunscreen should be used. An antioxidant (e.g. vitamin C, E) could be worn under sunscreen. There is good evidence for using a retinoid (prescription if tolerated) or non-prescription retinol (preferred to retinaldehyde) at highest tolerable concentration to maintain the skin. Clear instructions need to be given on the application of topical retinoids, gradually increasing the frequency to the limit of tolerance. AHAs or BHAs (depending on skin characteristics) can be used as a substitute for retinoids or in an alternating regime (retinoids, acids), guided by side effects and tolerability and oil content. Additional non-prescription de-pigmenting agents are also hugely helpful before and after laser and as maintenance regimes for patients with age/sun related dyschromia or melasma—such as those containing arbutin, kojic acid, ferulic acid, glycolic acid, tranexamic acid and glutathione. Finally, exciting new advances are occurring with the discovery of new anti-ageing peptides, and nanoparticles. Let us hope that appropriate clinical trials will be performed to arm us with evidence that they work.

Acknowledgements An acknowledgement is given to the Skin Care Bible, published by my colleague Dr. Anjali Mahto, that has assisted with some of the definitions outlined above, and the sections on moisturisers.

Disclaimers The information contained in Table 10.2 is the author's own personal view of cosmeceutical products. This is not an exhaustive list of helpful products and every attempt has been made to recommend products on the basis of evidence (if it exists), patient feedback and product performance during personal use—and not advertising or sponsorship.

References

1. Reuters.com. https://www.reuters.com/brandfeatures/venture-capital/article?id=30351. Accessed June 28 2019.
2. Zaleski-Larsen LA, Fabi SG. Laser-assisted drug delivery. Dermatol Surg. 2016;42(8):919–31.
3. Kricker A, Armstrong BK, English DR. Sun exposure and non-melanocytic skin cancer. Cancer Causes Control. 1994;5(4):367–92.
4. Oliveria SA, Saraiya M, Geller AC, Heneghan MK, Jorgensen C. Sun exposure and risk of melanoma. Arch Dis Child. 2006;91(2):131–8.
5. Lautenschlager S, Wulf HC, Pittelkow MR. Photoprotection. Lancet. 2007;370:528–37.
6. Sanchez G, Nova J, Rodriguez-Hernandez AE, Medina RD, Solorzano-Restrepo C, Gonzalez J, et al. Sun protection for preventing basal cell and squamous cell skin cancers. Cochrane Database Syst Rev. 2016;7:1–42.
7. Green AC, Williams GM, Logan V, Strutton GM. Reduced melanoma after regular sunscreen use: randomized trial follow-up. J Clin Oncol. 2011;29(3):257–63.
8. van der Pols JC, Williams GM, Pandeya N, Logan V, Green AC. Prolonged prevention of squamous cell carcinoma of the skin by regular sunscreen use. Cancer Epidemiol Biomark Prev. 2006;15(12):2546–8.
9. Jayaratne N, Russell A, van der Pols JC. Sun protection and vitamin D status in an Australian subtropical community. Prev Med. 2012;55(2):146–50.
10. Hughes MC, Williams GM, Baker P, Green AC. Sunscreen and prevention of skin ageing: a randomized trial. Ann Intern Med. 2013;158:781–90.
11. Mahmoud BH, Ruvolo E, Hexsel CL, Liu Y, Owen MR, Kollias N, et al. Impact of long-wavelength UVA and visible light on melanocompetent skin. J Invest Dermatol. 2010 Aug;130(8):2092–7.
12. Randhawa M, Seo I, Liebel F, Southall MD, Kollias N, Ruvolo E. Visible light induces melanogenesis in human skin through a photoadaptive response. PLoS One. 2015;10(6):e0130949.
13. Lim HW, Arellano-Mendoza M-I, Stengel F. Current challenges in photoprotection. J Am Acad Dermatol. 2017;76(3):S91–9.
14. Snell RS. The changes produced by infra-red irradiation in melanin pigmentation of the skin. Br J Dermatol. 1963;74:71–8.
15. Seo I, Baqer A, Kollias N. The effect of visible light and near-infrared radiation on constitutive pigment of patients with vitiligo. Br J Dermatol. 2010;163:208–34.
16. Kollias N, Baqer A. An experimental study of the changes in pigmentation in human skin in vivo with visible and near infrared light. Phtochem Photobiol. 1984;39:651–9.
17. Handel AC, Bartoli Miot LD, Miot HA. Melasma: a clinical and epidemiological review. An Bras Dermatol. 2014;89(5):771–82.
18. Moyal D. How to measure UVA protection afforded by sunscreen products. Expert Rev Dermatol. 2008;3(3):307–13.
19. Liebel F, Kaur S, Ruvolo E, Kollias N, Southall MD. Irradiation of skin with visible light induces reactive oxygen species and matrix-degrading enzymes. J Invest Dermatol. 2012;132:1901–7.
20. Sánchez G, Nova J, Rodriguez-Hernandez AE, Medina RD, Solorzano-Restrepo C, Gonzalez J, et al. Sun protection for preventing basal cell and squamous cellskin cancers (review) sun protection for preventing basal cell and squamous cell skin cancers. Cochrane Database Syst Rev. 2016;7:CD011161.
21. Matta MK, Zusterzeel R, Pilli NR, Patel V, Volpe DA, Florian J, et al. Effect of sunscreen application under maximal use conditions on plasma concentration of sunscreen active ingredients: a randomized clinical trial. JAMA. 2019;321(21):2082–91.
22. The Cosmetic Toiletry and Perfumery Association. http://www.thefactsabout.co.uk/skin-lightening-products/content/136. Accessed 26 July 2019.
23. Nordlund JJ. Hyperpigmentation: its historical treatment and the development of hydroquinone. Pigment Disord. 2015;2:221.
24. Ly F, Diousse P, Ndiaye C, Déme A, Diatta BA, Ndiaye MT, et al. Cutaneous squamous cell carcinomas (SCC) associated with cosmetic skin whitening: 8 cases reported in Senegal. Ann Dermatol Venereol. 2018;145(2):83–8.
25. McGregor D. Hydroquinone: an evaluation of the human risks from its carcinogenic and mutagenic properties. Crit Rev Toxicol. 2007;37(10):887–914.
26. O'Donoghue JL. Hydroquinone and its analogues in dermatology – a risk-benefit viewpoint. J Cosmet Dermatol. 2006;5(3):196–203.
27. Bandyopadhyay D. Topical treatment of Melasma. Indian J Dermatol. 2009;54(4):303–9.
28. Hamed SH, Sriwiriyanont P, de Long MA, Visscher MO, Wickett RR, Boissy RE. Comparative efficacy and safety of deoxyarbutin, a new tyrosinase-inhibiting agent. J Cosmet Sci. 2006;57:291–308.
29. Boissy RE, Visscher M, DeLong MA. DeoxyArbutin: a novel reversible tyrosinase inhibitor with effective in vivo skin lightening potency. Exp Dermatol. 2005;14:601–8.
30. Chawla S, de Long MA, Visscher MO, Wickett RR, Manga P, Boissy RE. Mechanism of tyrosinase inhibition by deoxy Arbutin and its second-generation derivatives. Br J Dermatol. 2008;159:1267–74.
31. Sarkar R, Chugh S, Garg VK. Newer and upcoming therapies for melasma. Indian J Dermatol Venereol Leprol. 2012;78(4):417–28.
32. Zhu W, Gao J. The use of botanical extracts as topical skin-lightening agents for the improvement of skin

pigmentation disorders. J Investig Dermatol Symp Proc. 2008;13(1):20–4.
33. Davis C. Review of the epidemiology, clinical features, and treatment options in skin of color. J Clin Aesthetic Dermatol. 2010;3(7):20–31.
34. Damevska. New aspects of melasma. Serbian J Dermatol Venereol. 2014;6(1):5–18.
35. Sarkar R, Arora P, Garg KV. Cosmeceuticals for hyperpigmentation: what is available? J Cutan Aesthet Surg. 2013;6(1):4–11.
36. Kimball AB, Kaczvinsky JR, Li J, Robinson LR, Matts PJ, Berge CA, et al. Reduction in the appearance of facial hyperpigmentation after use of moisturizers with a combination of topical niacinamide and N-acetyl glucosamine: results of a randomized, double-blind, vehicle-controlled trial. Br J Dermatol. 2010;162(2):435–41.
37. Villarama CD, Maibach HI. Glutathione as a depigmenting agent: an overview. Int J Cosmet Sci. 2015;27(3):147–53.
38. Watanabe F, Hashizume E, Chan GP, Kamimura A. Clinical cosmetic and investigational dermatology skin-whitening and skin-condition-improving effects of topical oxidized glutathione: a double-blind and placebo-controlled clinical trial in healthy women. Clin Cosmet Investig Dermatol. 2014;7:267–74.
39. Kanechorn N, Ayuthaya P, Niumphradit N, Manosroi A, Nakakes A. Topical 5% tranexamic acid for the treatment of melasma in Asians: a double-blind randomized controlled clinical trial. J Cosmet Laser Ther. 2012;14(3):150–4.
40. Banihashemi M, Zabolinejad N, Jaafari MR, Salehi M, Jabari A. Comparison of therapeutic effects of liposomal tranexamic acid and conventional hydroquinone on melasma. J Cosmet Dermatol. 2015;14(3):174–7.
41. Ebrahimi B, Naeini FF. Topical tranexamic acid as a promising treatment for melasma. J Res Med Sci. 2014;19(8):753–7.
42. Kim SJ, Park JY, Shibata T, Fujiwara R, Kang HY. Efficacy and possible mechanisms of topical tranexamic acid in melasma. Clin Exp Dermatol. 2016;41(5):480–5.
43. Berman B, Ellis C, Elmets C. Polypodium leucotomos – an overview of basic investigative findings. J Drugs Dermatol. 2016;15(2):224–8.
44. Wisniewski JD, Ellis DL, Lupo MP. Facial rejuvenation: combining cosmeceuticals with cosmetic procedures. Cutis. 2014;94(3):122–6.
45. Griffiths CE, Finkel LJ, Tranfaglia MG, Hamilton TA, Voorhees JJ. An in vivo experimental model for effects of topical retinoic acid in human skin. Br J Dermatol. 1993;129(4):389–94.
46. Mukherjee S, Date A, Patravale V, Korting HC, Roeder A, Weindl G. Retinoids in the treatment of skin ageing: an overview of clinical efficacy and safety. Clin Interv Ageing. 2006;1(4):327–48.
47. Griffiths CEM. The role of retinoids in the prevention and repair of aged and photoaged skin. Clin Exp Dermatol. 2001;26(7):613–8.
48. Dogra S, Kanwar AJ, Parsad D. Adapalene in the treatment of melasma: a preliminary report. J. Dermatol. 2002;29:539–40.
49. Levin J, Momin SB. How much do we really know about our favorite cosmeceutical ingredients? J Clin Aesthet Dermatol. 2010;3(2):22–41.
50. Rendon M, Berneburg M, Arellano I, Picardo M. Treatment of melasma. J Am Acad Dermatol. 2006;54:S272–81.
51. Rivers JK. The role of cosmeceuticals in antiageing therapy. Skin Therapy Lett. 2008;13(8):5–9.
52. Kornhauser A, Coelho SG, Hearing VJ. Applications of hydroxy acids: classification, mechanisms and photoactivity. Clin Cosmet Investig Dermatol. 2010;3:135–42.
53. Arif T. Salicylic acid as a peeling agent: a comprehensive review. Clin Cosmet Investig Dermatol. 2015;8:455–61.
54. Keen MA, I Hassan I. Vitamin E in dermatology. Indian Dermatol Online J. 2016;7(4):311–4.
55. Burke KE. Interaction of vitamins C and E as better cosmeceuticals. Dermatol Ther. 2007;20(5):314–21.
56. Decraene D, Smaers K, Gan D, Mammone T, Matsui M, Maes D, et al. A synthetic superoxide dismutase/catalase mimetic (EUK-134) inhibits membrane-damage-induced activation of mitogen-activated protein kinase pathways and reduces p53 accumulation in ultraviolet B-exposed primary human keratinocytes. J Invest Dermatol. 2004;122(2):484–91.
57. Antonio JR, Antonio CR, Cardeal IL, Ballavenuto JM, Oliveira JR. Nanotechnology in dermatology. An Bras Dermatol. 2014;89(1):126–36.
58. Pavicic T, Gauglitz GG, Lersch P, Schwach-Abdellaoui K, Malle B, Korting HC, et al. Efficacy of cream based novel formulations of hyaluronic acid of different molecular weights in anti-wrinkle treatment. J Drugs Dermatol. 2011;10:990–1000.
59. Schagen SK. Topical peptide treatments with effective anti-ageing results. Cosmetics. 2017;4(2):16.

Self-Assessment Questionnaire

11

Vishal Madan

1. Which one of the following is an ablative laser?
   (a) Er:YAG
   (b) Nd:YAG
   (c) Alexandrite
   (d) Ruby
2. Which laser/wavelength is most likely to remove red tattoo inks?
   (a) Alexandrite 755 nm
   (b) CO_2 10,600 nm
   (c) Q:S Nd:YAG 532 nm
   (d) Ruby 694 nm
3. The best age to treat port wine stains is
   (a) Pre-school
   (b) Teenage years
   (c) Adolescence
   (d) Adult life
4. Which parameter determines depth of penetration and absorption by a chromophore?
   (a) Spot size
   (b) Wavelength
   (c) Fluence
   (d) Power
5. Paradoxical hair growth is a complication of
   (a) IPL
   (b) Diode
   (c) Alexandrite
   (d) All
6. Which wavelength had deepest penetration in the skin?
   (a) Nd:YAG
   (b) Alexandrite
   (c) CO_2
   (d) Er:YAG
7. Most lasers which target pigments are Q: switched. True or False
8. Which of the following is the preferred wavelength for treating Naevus of Ota?
   (a) 1064 nm
   (b) 532 nm
   (c) 694 nm
   (d) 755 nm
9. Which would be the recommended *wavelength* to treat professional green tattoos?
   (a) 1064 nm
   (b) 532 nm
   (c) 694 nm
   (d) 755 nm
10. Of the following, which is the preferred laser for the management of recalcitrant melasma?
    (a) Fractional CO_2
    (b) Fractional 1550 nm
    (c) Low fluence QS Nd:YAG
    (d) Low fluence QS 532 nm

With contributions from all authors.

V. Madan (✉)
Consultant Dermatologist, Laser and Mohs Surgeon, Salford Royal NHS Foundation Trust, Stott Lane, Salford, UK
e-mail: vishal.madan@srft.nhs.uk

V. Madan (ed.), *Practical Introduction to Laser Dermatology*,
https://doi.org/10.1007/978-3-030-46451-6_11

11. Post-inflammatory hypopigmentation is a rare side effect of QS Nd:YAG laser treatment of pigmented lesions. Which one of the following is not considered a cause of this side effect?
    (a) Very high fluence
    (b) Excess overlapping
    (c) Use of small spot sizes
    (d) Longer wavelengths
12. Which device is the laser of choice in the treatment of lentigenes and ephilides?
    (a) QS 1064 nm
    (b) QS 532 nm
    (c) Fractional CO_2
    (d) 755 nm
13. What is the main advantages of the 1064 nm Nd:Yag laser over the 595 nm PDL Laser in treating some vascular anomalies?
    (a) Cheaper machine
    (b) Favourable side effect profile
    (c) Less painful treatments
    (d) Deeper penetration within the skin
14. A 14 year old girl developed this patch on her chest. This responded very well to PDL with complete clearance noted in two sessions. What is the most likely diagnosis?

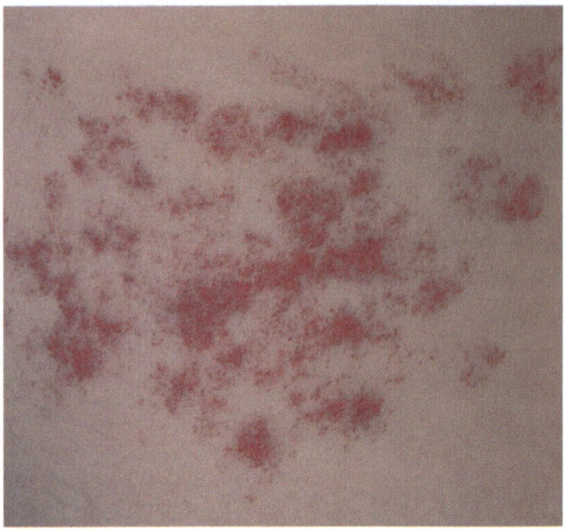

    (a) Port wine stain
    (b) Angioma Serpiginosum
    (c) Reticulate Vascular Naevus
    (d) Cutis marmorata Telangiectatica congenita
15. What would be the most appropriate treatment option for the pyogenic granuloma pictured below?

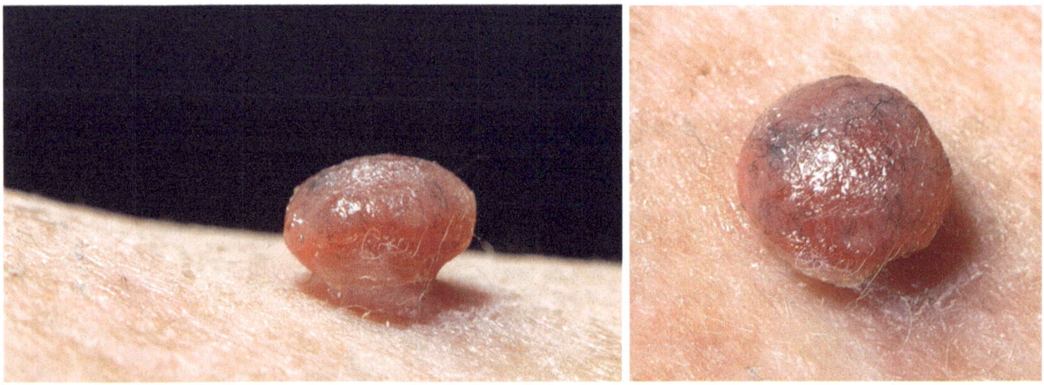

    (a) PDL
    (b) Nd:YAG laser
    (c) Surgical excision or curettage
    (d) Conservative management as it will resolve spontaneously
16. What is the commonest adverse effect from vascular laser therapy using PDL?
    (a) Purpura
    (b) Scabs
    (c) Pigmentation changes
    (d) Bleeding

17. Which laser is not suitable for management of vascular nodules arising in port wine stains?
    (a) Pulsed Dye laser
    (b) CO_2
    (c) QS 532 nm
    (d) Nd:YaG
18. Which of the following is an absolute contra-indication to fractional ablative laser treatment:
    (a) Isotretinoin 9 months ago
    (b) Pregnancy
    (c) Acne
    (d) Daily aspirin 75 mg
    (e) History of Polymorphic Light Eruption
19. Patient complains of tingling sensation on skin followed by the eruption of clusters of vesicles day 3–4 post-procedure. What is the likely diagnosis?
    (a) Herpes Zoster
    (b) Herpes Simplexc
    (c) Chicken Pox
    (d) Acne
20. Which type of acne scars are considered suitable for CO_2 laser resurfacing
    (a) Rolling
    (b) Icepick
    (c) Box car
    (d) Atrophic
21. Which mode on CO_2 laser would one use to treat milia?
    (a) Cutting
    (b) Resurfacing
    (c) Superpulse
    (d) Fractional
22. There is no need for protective eyewear for which of the lasers?
    (a) Alexandrite
    (b) CO_2
    (c) Q:S Nd:YAG
    (d) IPL
    (e) None
23. Absorption of Er:YAG beam by water is 16 times more than that of CO_2 beam, hence the deeper penetration. Is the statement—True or False
24. Which of the following is not an ablative device?
    (a) CO_2 laser
    (b) Er:YAG laser
    (c) Plasma
    (d) Er:YSGG
    (e) Alexandrite laser
25. Listed are the four most commonly used hair removal lasers. Which of these lasers is safest for the treatment of darker skin?
    (a) Ruby
    (b) Alexandrite
    (c) Diode
    (d) Nd:YAG
26. Considering all other parameters being constant, altering which of the following parameters will result in more thermal injury to the hair follicles?
    (a) Reducing pulse duration
    (b) Increasing wavelength
    (c) Increasing cooling
    (d) Reducing fluence
27. Which of the following is not a risk factor for paradoxical hypertrichosis after LHR?
    (a) Asian or Mediterranean descent
    (b) Treating vellus hair
    (c) Polycystic ovarian syndrome
    (d) Using Alexandrite laser
28. A patient presents for treatment of very fine, dark hair on her jawline and top lip. She is of South-Indian ancestry and has some very faint patches of pigmentation on her cheeks and forehead that darken during the summer months. All factors must be considered before proceeding with treatment except?
    (a) Use of lower fluence
    (b) Use of longer wavelength such as Nd:YAG
    (c) Treatment of pigmentation at the same time
    (d) Use of high factor sun protection
29. What measures must be employed prior to LHR?
    (a) Shave hair
    (b) Pluck hair
    (c) Wax hair
    (d) Leave hair long

30. One can undertake hair removal if the patient has a tattoo or semi-permanent make-up in the area. True or false?
31. A patient is taking a medication known to cause photosensitivity. This is an absolute contraindication. True or false?
32. What are the target chromophores in IPL photorejuvenation treatments?
    (a) Melanin
    (b) Haemoglobin
    (c) Water
    (d) Collagen
    (e) All of the above
33. Which pigmented lesions can be treated with IPL? Select one or more correct answers
    (a) Lentigo
    (b) Ephelides
    (c) Lentigo maligna
    (d) Melasma
    (e) Flat seborrhoeic keratosis
34. Which is best absorbs incident light the in vascular treatments?
    (a) Oxyhemoglobin—HbO_2
    (b) Melanin
    (c) Deoxyhaemoglobin—Hb
    (d) Met-haemoglobin—Met Hb
    (e) Myoglobin
    Answer: d. Met Hb has got 4.5 times more absorption of certain wavelengths than oxhaemoglobin and up to 20 times more than deoxyhaemoglobin.
35. Which one of the following circumstances will be more likely to cause problems following an IPL treatment?
    (a) Alcohol consumption before treatment.
    (b) Recent sunny holiday.
    (c) Concurrent oral antibiotics for a dental infection.
    (d) Planned holiday to Spain in four weeks.
    (e) Vegan diet.
36. Which are the active narrow bands on a vascular notch filter? Please select 2 answers
    (a) 500–1200 nm
    (b) 530–650 nm
    (c) 560–590 nm
    (d) 900–1200 nm
    (e) 650–900 nm
37. Radiofrequency devices use electromagnetic radiation to deliver to tissues
    (a) Sound energy
    (b) Nuclear energy
    (c) Thermal energy
    (d) Chemical energy
38. The first radiofrequency devices used in aesthetic medicine were
    (a) Monopolar RF
    (b) Bipolar RF
    (c) Unipolar RF
    (d) Microneedling RF
39. Which RF device applies minimally invasive microneedles or electrode pins to achieve targeted dermal injury with minimal superficial involvement
    (a) Bipolar
    (b) Monopolar
    (c) Fractional
    (d) ELOS (electro-optical synergy)
40. Therapeutic indications of fractional radiofrequency include
    (a) Skin tightening
    (b) Acne scars
    (c) Axillary hyperhidrosis
    (d) All of the above
41. Most frequent complications of Radiofrequency treatments are
    (a) Pain, haematoma, hyperpigmentation
    (b) Pain, erythema, oedema
    (c) Hyperpigmentation, scarring, erythema
    (d) Burns, dysesthesia, oedema
42. Which of the following best describes a cosmeceutical?
    (a) A prescription topical
    (b) A lipstick
    (c) A topical that is sold as a cosmetic item but is reported by the manufacturer to have properties that alter the skin
    (d) A cream that has been dermatologically tested
43. Regarding sun protection which of the following statements is CORRECT:
    (a) There are two scales for sunscreen testing: SPF and UVA-PF and both of these are in vitro.
    (b) SPF is a measure of UVA protection and measures persistent pigment darkening.
    (c) The standardised scale for visible light (VL) protection measures the production of reactive oxygen species.

(d) After exposure, both UVA and UVB produce immediate pigment darkening.

44. Which of the following would NOT be useful as an anti-pigmentation agent:
    (a) Arbutin
    (b) soy isoflavine
    (c) *N*-acetyl-4-*S*-cysteaminylphenol (NCAP)
    (d) Tranexamic acid
    (e) Glabridin
45. The action of retinoids include all of the following EXCEPT:
    (a) Thickening of the epidermis
    (b) Compaction of the stratum corneum
    (c) Increase in the production of hyaluronic acid
    (d) Increase in the production of collagenases
46. Which of the following is likely to be the most efficacious retinoid?
    (a) 0.5% retinaldehyde
    (b) 1% retinol
    (c) 2% retinyl acetate
    (d) 1% retinyl palmitate
    (e) 0.05% tretinoin
47. Which of the following is NOT an anti-oxidant?
    (a) Ascorbyl-6-palmitate
    (b) Tocopherol
    (c) Zinc oxide
    (d) Ferulic acid
    (e) Niacinamide
48. In the context of lasers, gain medium can be
    (a) Solid
    (b) Gas
    (c) Liquid
    (d) Semiconductors
    (e) All
49. Picodecond lasers for treatment of pigmented lesions produce one of the following effect
    (a) Photothermal
    (b) Photomechanical
    (c) Phototodynamic
    (d) Photochemical
50. The Extended Theory of Selective Photothermolysis explains desctruction of whic of the chromophores by lasers?
    (a) Water
    (b) Melanin
    (c) Hair
    (d) Haemoglobin

Answers

1. Answer: a

   Other ablative lasers include carbon dioxide and Er:YSSG 2790-nm, Er:YSGG erbium:yttrium-scandium-gallium-garnet lasers.
2. Answer: c

   The QS Nd:YAG laser at 532 nm emits in the green spectrum, so is best suited to treat red coloured tattoos.
3. Answer: a

   Earlier treatment of port wine stains is likely to result in better outcomes, when compared to treatment undertaken later in life.
4. Answer: b

   Besides determining depth of penetration, wavelength determines the 'colour' of the laser beam.
5. Answer: d

   Paradoxical hair growth is thought to affect 0.6–10% of all patients undergoing laser hair reduction treatments. Paradoxical growth has been reported with all types of laser and IPL devices.
6. Answer: a
7. Answer: True
8. Answer: a

   The pigment in Naevus of Ota is dermal, so the wavelength of choice is 1064 nm QS Nd:YAG laser
9. Answers: c and d

   Green and blue colours are difficult to treat with nanosecond lasers and the wavelengths used include QS 694 and 755 nm Alexandrite lasers.
10. Answer: c

    Lasers should not be routinely used in the treatment of melasma. Current evidence supports use of fractional non-ablative lasers, IPL and QS Nd:YAG for melasma and are FDA approved for this indication. Low fluence multi pass technique which is also known as laser toning has gained popularity and is generally the preferred option in recalcitrant melasma. This is based on the concept of sub-cellular selective photothermolysis where in the melanosomes are targeted in the melanocytes, keratinocytes and macrophages while sparing those cells form destruction.

This is due to photoacoustic rather than photothermal destruction of melanosomes.

11. Answer: d

    For darker skin phototypes it is best to use longer wavelengths and larger spots to avoid risk of post inflammatory hypopigmentation.

12. Answer: b

    Lentigines are epidermal lesions which readily respond to QS 532 nm Nd:YAG laser. Usually only 1 or 2 sessions are sufficient. Recurrences are common though and continued sun protection is often beneficial

13. Answer: d

    Nd:YAG laser at 1064 nm has a deeper depth of penetration as compared to PDL.

14. Answer: b

    Angioma Serpiginosum is a rare vascular anomaly comprising of small red non-blanching punctate lesions in the upper dermis due to capillary dilatation which arrange themselves in a serpiginous pattern. 2–4 PDL treatments result in a good clinical improvement in most patients.

15. Answer: c
16. Answer: a
17. Answer: c
18. Answer: b

    Pregnancy is an absolute contraindication to elective laser treatment.

    Isotretinoin usage more than 6 months previously is unlikely to continue to pose a threat of poor wound healing/keloid scarring.

    Acne control should be optimised in advance, and treatment of active disease sites should be avoided. Acneiform reactions during recovery are more likely and the practitioner should be ready to treat this if necessary.

    If possible, blood thinners should be stopped in advance of therapy such that its action has ceased by the time of treatment. If this is not possible, careful test patches are required and patients consented for increased risk of petechiae/purpura.

    The wavelength of light is unlikely to trigger Polymorphic Light Eruption

19. Answer: b

    Herpes Simplex infection. Ideally this would have been pre-empted at the pre-operative visit and covered with prophylactic antivirals, but once suspected, take viral swabs and start treatment dose antivirals e.g. acyclovir 400 mg 5 × day 1 week.

20. Answer: c

    Box car scars. Rolling scars respond to subcision or dermal fillers, while ice-pick scars are best treated by punch excision/punch elevation or TCA cross peel.

21. Answer: c

    Superpulse mode. The high peak power packed in ultra-short pulses limit thermal damage to the lesion and reduce risk of scarring.

22. Answer: e

    None. Eye protection is mandatory for all class 4 lasers and IPL devices

23. Answer: False

    Higher absorption of Er:YAG beam limits the depth of penetration of this wave length in the dermis.

24. Answer: e

    Alexandrite laser

25. Answer: d

    The lasers used for hair removal are Ruby, Alexandrite, Diode and Nd:YAG (IPLs are also commonly used, but are intense light sources rather than lasers). These lasers are all 'long-pulsed' as opposed to Q-Switch, working via a photo-thermal response. The longer the wavelength (over this particular wavelength range), the smaller the absorption co-efficient in melanin, meaning that less absorption, occurs in the melanin present in the hair follicle and the skin. The effect of the reduced absorption is that less heat is produced both in the hair follicle and also in the skin. This means that the Nd:YAG laser at 1064nm is less likely to cause thermal injury when used in darker skin types.

26. Answer: a

    If the energy applied is constant, decreasing the pulse duration will increase the power applied, resulting in high peak temperatures in the hair follicles, and effective treatment of fine and fair hairs. Increasing the pulse duration reduces peak temperatures and makes the treatments less aggressive and therefore safer for the treatment of darker skin types.

27. Answer: d

Sometimes known as reactive hair growth, a rare but notable side effect of laser / light hair removal treatment, is the appearance of excess hair in or around the previously treated area. This is reportedly more common in women of Asian or Mediterranean descent, and usually occurs in the neck / jaw-line areas whilst treating fine, vellus hair. Underlying hormonal issues such as Polycystic Ovarian Syndrome may be a contributing factor, however, it has also been reported in men, usually on the back and shoulders.

28. Answer: c

Treatment of very fine hair can present difficulties, and generally requires shorter wavelengths, high fluences and short pulse durations. However, the darker skin type of this patient necessitates the use of less aggressive settings in order to avoid skin trauma, which may impact on the clearance that can be achieved. The patches of hyperpigmentation are indicative of melasma, and the inflammatory response caused by hair removal in this area may cause a worsening or spreading of the pigmentation. Paradoxical hypertrichosis is also an increased risk due to the patient's ethnicity. Proceed with caution (if at all).

29. Answer: a

When carrying out hair removal treatments, the melanin within the hair shaft absorbs the light and creates heat. This heat then diffuses into the follicle and damages the stem cell to prevent regrowth. The hair shaft is therefore acting as the conduit for the heat transfer into the follicle and it's essential that the hair isn't plucked or otherwise removed from the hair follicle. However, if the hair has not been shaved, then the light will be absorbed in the hair above the skin surface, which will not contribute to heating the follicle, and the resultant frazzled hair can result in skin burns.

30. Answer: False

One should never treat over a tattoo or semi-permanent make-up. The IPL/LASER will be absorbed by the pigment, resulting in burning and blistering of the patient, damage to tattoo, or in the case of semi-permanent make-up, potentially cause a colour shift. An area of at least one centimetre must be left around any tattoo or semi -permanent makeup.

31. Answer: False

Photosensitivity reactions normally occur upon to exposure to UV radiation; it is exceptionally rare for a photosensitizing medication to cause a reaction to light above 500nm, and all laser/light sources used for hair removal use longer wavelengths than this. If a patient is taking a known photosensitizing medication, the advice is to test patch and wait a week before proceeding with treatment.

Certain medications however, should be avoided; these include oral retinoids and high-dose oral steroids (due to wound healing impairment); amiodarone and minocycline (risk of pigmentation change); St John's Wort and drugs used for Photo-Dynamic Therapy (risk of photosensitivity).

32. Answer: e

IPL emits broadband light: the 560 and 590 nm filters used in the treatment of photoageing will allow for targeting melanin, haemoglobin, water and collagen.

33. Answer: a, b, d, e

This is a question about safety. All the above lesions can be treated safely with IPL except lentigo maligna. Melasma will need a combination of topical, sometimes oral and rarely energy based treatments. Flat SKs are safe to treat but the response is often poor. Lentigos and ephelides respond well to IPL, and are safe to treat. Lentigo maligna, melanoma and any uncertain or undiagnosed pigmented lesion should never be treated with a laser or IPL.

34. Answer: d

For certain wavelengths Met Hb absorption is 4.5 that of oxyhaemoglobin and up to 20 times more than deoxyhaemoglobin.

35. Answer: b

Alcohol can increase the risk of bruising, and also reduce hydration levels which can have minor effect in the efficacy of the treatment. If in doubt, the BNF or other local formularies can provide more information about a particular antibiotic if the practitioner is not familiar with it. After 4 weeks, light sensitivity should be back to normality, so going on a holiday should not be a problem. Vegan, vegetarian, kosher, halal or any other diets have no effect on the IPL treatments.

A patient who has just come back from a holiday may not look excessively tanned but the melanocytes will be stimulated and often there is increased light sensitivity. The unspecific heating of epidermal melanin is the reason for most side effects. In UV-stimulated melanocytes, there is a risk of causing permanent damage to melanocytes leading to persisting hypo- or depigmentation of the skin. Irradiation of pigmented epidermis with excessive energy densities leads to burns with the formation of vesicles, blisters, erosions, crusts and the potential risk of infections and post-inflammatory pigmentation changes.

36. Answers: b, d

    A is the normal total output of an IPL, without using any filters. C are the usual wavelengths used in photorejuvenation. E is one the ranges of wavelengths which are attenuated in this filter as there is very little absorption of light by Hb in those wavelengths. The other one will be 500–530 nm.

37. Answer: c

    RF medical devices conduct electric current to tissues in repetitive pulses. The energy delivered causes oscillation and vibration of charged particles against tissue's resistance (impedance). This kinetic energy is converted to thermal energy.

38. Answer: a

    In 2002, the Food and Drug Administration (FDA) approved the first monopolar RF device Thermage Thermacool TC (Solta Medical Inc., Hayward, Calif., USA) for the treatment of periorbital wrinkles.

39. The correct answer is c

    Fractional Radiofrequency uses minimally invasive microneedles or electrode pins to achieve targeted dermal injury with minimal superficial involvement. The thermal injury results in denaturated fibrils of collagen and initiates a wound healing response.

40. The correct answer is d

    Reported indications of fractional radiofrequency include: skin tightening, acne scars, axillary hyperhidrosis, cellulite, striae distensae.

41. The correct answer is b

    Although complications potentially vary between different devices, generally mild adverse events, such as pain, erythema and oedema, commonly occur but usually resolve within few hours.

42. The correct answer is c
43. The correct answer is a
44. The correct answer is b
45. The correct answer is d
46. The correct answer is e
47. The correct answer is c
48. The correct answer is e

    The gain medium, also known as active medium is the collection of atoms or materials that can be excited to gain and amplify optical energy. A gain medium may be a:

    - Solid e.g. Nd:YAG crystal, also known as solid-state
    - Gas e.g. CO_2
    - Liquid e.g. organic dye
    - Semiconductor materials, e.g. diodes and ceramics.

49. The correct answer is b

    The pulses emitted by nanosecond (ns) and picosecond (ps) lasers induce a number of photomechanical interactions in soft tissue or fluids depending upon incident wavelength and pulse characteristics

50. The correct answer is c

    The extended theory of selective photothermolysis distinguishes between an absorber or heater chromophore (e.g. melanin in the hair shaft having a high absorption coefficient in the UV and visible spectrum) and a distant target (e.g. the stem cells of isthmus of hair with a low absorption coefficient with unknown absorption spectra).

Index

A

Ablative carbon dioxide (CO_2), 163
Ablative laser, 143
  acne scarring, 159
  CO_2 laser, 143, 144
  complications, 157, 158
  cutting mode
    ear keloids, 155, 156
    hidradenitis suppurativa, 154, 156
    neurofibromas, 155
  Erbium, YSGG laser, 144
  indications, 145
  post-treatment care, 155, 157
  rhinophyma, 159, 160
  sebaceous gland hyperplasia, 159–161
  technique and indications
    acne scarring, 146, 147
    actinic cheilitis, 148, 150
    actinic keratoses and Bowen's disease, 150
    anaesthetic considerations, 145
    comedones, 153
    consent, 145
    cylindromas and benign cutaneous tumours, 151, 153
    Darier's and Hailey-Hailey disease, 151
    dermatosis paulosa nigra, 153, 155
    epidermal and congenital melanocytic naevi, 150, 151
    laser precautions, 146
    milia, 154
    neurofibromas, 150, 152
    post-ablative laser treatment care, 146
    preparation, 145
    pre-treatment preparation, 146
    rejuvenation/rhytides, 147, 148
    rhinophyma, 148, 149
    sebaceous gland hyperplasia, 153, 155
    seborrhoeic keratoses, 148, 149
    steatocystoma multiplex, 151, 154
    syringomas, 154
    warts, 151, 152
Ablative therapy, 167
Absorption, 37
Acne
  LLLT, 209
  radiofrequency systems, 188
Acne scarring, 146, 147
  ablative laser, 159
  monopolar devices, 183
Acne scars, 251
  bipolar devices, 184
  fractional radiofrequency, 187, 191, 195
Acne vulgaris, 180, 209
  bipolar devices, 184
  fractional radiofrequency, 187
  monopolar devices, 183
Acneiform eruptions, fractional laser technology, 168
Actinic cheilitis, ablative laser, 148, 150
Actinic keratoses, 150, 232
Active 'Q' switching, 32
Adult vascular indications
  applications, 73
  Cherry angiomas, 76, 79
  complications, 81
  diffuse erythema, 76
  erythema, 74
  facial spider naevus, 82
  facial telangiectases, 73, 75
  hypertrophic scars, 79
  leg telangiectases, 74, 78
  mature port wine stains, 73
  truncal angiokeratomas, 80
  vascular lasers in inflammatory skin conditions, 81
  venous lake, 79
  warts, 76
Adverse skin reactions, 133
Age defying laser, 169
Alcohol, 255
Alexandrite lasers, 123, 132, 139, 251, 254
Alpha-hydroxy acids (AHAs), 243
Alpha-tocopherol, 244
Aminolevulinic acid photodynamic therapy (ALA-PDT), 209
Amplitude, 7
Amputees, limb prosthetics in, 128, 129
Anagen, 121
Angioma serpiginosum, 66, 250
Antioxidants, 242, 244, 245

V. Madan (ed.), *Practical Introduction to Laser Dermatology*,
https://doi.org/10.1007/978-3-030-46451-6

Arbutin, 240
Argireline, 245
Articulated arm, 18, 19
Axillae, laser hair removal in, 128
Axillary hyperhidrosis, fractional radiofrequency, 187
Azelaic acid, 243

B
Bacterial infection, radiofrequency systems, 188
Basal cell carcinoma, Mohs surgery for, 171
Beam area, 28
Beam scanning technologies, 20
Bearberry, 240
Becker's naevus, 106
Benign cutaneous lesions, 153
Beta-hydroxy acids (BHAs), 243, 244
Bipolar devices
  acne vulgaris and acne scars, 184
  cellulite, 181, 185
  hair removal, 185
  skin rejuvenation, 182, 184
Bipolar radiofrequency
  advantages and disadvantages, 179
  devices and technique of administration, 177
  mechanism of action, 176, 177
Bleeding, radiofrequency systems, 188
Blistering, 132, 133
Blue and red light, photodynamic therapy using, 209
Blue light irradiation, 209
Botanical/vegan, 237
Botanically derived anti-oxidants, 244
Bowen's disease, 150
Box car scars, 254
Bruising, radiofrequency systems, 188
Burning, 132, 133

C
Café-au-lait macules (CALM), 92, 99, 112
Calaguala, 242
Carbon dioxide laser, 144
Catagen, 121
Cellulite, 180
  bipolar devices, 181, 185
  fractional radiofrequency, 187
Cherry angiomas, 79
Chromophores, 38, 175, 249
Chronic wound, 205
Classification of lasers, 46
Cleansers, 238
Clinically proven, 236
CO_2 laser
  ablative lasers, 143, 144
Comedones, 153
Concept of thermal relaxation time, 42, 43
Congenital haemangiomas, 70
Congenital melanocytic naevi, 150, 151
Connexin 43 (Cx43), 207
Contact dermatitis
  ablative laser, 158
  fractional laser technology, 168
Cosmeceuticals, 231, 236, 237, 252
  effective depigmenting ingredients in, 240
  sun protection, 232
Cosmetic, 236
Cutis Marmorata Telangiectatica Congenita (CMTC), 61, 63, 64
Cylindromas, 151, 153

D
Darier's and Hailey-Hailey disease, 151
Décolletage, 180
  fractional radiofrequency, 186
Deeper penetration within the skin, 250
Deoxyarbutin, 241
Dermatologically tested, 236
Dermatosis paulosa nigra, 153, 155
Dichroic mirrors, 25
Diffuse erythema, 76
Diode lasers, 123
Disability Life Quality Index score (DLQI, 127
Dissecting cellulitis, 131
Dosimetry, 214
Dysmorphophobia, 157
Dyspigmentation
  ablative laser, 158
  fractional laser technology, 168, 169

E
Ear keloids, ablative laser, 155, 156
Elastosis perforans serpiginosa, 84
Electromagnetic (EM) spectrum, 2, 4
Electromagnetic radiation, 4, 173
  radiofrequency devices use, 252
Electromagnetic radiation (EMR), 2
Emollients, 238
Energy density, 122
Ephilides, 250
Epidermal lesions, 99
Epidermal melanocytic naevi, 150, 151
Epilation lasers, 119
  hair growth cycle, 121, 122
  hair removal laser treatments, complications of, 132
    adverse reaction, causes of, 135, 136
    burning, blistering and scarring, 132, 133
    leukotrichia, 134
    paradoxical Hypertrichosis, 134, 135
    pigmentation changes, 133, 134
  hair removal lasers and light sources
    Alexandrite lasers, 123
    diode lasers, 123
    intense light sources, 123, 124
    neodymium YAG lasers, 123
    ruby laser, 123
  hair structure, 121
  home-use devices, 136, 137

iMedical Indications
amputees, limb prosthetics in, 128, 129
axillae, laser hair removal in, 128
dissecting cellulitis, 131
folliculitis decalvans, 131
hair-bearing skin flaps and grafts, 131
hair follicle pathology, 128, 129
hair restoration surgery, redesign frontal hairline, 132
hairy intraoral flaps, 131
hidradenitis suppurativa, 130
hirsutism, 127, 128
PCOS, 128
peristomal hair growth, 132
pilonidal sinus, 130
pseudofolliculitis barbae, 131
transgender laser hair removal and genital gender affirming surgery, 131
trichostasis spinulosa, 131
mode of action, 119, 120
pain-free hair removal, 136
photoepilation, lasers and light sources used for, 122
fluence, 122
pulse duration, 122, 123
wavelength, 122
pre-treatment preparation and precautions, 125
contraindications, 125, 126
informed consent, 126
test-patching, 126, 127
Er:YAG beam, 251
Er:YAG lasers, 144
Er:YSSG 2790-nm, 253
Erbium laser, 144
Erythema, 74
ablative laser, 157
Erythemotelangiectatic rosacea (ETR), 73
Eutectic mixture of local anaesthetic (EMLA), 95
Exillis, 176
Extended theory of selective photothermolysis, 43
Eye protection, 95, 254

F
Face and neck, fractional radiofrequency, 186
Facial hair removal, 138
Facial pigmentation and rejuvenation, 169
Facial rejuvenation, radiofrequency systems, 190, 192, 193
Facial spider naevus, 82
Facial telangiectasia, 73, 74, 227
Ferulic acid, 244
Fitzpatrick skin type 5, 137
Flashlamps, 24
Fluence, 122
Folliculitis, radiofrequency systems, 188
Folliculitis decalvans (FD), 131
Fractional ablative treatments, 170
Fractional beam technologies, 20
Fractional laser technology, 163, 164
complications, 167
acneiform eruptions, 168
contact dermatitis, 168
dyspigmentation, 168, 169
infection, 168
koebnerisation, 169
LADD, 169
prolonged erythema, 168
scarring, 169
fractional ablative and non-ablative devices, 165
fractional devices/wavelengths, 165
fractionated laser indications, 164
post treatment care, 167
pre-treatment preparation and precautions, 165, 166
skin treated with fractional ablative CO2 laser, 164
skin treated with fractional non ablative device, 165
technique, 166, 167
Fractional radiofrequency, 252, 256
acne scars and acne vulgaris, 187, 191, 195
advantages and disadvantages, 179
axillary hyperhidrosis, 187
cellulite, 187
décolletage, 186
devices and technique of administration, 178
face and neck, 186
facial rejuvenation, 190, 192–194
mechanism of action, 177
periorbital area, 185
post-traumatic scars, 190
striae distensae, 187
teleangiectatic haemangioma, 191
Fragrance-free, 237
Fraxel™ device, 163
Freckles, 99
Full width at half maximum (FWHM), 29

G
Gain medium, 13
Genital gender affirming surgery (GAS), 131
Glutathione, 241
Grouped box car scars, 146

H
Haemangiomas, 68, 69
Haemoglobin, 38
Hair-bearing skin flaps and grafts, 131
Hair follicle pathology, 128, 129
Hair growth, 207
cycle, 121, 122
LLLT, 204, 206
Hair removal lasers
bipolar devices, 185
and light sources
Alexandrite lasers, 123
diode lasers, 123
intense light sources, 123, 124
neodymium YAG lasers, 123
ruby laser, 123

Hair restoration surgery, redesign frontal hairline, 132
Hair, structure, 121
Hairy intraoral flaps, 131
Hands, monopolar devices, 183
Heat shock proteins (HSP), 174
Herpes simplex infection, 251, 254
Hidradenitis suppurativa (HS), 130
ablative laser, 154, 156
Hirsutism, 127, 128
Home-use devices, epilation lasers, 136, 137
Hyaluronic acid (HA), 237
Hydroquinone, 239
compounds related to, 240, 241
Hyper pigmentation, 133, 134
Hyperkeratotic cryotherapy resistant plantar verruca vulgaris, 152
Hypertrophic, LLLT, 212
Hypertrophic acne scarring, 147
Hypertrophic scarring, 158
Hypertrophic scars, 79, 146, 212
Hypo pigmentation, 133, 134
Hypoallergenic, 237

I

Immediate pigment darkening (IPD), 233
Infections
ablative laser, 157
fractional laser technology, 168
Informed consent, 126
Intense light practitioners, 50
Intense light sources (ILS), 19, 123, 124
components, 24
Intense pulsed light (IPL), 123
complications, 226
during treatment, 225
facial port wine stain, 228
facial telangiectasia, 227
following treatment, 225, 226
hair removal treatments, 226
handpiece, 219
indications and techniques, 220, 221
inflammatory lesions, 227
laser *vs.*, 220
leg veins, treatment of, 223, 224
lentigines, 228
melasma, 224
photoepilation, 224
photorejuvenation, 222
chromophores in, 252
notch filters, 223
photoageing, photofractional treatment for, 223
PIH, 224, 225
preparation prior to treatment, 225
pulses and delays, 220
rosacea, 220, 221
classification and clinical presentation, 221
treatment protocol, 221, 222
treatment, contraindications for, 225
INTRAcel, 188

K

Keloids, 212
Kirby-Desai scale, 111
Koebnerisation, fractional laser technology, 169
Kojic acid, 241

L

L-ascorbic acid, 244
Laser
amplitude, 7
beam area, 28, 29
beam delivery methods, 18–21
beam quality, 15, 16
classification, 45
electromagnetic wave, 2, 4
equipment, 46
excitation mechanism, 13
frequency, 5
frequency doubling, 6
gain medium, 13
historical development, 1, 2
intense light sources, 23, 25
light as a particle, 5
light emitting diodes, 21
light tissue interactions, 34, 38, 40, 41
modes, 15, 16
optical resonator, 14
procedure, 96
producing pulsed outputs, 31–33
pulsed laser output, 29, 31
radiant energy, 26
radiant power, 27
selective photothermolysis, 41
spontaneous emission of light, 8
stimulated emission of light, 10, 12
technique, 97
velocity, 7
wavelength, 5
Laser-assisted drug delivery (LADD), fractional laser technology, 169
Laxity, uniopolar devices, 184
Leg telangiectases, 74
Leg veins, treatment of, 223, 224
Lentigines, 99, 228
Leukotrichia, 134
Lichen planus pigmentosus (LPP), 107
Light-assisted hair removal, 119, 123
Light emitting diode red light (LED-RL), 203
Light-emitting diodes (LEDs), mechanism of action, 201, 203
Limb prosthetics, amputees, 128, 129
Low level laser therapy (LLLT), 23
complications, 215
contraindications of, 214
dermatology, indications in, 203
acne, 209
blue and red light, photodynamic therapy using, 209, 210
for hair growth, 204, 206

hypertrophic and keloid, 212
photoprotection, 212, 214
psoriasis, 210, 211
skin rejuvenation, 206, 208, 209
vitiligo, 211, 212
wound healing, 203, 204
indications of, 213–214
mechanism of action, 201, 202
post treatment care advice and plan, 215
pre-treatment preparation and precautions, 214, 215
treatment technique, 215
Lower eyelids, 191
Lumina IPL system, 137, 138
Lymphatic malformations, 63
Lymphovenous malformation, 83

M
Mat telangiectases, 61
Mature port wine stains, 73
Medical device regulation (MDR), 44
Medical laser systems, 17–18
Melanoma, 232
Melasma, 103, 224, 249, 255
Mequinol, 241
Met Hb absorbtion, 255
Methyl aminolevulinate photodynamic therapy (MAL-PDT), 209
Microneedle radiofrequency, 193, 194
Microneedle radiofrequency devices, 179
Microneedle radiofrequency system, 178
Microneedle therapy system (MTS), 177
Micronised minerals, 234
Microsclerotherapy, 223
Middle-lower face and neck, monopolar devices, 182
Milia, 154, 251
ablative laser, 158
Mode hopping, 15
Mode-locked lasers, 33
Mohs surgery, for basal cell carcinoma, 171
Monochromatic infrared energy (MIRE), 203
Monochromaticity, 16
Monopolar devices
acne vulgaris and acne scarring, 181, 183
body, 183
hands, 183
middle-lower face and neck, 180, 182
periorbital area, 182
Monopolar radiofrequency, 196
advantages and disadvantages, 178
devices and technique of administration, 175, 176
mechanism of action, 175
Multiple fractional laser beams, 163, 177
Mycoplasma, 168

N
N-acetyl glucosamine (NAG), 241
N-acetyl-4-S-cysteaminylphenol (NCAP), 241
Naevus of Ota, 101
Naevus of Ota with scar, 113
Naevus spilus, 100
Nanoparticles, 245
Nd:YAG, 251
Neodymium YAG lasers, 123
Neurofibromas, ablative laser, 150, 152, 155
Nevocellular naevi, 106
Niacinamide, 244
Non-comedogenic, 237
Non-involuting congenital haemangiomas (NICH), 70
Non-melanoma skin cancer (NMSC), 232
Notch filters, 25, 223
Novel cosmeceutical peptides, 245, 246

O
Optical fibres, 18
Optical radiation hazards, 47
Oral retinoids, 95

P
Paediatric vascular indications
adverse effects, 72
angioma serpiginosum, 66
assessment shots on normal skin, 56
congenital haemangiomas, 70
Cutis Marmorata Telangiectatica Congenita, 61
haemangiomas, 68, 69
laser applications, 58
laser technique, 55, 57
lymphatic malformations, 63, 65
mat telangiectases, 61
photoablative, 53
photochemical properties, 53
photodisruptive, 53
photothermal, 53
pyogenic granulomas, 70
recalcitrant lesions, 71, 72
spider naevi, 60
test patch on Port Wine Stain, 56
tufted angiomas, 71, 72
vascular anomalies, 57
verrucous vascular malformations, 66, 67
Pain-free hair removal, epilation lasers, 136
Paradoxical hair growth, 249, 253
Paradoxical hypertrichosis, 134, 135
Partially involuting congenital haemangiomas (PICH), 70
Passive Q switching, 33
PDL Laser, 250
Perinasal telangiectases, 77
Perioral rhytides, 170
Periorbital area
fractional radiofrequency, 185
monopolar devices, 180, 182
Periorbital rejuvenation, 190
Peristomal hair growth, 132
Periungual warts, 81
Permanent hair reduction, 119

Persistent pigment darkening (PPD), 233
Personal protective equipment (PPE), 34
Pharmaceutical, 236
Photoablation, 40
Photoageing, 148
  photofractional treatment for, 223
Photobiomodulation, 23, 201, 206
PhotoBioModulation (PBM), 41
Photochemical interactions, 40
Photodamage, 194
Photodisruption, 41
Photodynamic therapy, using blue and red light, 209, 210
Photoepilation, IPL, 224
Photoepilation, lasers and light sources used for, 122
  fluence, 122
  pulse duration, 122, 123
  wavelength, 122
Photomechanical interactions, 41
Photomodulated light emitting diode yellow light (LED-YL), 203
Photoprotection, LLLT, 212, 214
Photorejuvenation, IPL, 222, 223
Photosensitivity, 255
Photothermal interactions, 40
Photothermolysis, 41, 120
Picosecond lasers, 112
Pigmentation, treatment of, 251
Pigmented lesions
  anesthesia, 95
  Becker's naevus, 106
  blue naevi, 103
  Café au lait macules, 99, 112
  Congenital melanocytic naevi, 106
  counseling, 95
  dermal lesions, 101
  dermatosis papulosa nigra, 100
  epidermal lesions, 99
  eye protection, 95
  freckles, 99
  hair over, 96
  laser basics and systems, 91, 92
  laser procedure
    endpoint of treatment, 96
    fluence, 96
    spot size, 96
  laser technique, 97
  lentigines, 99
  melasma, 103
  naevus of Ota, 101
  naevus of Ota with scar, 113
  naevus spilus, 100
  nevocellular naevi, 106
  oral retinoids, 95
  patient selection, 95
  picosecond lasers, 112
  postinflammatory hyperpigmentation, 107
  postoperative instructions, 108
  quality switch, 92–94
  seborrheic keratoses, 101
  sun protection, 95
  tattoos, 110
  test patch, 95
Pilonidal sinus (PNS), 130
Plasma-induced ablation, 41
Poat-traumatic scars, fractional radiofrequency, 190
Polycystic ovarian syndrome (PCOS), 128
Polymorphous light eruption (PLE), 213
Polypodium leucotomos, 242
Port wine stains (PWS), 58, 59, 253
Post inflammatory hyper-pigmentation (PIH), 232
Post-ablative laser treatment care, 146
Post-burn hypertrophic scars, 213
Post-inflammatory hyperpigmentation (PIH), 107, 224, 225
Pregnancy, 251
Preservative-free, 237
Professional green tattoos, wavelength, 249
Prolonged erythema, fractional laser technology, 168
Pronounced follicular erythema, 127
Pseudofolliculitis barbae (PFB), 131
Psoriasis, LLLT, 210, 211
Pulse duration, 122, 123
Pulses, IPL, 219, 220
Purpura, 250
Pyogenic granulomas (PG), 70, 250

Q

Q switching, 92
QS 532nm, 251
QS Nd:YAG laser, 253

R

Radiant energy, 27
Radiofrequency, complications of, 252
Radiofrequency devices, aesthetic medicine, 252
Radiofrequency systems
  advantages and disadvantages, 178, 179
  in aesthetic medicine, 175
  bipolar radiofrequency
    devices and technique of administration, 177
    mechanism of action, 176, 177
  body treatments, 190
  complications and pitfalls and how to identify and avoid, 189
  cosmetic interventions, substantial increase of, 189
  EBM, 190
  electromagnetic radiation, 173
  fractional radiofrequency
    acne scars, 191, 195
    devices and technique of administration, 178
    facial rejuvenation, 190, 192–194
    mechanism of action, 177
    post-traumatic scars, 190
    teleangiectatic haemangioma, 191
  in aesthetic medicine, 175
  indications, 179–181
    bipolar devices, 181, 182, 184, 185

fractional radiofrequency, 185–187
monopolar devices, 180–183
uniopolar devices, 183, 184
monopolar radiofrequency
devices and technique of administration, 175, 176
mechanism of action, 175
periorbital rejuvenation, 190
post-treatment care advice and plan, 189
pre-treatment preparation and precautions, 183, 188
skin thermal interactions, 173–175
unipolar radiofrequency
devices and technique of administration, 176
mechanism of action, 176
Rapidly involuting congenital haemangiomas (RICH), 70
Reactive oxygen species (ROS), 233
Recalcitrant lesions, 71, 72
Red light therapy, 209
Refraction, 35
Rejuvenation/rhytides, ablative laser, 147, 148
Residual thermal damage (RTD), 144
Resorcinol, 241
Reticulate vascular naevi (RVN), 62
Retinoids, 242, 243
RF medical devices, 256
Rhinophyma, 148, 149
ablative laser, 159, 160
Rhytides, uniopolar devices, 184
Rosacea, IPL, 220, 221
classification and clinical presentation, 221
treatment protocol, 221, 222
Ruby lasers, 119, 123
Rucinol, 241

S
Scarring, 132, 133
ablative laser, 158
fractional laser technology, 169
Scattering, 35
Scrotal angiokeratomas, 80
Sebaceous gland hyperplasia, ablative laser, 153, 155, 159–161
Seborrhoeic keratoses, 148, 149
Shave hair, 251
Skin moisturisers, 237, 238
Skin rejuvenation, 210
bipolar devices, 184
LLLT, 206, 208, 209
Skin scali, radiofrequency systems, 188
Skin thermal interactions, 173–175
Skincare products, 237–239
Small angiomas, 76
Soy isoflavine, 253
Spider naevi, 60
Spontaneous emission of light, 8
Steatocystoma multiplex, 151, 154
Stimulated emission of light, 10
Striae distensae, 181
fractional radiofrequency, 187
Sublation, 177
Sun protection, 232, 236
practical advice, 233, 234
Sun protection factor (SPF), 233
Sunlight, 232
Sunscreen, 234
Superficial box car acne scarring, 170
Superpulse mode, 254
Surgical scars, 171
Syringomas, ablative laser, 154

T
Tardive involuting congenital haemangiomas (TICH), 70
Tattoos, 110
Tazoratene, 243
Teleangiectatic haemangioma, 191
Telogen, 121
Test-patching, 126, 127
ThermaCool NXT system, 176
Thermage, 191
Thermal damage time (TDT), 43
Thermal energy, 196
Thermal relaxation time (TRT), 42
Toners, 238
Topical agents
AHAs, 243
antioxidants, 244, 245
BHAs, 243
cleansers, toners and wash off-products, 238
depigmenting and pigment control agents, 238
antioxidants, 242
BHAs, 244
botanicals, 241
compounds related to hydroquinone, 240, 241
glutathione, 241
hydroquinone, 239
kojic acid, 241
NAG, 241
NCAP, 241
polypodium leucotomos, 242
retinoids and cosmeceutical peeling agents, 243
tranexamic acid, 242
moisturisers, 237, 238
nanoparticles, 245
novel cosmeceutical peptides, 245, 246
post-treatment applications, 246
retinoids and cosmeceutical peeling agents, 242, 243
skincare products, 237–239
Training for laser, 49
Tranexamic acid, 242
Transgender laser hair removal, 131
Tretinoin, 253
Tricholetheliomas, 153
Trichostasis spinulosa, 131
Triple pass therapy, 71
Tripolar systems, 177
Truncal angiokeratomas, 80
Tufted angiomas, 71, 72

U
Ubiquinone, 244
Uniopolar devices
  cellulite, 183
  rhytides and laxity, 184
Unipolar radiofrequency
  advantages and disadvantages, 179
  devices and technique of administration, 176
  mechanism of action, 176
Upper eyelids, 190
UVA, 233
UVB, 233

V
Velocity, 7
Venous lake, 79
Verrucous vascular malformations (VVMs), 66, 67
Vitamin C, 244
Vitamin E, 244
Vitiligo, LLLT, 211, 212
Visible light (VL), 233
VR, 233

W
Warts, 76
  ablative laser, 151, 152
Wash off-products, 238
Wavelength, 5, 249
  photoepilation, lasers and light sources, 122
Wine stains, 249
Wound healing, LLLT, 203, 204

X
Xenon flashlamp, 124

The manufacturer's authorised representative in the EU is Springer Nature Customer Service Centre GmbH, Europaplatz 3, 69115 Heidelberg, Germany. If you have any concerns regarding our products, please contact ProductSafety@springernature.com

Printed and bound by CPI Group (UK) Ltd, Croydon, CR0 4YY
30/09/2026
02225504-0019